DEVELOPMENTAL SCIENCE AND PSYCHOANALYSIS

Developments in Psychoanalysis Series

Peter Fonagy, Mary Target, & Liz Allison (Series Editors)

Published and distributed by Karnac Books

DEVELOPMENTAL SCIENCE AND PSYCHOANALYSIS
Integration and Innovation

Celebrating the Renewal of the Collaboration of the Yale Child Study Center and the Anna Freud Centre in Promoting Psychoanalytic Developmental Research

Edited by
Linda Mayes, Peter Fonagy, & Mary Target

Routledge
Taylor & Francis Group
LONDON AND NEW YORK

First published 2007 by Karnac Books Ltd.

2 Park Square, Milton Park, Abingdon, Oxfordshire OX14 4RN
52 Vanderbilt Avenue, New York, NY 10017

Routledge is an imprint of the Taylor & Francis Group, an informa business

First issued in hardback 2019

British Library Cataloguing in Publication Data

A C.I.P. for this book is available from the British Library

ISBN: 978-1-85575-440-9 (pbk)
ISBN: 978-0-367-32406-9 (hbk)

Edited, designed, and produced by Communication Crafts

CONTENTS

ACKNOWLEDGEMENTS

Chapter 3: James F. Leckman, Ruth Feldman, James E. Swain, and Linda C. Mayes thank Virginia Eicher and Nancy Thompson for their dedicated efforts in advancing this area of study at the Child Study Center, as well as their comments on this manuscript. Aspects of this work were presented at a joint meeting of the Anna Freud Centre and the Child Study Center at the University College London, January 2004, and have appeared in earlier publications (Leckman, Mayes, & Cohen, 2002; Leckman et al., 2004, 2006).

Chapter 8: V. Robin Weersing thanks the collaborators on the empirical investigations described in the chapter, most notably John Weisz, David Brent, and John Hamilton.

Figure 8.1 reprinted by permission from V. R. Weersing & J. R. Weisz (2002), "Community Clinic Treatment of Depressed Youth: Benchmarking Usual Care against CBT Clinical Trials." *Journal of Consulting and Clinical Psychology, 70:* 299–310. Copyright 2002 by the American Psychological Association.

Chapter 10, "Psychoanalytic Responses to Violent Trauma: The Child Development–Community Policing Partnership", reprinted by permission from: B. Tremlow, S. W. Skalrew, & S. M. Wilkinson (Eds.), *Analysts in the Trenches: Streets, Schools, War Zones* (Hillsdale, NJ: Analytic Press, 2004), pp. 211–236.

Chapter 12: Robert A. King, Alan Apter, and Ada Zohar would like to acknowledge the collaboration of Shmuel Kron, MD; Anat Dycian, PhD; and Avi Bleich, MD.

SERIES FOREWORD

Peter Fonagy, Mary Target, & Liz Allison

After the first hundred years of its history, psychoanalysis has matured into a serious, independent intellectual tradition, which has notably retained its capacity to challenge established truths in most areas of our culture. Above all, psychoanalytic ideas have given rise to an approach to the treatment of mental disorders and character problems—psychodynamic psychotherapy—which has become a thriving tradition in most countries, at least in the Western world.

The biological psychiatrist of today is called to task by psychoanalysis, much as was the specialist in nervous diseases of Freud's time, in turn-of-the-century Vienna. Today's cultural commentators, regardless of whether they are for or against psychoanalytic ideas, are obliged to pay attention to considerations of unconscious motivation, defences, the formative impact of early childhood experience, and the myriad other discoveries that psychoanalysts brought to twentieth-century culture. Twenty-first century thought implicitly incorporates much of what was discovered by psychoanalysis in the last century. Critics who try to pick holes in or even demolish the psychoanalytic edifice are often doing this from ramparts constructed on psychoanalytic foundations. A good example of this would be the recent attacks by some cognitive behaviour therapists on psychodynamic approaches. Vehement as these are, they have to give credit to psychoanalysis for its contribution to cognitive therapeutic theory and technique. These authors point to the advances they have made in relation to classical ideas but rarely acknowledge that the psychodynamic approach has also advanced. An unfortunate feature of such debates is that often attacks on psychoanalysis are addressed to where the discipline was 50 or even 75 years ago.

Both the epistemology and the conceptual and clinical claims of psychoanalysis are often passionately disputed. We see this as a sign that psychoanalysis may be unique in its capacity to challenge and provoke. Why should this be? Psychoanalysis is unrivalled in the depth of its questioning of human motivation, and whether its answers are right or wrong, the epistemology of psychoanalysis allows it to confront the most difficult problems of human experience. Paradoxically, our new understanding of the physical basis of our existence—our genes, nervous systems, and endocrine functioning—has, rather than finally displacing psychoanalysis, created a pressing need for a complementary discipline that considers the memories, desires, and meanings that are beginning to be recognized as influencing human adaptation even at the biological level. How else, other than through the study of subjective experience, will we understand the expression of the individual's biological destiny within the social environment?

It is not surprising, then, that psychoanalysis continues to attract some of the liveliest intellects in our culture. These individuals are by no means all psychoanalytic clinicians, or psychotherapists. They are distinguished scholars in an almost bewildering range of disciplines, from the study of mental disorders with their biological determinants to the disciplines of literature, art, philosophy, and history. There will always be a need to explicate the meaning of experience. Psychoanalysis, with its commitment to understanding subjectivity, is in a leading position to fulfil this intellectual and human task. We are not surprised at the upsurge of interest in psychoanalytic studies in universities in many countries. The books in this series will aim to address the same intellectual curiosity that has made these educational projects so successful.

The theme of our series is a focus on advances in psychoanalysis: hence our series title, "Developments in Psychoanalysis". In our view, while psychoanalysis has a glorious and rich history, it also has an exciting future, with dramatic changes and shifts as our understanding of the mind is informed by scientific, philosophical, and literary enquiry. Our commitment is to no specific orientation, to no particular professional group, but to the intellectual challenge to explore questions of meaning and interpretation systematically, and in a scholarly way. Nevertheless, we would be glad if this series particularly spoke to the psychotherapeutic community—to those individuals who use their own minds and humanity to help others in distress.

Our focus in this series is to communicate some of the intellectual excitement that we feel about the past, present, and future of psychoanalytic ideas, and which we enjoy seeing in our students each year. We hope that our work with the authors and editors in the series will help to make these ideas accessible to an even larger group of students, scholars, and practitioners worldwide.

University College London
January 2007

ABOUT THE EDITORS AND CONTRIBUTORS

Editors

Linda C. Mayes, MD, is the Arnold Gesell Professor of Child Psychiatry, Psychology, and Psychiatry at the Yale Child Study Center in New Haven, Connecticut, and the chairman of the directorial team of the Anna Freud Centre in London. Dr Mayes is trained as a developmental paediatrician and an adult and child psychoanalyst. Her research focuses on the long-term impact of early stressful events during pregnancy and early preschool years on children's neurocognitive and emotional development.

Peter Fonagy, PhD FBA, is Freud Memorial Professor of Psychoanalysis and Director of the Sub-Department of Clinical Health Psychology at University College London. He is Chief Executive of the Anna Freud Centre, London. He is consultant to the Child and Family Program at the Menninger Department of Psychiatry at Baylor College of Medicine. He is a clinical psychologist and a training and supervising analyst in child and adult analysis in the British Psycho-Analytical Society. His clinical interests centre around issues of borderline psychopathology, violence, and early attachment relationships. His work attempts to integrate empirical research with psychoanalytic theory. He holds a number of important positions, which include co-chairing the Research Committee of the International Psychoanalytic Association, and Fellowship of the British Academy. He has published over 300 chapters and articles and has authored or edited several books.

Mary Target, PhD, is reader in psychoanalysis at University College London and a Fellow of the British Psycho-Analytical Society. She originally trained as a clinical psychologist. She is Professional Director of the Anna Freud Centre. She is Chair of the British Psychological Society's Psychotherapy Section. She has been a member of the Curriculum and Scientific Committees, and Chair of the Research Committee of the British Psychoanalytic Society, and former Chair of the Working Party on Psychoanalytic Education of the European Psychoanalytic Federation. She is a member of the Research Committee (Conceptual Research) of the International Psychoanalytic Association. She is Course Organizer of the UCL MSc in Psychoanalytic Theory and Academic Course Organizer of the UCL/Anna Freud Centre Doctorate in Child and Adolescent Psychotherapy. She is Joint Series Editor for Karnac's new "Developments in Psychoanalysis" series. She has active research collaborations in many countries in the areas of developmental psychopathology, attachment, and psychotherapy outcome. She is Consultant to the Child and Family Programme at the Menninger Department of Psychiatry at Baylor College of Medicine.

Contributors

Alan Apter, MD, is Director of the Feinberg Child Study Center in Schneider's Children's Medical Center of Israel. He is also Professor of Psychiatry in the Sackler School of Medicine at the University of Tel Aviv.

Eia Asen, MD, FRCPsych, is both a consultant child and adolescent psychiatrist as well as a consultant psychiatrist in psychotherapy. He grew up in Berlin, where he also studied medicine. He came to the United Kingdom in the early 1970s, and he then started his psychiatric training at the Maudsley Hospital in London. He is now the Clinical Director of the Marlborough Family Service (CNWL Mental Health NHS Trust), which is a publicly funded (NHS) integrated CAMHS and Adult Psychotherapy service in Central London, predominantly with a systemic orientation. Until 2002 he also worked as a consultant psychiatrist at the Maudsley Hospital, as well as being a senior lecturer at the Institute of Psychiatry. He is the author and co-author of seven books, as well as of many scientific papers and book chapters. He lectures all over Europe, and he is and has been involved in a number of research projects on depression, eating disorders, family violence, and educational failure.

Anthony W. Bateman, MA, FRCPsych, is consultant psychiatrist in psychotherapy (Haringey), Halliwick Unit, Barnet, Enfield, and Haringey Mental Health Trust, visiting professor at University College, London, and visiting consultant at the Menninger Clinic, Baylor College of Medicine, Houston, Texas. He is clinical tutor in Haringey for Education, Chief Examiner of the Royal College of Psychiatrists, and was formerly Chair of the Psychotherapy Training Committee for the United Kingdom. His clinical and research interest is in the treatment of personality disorder. He was a member of the Department of Health Expert Committee on the Treatment of Personality Disorder, is an executive member of the British and Irish Group for Study of Personality Disorder, and is an expert member of National Institute for Clinical Excellence development group for treatment guidelines for borderline personality disorder. He has authored several books, including (with Peter Fonagy) *Psychotherapy for Borderline Personality Disorder: Mentalization-based Treatment*, as well as numerous chapters and many research articles on personality disorder and the use of psychotherapy in psychiatric practice.

Efrain Bleiberg, MD, is a native of Monterrey, Mexico, where he graduated from the School of Medicine of the University of Nuevo Leon and the School of Psychology at the University of Monterrey. He completed his training in psychiatry and child and adolescent psychiatry at The Menninger School of Psychiatry in Topeka, Kansas. He has currently the Alicia Townsend Friedman Professor of Psychiatry and Developmental Psychopathology. He is the Vice Chairman of The Menninger Department of Psychiatry and Behavioral Sciences at Baylor College of Medicine; Director, Division of Child and Adolescent Psychiatry, at The Menninger Department of Psychiatry; and Medical Director, Professionals in Crisis Program at The Menninger Clinic. He is also Training and Supervising Psychoanalyst at the Houston–Galveston Psychoanalytic Institute.

Ruth Feldman is an associate professor and chair of the Child Clinical Program at the Department of Psychology and the Gonda Brain

Sciences Center, Bar-Ilan University, Israel. Her research interests include the parent–infant relationship, infants' social–emotional development in normative and high-risk populations, and the biological basis of parenting, close bonds, and emotional development in young children.

György Gergely received his undergraduate degree in social psychology in 1978 at the London School of Economics, and his MPhil degree in psychology in 1980 at University College London. In 1986 he received his PhD in psychology at the experimental psycholinguistics programme of Columbia University, New York. He was a post-doctoral fellow at Stanford University and spent a year as a visiting assistant professor at Rochester University. In 1977 he completed a second PhD in clinical child psychology at the Semmelweis Medical University in Budapest. He trained as a psychoanalyst at the Hungarian Psychoanalytic Association. In 2002 he received the DSc Degree in Psychology at the Hungarian Academy of Sciences, and in 2006 he was awarded the Dr Habil Title at the Cognitive Neuroscience Doctoral Programme of the Budapest University of Technology and Economics, Hungary. Professor Gergely has published widely in peer-reviewed journals of experimental psychology and psychoanalysis. He has published two scholarly books and is working on a third. Professor Gergely is currently Head of the Department of Developmental Research of the Institute for Psychological Research of the Hungarian Academy of Sciences and is a Professor of the graduate school at the Cognitive Neuroscience Doctoral Programme of the Budapest University of Technology and Economics, Hungary. He has also been visiting professor at University College London and senior research consultant both at the Anna Freud Centre in London, and at the Child and Family Center of the Menninger Clinic at the Baylor School of Medicine in Houston, Texas.

Kay Henderson is course tutor for the UCL/AFC MSc in Psychoanalytic Developmental Psychology and a research psychologist working in adoption and parenting skills training.

Jonathan Hill is professor of child and adolescent psychiatry, University of Manchester, and honorary consultant child psychiatrist at the Central Manchester and Manchester Children's University Hospitals NHS Trust, and at the Tavistock and Portman NHS Trust, London. His research focuses on the causes and treatment of conduct problems in young children, the impact of maltreatment on development, and on the developmental origins of personality disorders. His measure—the Adult Personality Functioning Assessment—has been used extensively to explore social domain dysfunction and personality disorder. He is about to start a study of the earliest origins of conduct problems from pregnancy onwards.

Saul Hillman, MSc, is a research officer, honorary lecturer at University College London, and research coordinator for the MSc in Psychoanalytic Developmental Psychology at the Anna Freud Centre/University College London. He also coordinates and runs trainings in the use of the Story Stem Assessment Profile (SSAP).

Jill Hodges, MD, is consultant child psychotherapist in the Child and Adolescent Mental Health Service, Great Ormond Street Hospital for Sick Children, honorary senior lecturer in the Brain and Behavioural Sciences Unit, Institute of Child Health, and a senior research Fellow at the Anna Freud Centre. She works clinically in the areas of child maltreatment and post-protection work on the sequelae of earlier maltreatment. She continues to carry out research in the areas of attachment, adoption, and the impact of earlier adversities upon children's development.

Warren Jones is currently completing his PhD in neuroscience at the Yale University School of Medicine, Interdepartmental Neuroscience Program. His research interests focus on mechanisms of social development and disruptions of these processes in autism spectrum disorders. Together with Ami Klin, he has been pursuing novel methods to visualize and quantify visual engagement with the surrounding social environment.

Jeanne Kaniuk has been Head of the Coram Adoption Service for 26 years. Coram specializes in placing older children who have suffered abuse and/or neglect and who are in public care in adoptive families. Jeanne has a longstanding interest in the emotional needs of this population of children and a commitment to ensuring that they can experience nurturing and reparative care in adoptive families. She has been active in promoting the application of insights from attachment theory by adoption agencies in the United Kingdom. She has also participated in a research project that developed a parenting skills training course for adopters, based on the Incredible Years programme developed by

Carolyn Webster Stratton but modified to incorporate themes particularly relevant to parents of adopted children.

Alan E. Kazdin, PhD, is John M. Musser Professor of Psychology and Child Psychiatry at Yale University and Director of the Yale Parenting Center & Child Conduct Clinic, an outpatient treatment service for children and their families. Prior to coming to Yale he has held positions at The Pennsylvania State University and The University of Pittsburgh School of Medicine. His research focuses primarily on the development, treatment, and clinical course of oppositional, aggressive, and antisocial child behaviour. He teaches and supervises graduate and undergraduate students. He has authored or edited over 600 articles, chapters, and books. His 43 books focus primarily on child and adolescent psychotherapy, aggressive and antisocial behaviour, and research methodology.

Robert A. King, MD is a professor of child psychiatry at Yale Child Study Center in Yale University School of Medicine. He is a faculty member of the Western New England Psychoanalytic Institute and is Managing Editor of *The Psychoanalytic Study of the Child.*

Ami Klin is the Harris Associate Professor of Child Psychology and Psychiatry and Director, Autism Program, at the Yale Child Study Center. He received his PhD in psychology at the University of London and completed post-doctoral fellowships in Clinical Psychology and Developmental Psychopathology at the Yale Child Study Center. His research interests focus on mechanisms of social development and disruptions of these processes in autism spectrum disorders. Together with Warren Jones, he has been pursuing novel methods to visualize and quantify visual engagement with the surrounding social environment.

James F. Leckman, MD, is the Neison Harris Professor of Child Psychiatry, Paediatrics, and Psychology and Director of Research at the Child Study Center, Yale University. He is an academic child psychiatrist with training in psychoanalysis at The Western Psychoanalytic Institute. Dr Leckman's specific research interests include the interaction of genes and environment in the pathogenesis of Gilles de la Tourette's syndrome and obsessive-compulsive disorder (OCD). His research on these disorders is well known and multifaceted, from phenomenology and natural history to neurobiology (neuroimaging, electrophysiology, neuroendocrinology, neuroimmunology) to genetics, to risk factor research (perinatal factors are important), to treatment studies. His interest in the evolutionary origins of OCD led him to focus with his colleagues at Yale on the heightened parental preoccupations seen in new parents that were vividly described by Donald Winnicott in the 1950s. Dr Leckman is the author or co-author of over 300 original articles published in peer-reviewed journals, seven books, and 120 book chapters. He has written, edited or co-edited seven books. In 2002 he was identified by American Society for Information, Science and Technology as a "Highly Cited Researcher"—one of the world's most cited authors in psychology and psychiatry—in the top half of the top one percent of all publishing researchers.

Steven R. Marans, MD, Professor of Child Psychiatry and Psychiatry at the Yale Child Study Center and Department of Psychiatry, is the director of the National Center for Children Exposed to Violence (NCCEV), established by the White House and the US Department of Justice in 1999, and founder of the Child Development Community Policing (CD–CP) Program, a pioneering collaboration between mental health and law enforcement professionals providing collaborative responses to children and families exposed to violence that occurs in homes, neighbourhoods, and schools. Dr Marans joined the faculty of the Yale Child Study Center in 1984, after completing his training in child and adolescent psychoanalysis at the Anna Freud Centre in London. He received his master's degree in clinical social work from Smith College and his PhD in psychology from University College at London University. He is on the faculty of the Western New England Institute of Psychoanalysis, where he received his training in adult psychoanalysis. Dr Marans is on the editorial boards of the Psychoanalytic Study of the Child and the International Journal of Applied Psychoanalytic Studies and is a member of the Steering Committee and Advisory Board of the National Childhood Traumatic Stress Network. Additionally he is a member of the advisory boards of Lawyers for Children, America, and the Center for Social Emotional Education. His publications include *Listening to Fear: Helping Kids Cope, from Nightmares to the Nightly News* (2005).

Duncan J. McLean is an adult and child psychoanalyst. He is an Associate Member of the British Psychoanalytic Society and consultant psychiatrist in psychotherapy at the Maudsley Hospital. He is a psychiatrist at The Anna Freud Centre London.

David R. Shanks is Professor of Psychology and Head of the Psychology Department at University College London, England. He received his training in Cambridge and San Diego. He conducts research in cognitive psychology and has wide interests in many aspects of learning, memory, and decision making. His most recent book (co-authored with B. Newell and D. Lagnado) is *Straight Choices: The Psychology of Decision Making*.

Arietta Slade, PhD, is professor of clinical and developmental psychology at the City University of New York, and associate research scientist at the Yale Child Study Center. A clinician, teacher, and researcher, she has published widely in a number of areas, including the clinical implications of attachment theory and research, the interface between psychoanalysis and attachment theory, the development of the parent–child relationship and parental representations of the child, the relational contexts of play and early symbolization, and—most recently—the development of parental reflective functioning. She is on the editorial board of *Attachment and Human Development* and the *Journal of Infant, Child, and Adolescent Psychotherapy* and is editor, with Elliot Jurist and Sharone Bergner, of *Reflecting on the Future of Psychoanalysis* (forthcoming) and, with Dennie Wolf, of *Children at Play: Developmental and Clinical Approaches to Meaning and Representation*. She has also been in private practice for 25 years, working with children and adults, and has for the past five years been involved in developing early-intervention programmes for high-risk families and their children at the Yale Child Study Center.

Mark Solms, PhD, is Professor in Neuropsychology at the University of Cape Town, Honorary Lecturer in Neurosurgery at the St Bartholomew's & Royal London School of Medicine, and Lecturer in Psychology at University College London. He is also Director of the Arnold Pfeffer Center for Neuro-Psychoanalysis, New York. He is an Associate Member of the British Psychoanalytical Society, Honorary Member of the New York Psychoanalytic Society, Member of the British Neuropsychological Society, and Founding Co-chairman of the International Neuro-Psychoanalysis Society. With Edward Nersessian, he also founded, in 1999, the journal *Neuro-Psychoanalysis*.

Howard Steele is Associate Professor and Director of Graduate Studies in Psychology at the New School for Social Research in New York City. He is Founding and Senior Editor of the international quarterly journal, *Attachment & Human Development*, where review papers, clinical reports, and empirical studies appear that represent and extend the reach of attachment theory. Dr Steele's authored work addresses topics that include intergenerational patterns of attachment, reflective functioning, children's understanding of emotion, attachment and dementia, attachment issues in adoption, and the interface between attachment theory and other psychoanalytic theories. Currently, Dr Steele is completing an edited book project on clinical applications of the Adult Attachment Interview.

Miriam Steele, PhD, is currently an associate professor and Assistant Director of Clinical Psychology in the Graduate Faculty at the New School University. While training as a child psychoanalyst at the Anna Freud Centre in London, Miriam Steele received her PhD from the Department of Psychology at University College London. Her interest has been in bridging the world of psychoanalytic thinking and clinical practice with contemporary research in child development. Her research began with the study of "Intergenerational Patterns of Attachment", which embodied one of the first prospective longitudinal studies incorporating the Adult Attachment Interview and Strange Situation paradigms. This study has followed 100 families into the children's 17th year of life. The study was important in initiating the concept of "reflective functioning" and providing empirical data to demonstrate the importance of parental states of mind in the social and emotional development of their children. More recently, Dr Steele has become interested in the field of adoption and foster care with a view to understanding the impact of attachment representations from both the adopters and the children's perspectives. In a large longitudinal study of previously maltreated children who had been recently adopted, she demonstrated the utility in employing state of the art measures of attachment representations in understanding issues of matching adopter's and children's characteristics, the resolution of trauma, and change in the internal worlds of the children as a result of the dramatic intervention of the adoptive process.

Lane Strathearn, MD, is a developmental paediatrician who received his undergraduate and medical education at the University of Queensland, Brisbane, Australia. He did a fellowship in child protection and neurodevelopment at the Mater Children's Hospital in Brisbane before coming, in 2001, to Baylor College of Medicine, Houston, Texas, for a fellowship in developmental paediatrics. He is currently an assistant professor in paediatrics and research fellow at the Human Neuroimaging Laboratory. His research focuses on environmental factors associated with infant neurodevelopment, such as prenatal drug exposure, mother–infant attachment, and child maltreatment. He is currently the Principal Investigator in a longitudinal study of mothers and babies, funded by the National Institutes of Health, examining maternal brain responses to infant cues using functional MRI.

James E. Swain is a clinician—scientist doing neuroimaging research aimed at understanding the physiological and psychological basis of the parent–infant bond—critical to family functioning and the long-term health of the infant. After basic training in neuroscience, James completed a basic science doctorate on mechanisms nerve cell communication at the University of Toronto. Following this, he completed medical school in Toronto and followed his interest in neurons, brains, and behaviour through a psychiatry residency at the University of Ottawa. The impact of development and early life events drew him to also complete child psychiatry training, which is his current area of clinical practice. After scientific and clinical training in Canada, he completed a clinical research fellowship at the Yale Child Study Center. After gaining private foundation support from the Institute for Unlimited Love and the National Alliance for Research on Schizophrenia and Depression, he joined the faculty in 2005 to help lead a new developmental neuropsychiatry program in risk, resiliency, and recovery.

V. Robin Weersing, PhD, is an assistant professor in the Joint Doctoral Program in Clinical Psychology between San Diego State University and the University of California at San Diego. She has honorary faculty appointments at the Yale University Child Study Center and in psychiatry at the University of Pittsburgh Medical School. She also serves as the co-director of the Treatment Effectiveness and Dissemination Unit of the Pittsburgh-based Advanced Center for Interventions and Services Research for Early-Onset Mood and Anxiety Disorders. She received her doctorate in clinical psychology with a secondary concentration in quantitative methods in 2000 at the University of California, Los Angeles, and her dissertation was awarded the Michael J. Goldstein Distinguished Dissertation Award by the department. Dr Weersing has been a postdoctoral fellow in the Klingenstein Third Generation Foundation Program in Child Depression and is currently a faculty fellow of William T. Grant Scholars Program, a 2006 fellow of the Beck Institute for Cognitive Therapy and Research, and an awardee in the Robert Wood Johnson Depression in Primary Care program. Dr Weersing's work focuses on testing the effectiveness of psychosocial interventions for mood and anxiety disorders in youth in real-world clinical service settings and on understanding the mechanisms of action of behavioural health treatments.

Ada Zohar, PhD, is an associate professor of psychology and chair of the Department of Behavioral Sciences at Ruppin Academic Center in Israel. She was educated in clinical psychology and behaviour genetics at the Hebrew University of Jerusalem, received her postgraduate training in clinical psychology at the Hadassah Medical Center Jerusalem, and, on completing her PhD and qualifying as an expert clinical psychologist, spent two years as a postdoctoral fellow at the Yale Medical School Child Study Center, where she was honoured to collaborate with several prominent psychoanalysts, in addition to her focus on psychiatric genetics. On her return to Israel, her research interests have been the behaviour genetics of Gilles de la Tourette syndrome, obsessive-compulsive disorder, attention deficit hyperactive disorder, anorexia nervosa, and the role of personality as an endophenotype for psychopathology. In the autumn of 2006 she launched a large-scale study of personality and health in collaboration with Professor Robert Cloninger of George Washington University. In addition, she is an evidence-based interpersonal clinical psychologist, with a very active practice. A large proportion of her time is dedicated to the teaching of academic psychology and to training clinical psychology professionals.

Introduction

Linda C. Mayes, Peter Fonagy, & Mary Target

This volume marks the renewal of a past tie between two institutions historically dedicated to the well-being of children and their families—the Anna Freud Centre in London and the Yale Child Study Center. Both institutions have their beginnings with individuals who were leaders in the science of child development and children's mental health. The Anna Freud Centre, formally established a half-century ago, actually began with Anna Freud's commitment to the traumatized and orphaned children of London and the surrounding English countryside during World War II. From her and her colleagues' clinical experience, gained literally at the front lines, she established a world-renowned centre for the treatment and study of children with a range of serious developmental and psychological disorders. Her collaborations with Yale were extensive, involving the medical and law school as well as various colleagues in the community and clinical faculty. She spent much time at the Yale School of Medicine, working with Albert Solnit in the Child Study Center around innovative collaborations for children in the legal system. To this day, the volumes emerging from the Freud–Solnit–Goldstein collaborations are standards in the field of jurisprudence involving children. And there are a number of programmes at the Yale Child Study Center that show the influence of these bridge-building collaborations—those that take the most refined of clinical skills into the streets and the community to help children where they live.

At the same time Anna Freud was developing her methods for observing children's development, Arnold Gesell, the first director of the Child Study Center, was doing the same in New Haven. The Child Study Center began in 1911 with Gesell's studies of the benchmarks of normal development in a closely studied sample of New Haven children. While there is no record that Gesell and Anna Freud met, we know that he was invited to her lecture at Clark University when she came to commemorate her father's work. Gesell established the Child Study Center as a place where scholars interested in children and child development might come together—and his successors, Milton Senn, Albert Solnit, and Donald Cohen, continued and expanded that tradition. Today the Child Study Center is one of the Yale School of Medicine's most valued departments. It is nationally and internationally recognized for leadership in the scholarship and research in children's mental health. It trains the future clinical and investigative leaders in the field and sets much of the research agenda for child psychiatry and related disciplines.

The ties between these two institutions continued with the leadership of Donald Cohen, who, like Solnit, was a member of the board of trustees of the Anna Freud Centre. Alan Kazdin, the current director of the Child Study Center, was also involved over a decade ago with the first retrospective study of child psychoanalysis based on accumulated data from the Anna Freud Centre. Thus, the ties between the Child Study Center and Anna Freud Centre have a long history of colleagueship from leaders at the Child Study Center being involved collegially with scholars at the Anna Freud Centre. This new bridge, building on the years of good will and marked by the contributions to this volume, is another step forward. The programme is multidisciplinary, it bridges basic and clinical science, brings psychoanalytic perspectives to a range of treatment modalities, encourages young scholars to be interested in psychodynamically informed research perspectives, and nurtures new and integrative scholarship in psychoanalytic theory. The programme provides a model for how two institutions related in purpose and history can build an international programme that combines the best of the two individual centres.

A word about developmental psychoanalysis—the theme of this joint programme. As a discipline, psychoanalysis began at the interface of mind and brain and has always been about those most basic questions of biology and psychology: loving, hating, what brings us together as lovers, parents, and friends and what pulls us apart in conflict and hatred. These are the enduring mysteries of life and especially of early development—how young children learn the language of the social world with its intertwined biological, genetic, and experiential roots and how infants translate thousands of intimate moments with their parents into a genuine, intuitive, emotional connection to other persons. Basic developmental neuroscience and psychology has also of late turned to these basic questions of affiliation: of how it is that as humans our most basic concerns are about finding, establishing, preserving, and mourning our relationships. These are key areas to understanding our capacities for resilience across life or our vulnerability to life's hardships. These areas in broad strokes are also the substance of mind and brain, and the last decade has brought much new science to the biology of attachment, love, and aggression. These are areas that practicing psychoanalysts have long been immersed in and have much to say about—and contemporary neuroscientists and developmentalists are recognizing the importance of understanding these basic issues at a deeper, and more subjective experiential level. Implicitly and explicitly, this new programme is bringing together psychoanalysts and developmental cognitive and neuroscientists so that we may address these most basic mind–brain, body-and-mind issues with shared perspectives. The challenges before us are how to facilitate open discourse and collaborations among these perspectives and practitioners that often work at very different levels of discourse. But old boundaries are made seamless by a willingness to engage playfully with an idea and a shared focus—clinicians and scientists imagining side by side. We hope this volume is not only a first step in that process but also, through the themes of the chapters and the pairing of discussants, a beginning illustration of how the cross-disciplinary discourse might work.

CHAPTER ONE

Embodied psychoanalysis? Or, on the confluence of psychodynamic theory and developmental science

Ami Klin & Warren Jones

Background

What is the common ground between psychodynamic theory and developmental science? Some years ago, any attempt to address this question might have resulted in the excommunication of the attempter in both camps. And yet, there are many productive ways in which psychoanalysis and developmental science could interact, in a mutually beneficial manner, to fill in conceptual and methodological gaps in both.

Some reluctance to address potential areas of confluence comes from the attitude that these different approaches to the emergence and functioning of the human mind operate at different levels of discourse (e.g., the emotional mind vs. the cognitive mind, the clinical approach vs. the experimental approach, or the irrational psyche vs. brain-based mechanisms of information processing). This hesitation might be misplaced, however, since there are at least two reasons why these divides might be more artificial than real, and more reflective of a needless cultural battle rather than based on irreconcilable constructs and approaches: (a) The adoption of different levels of discourse was never an obstacle in cognitive science. For example, the powerful computer metaphor separating brain and mind into "hardware" and "software" processes (Gardner, 1985; Winograd, 1975) has allowed, for several decades, cognitive scientists to generate "software" models of information processing and then seek reification of their hypotheses in the brain through experiments, computer simulations, and, more recently, in functional neuroimaging studies (for a critical history of this effort in the artificial intelligence field, see Winograd & Flores, 1986). (b) A long-ignored approach to cognitive neuroscience is making an important comeback in the past few years (see Clark, 1999; Varela, Thompson, & Rosch, 1991). Variably called "embodied cognition" or "enactive mind", its main tenet is that any separation between mind and brain, or between cognition on the one hand and actions or bodily sensations on the other hand, is an artificial artefact of the cognitivist approach adopted in neuroscience since the advent of the computer metaphor. This approach states that to render cognitive processes independent of the body, in the same way as computer software is largely independent of computer hardware, is to make the psyche a "ghost" entity. This ghost hovers over an individual's bodily reality in some artificial theoretical space very much like software hovers over the computer circuitry. The computer metaphor makes Meaning—or how something means something to someone—an inscrutable mystery. We know where the meaning of software comes from—namely, from the mind of the programmer. But how do human cognitive processes (our software) mean anything to our sensations, actions, and feelings (our intimate hardware)? In our cognitive models of ourselves we typically have arrows connecting our various modules, or how sensory data feed into perception that feed into cognition and prompt action. However, we know very little what these arrows really are (Putnam, 1973) and whether it makes any sense to divide our minds and bodies into such distinct systems—not unlike a textbook that needs to be divided into chapters, ranging from more basic to more complex ones (e.g., from sensations to higher cognitive functions).

Psychoanalysis never made this divide. In this approach, the mind is, in many ways, a result of the developmental experiences of the body. Clearly, the psyche can elevate itself to great heights of symbolism and symbolic processing, but it is never free of its primordial generating forces—namely, the bodily experiences. But paradoxically, although psychoanalysis focuses a great deal on instinctual needs and responses to the world, it shies away from dealing with the basic unit of its philosophy—that is, how bodily sensations and experiences become symbolic tools. In fact, psychoanalysis deals almost exclusively with the (irrational) transactions of symbols and what they stand for. Just as in cognitivist psychology, there is a reluctance to bring mind and body together, and there is a clear preference for the mind. In this sense, the only contrast is that the former prefers the irrational mind, whereas the latter prefers the rational one. But there is an important difference. In contrast to cognitivist psychology and its software constructs, the mind in psychoanalysis is never a ghost: it is an immediate experience, a sensation, a motivation, an action, or a perception, all rooted in the body and its developmental experiences. In this sense, psychoanalysis is much closer to the emerging neuroscience approach of embodied cognition than it is to traditional cognitive psychology. Thus it may contribute to developmental science by dispelling the cognitive ghosts and transforming them into embodied pieces of meaning. And yet, psychoanalysis may benefit from developmental science by making its most fundamental theoretical unit—how bodily sensations become symbols and symbolic transactions—more available to systematic study.

Piaget: "the affective unconscious and the cognitive unconscious"

It is very reassuring that prior to this book and its brave contributors, some three decades ago, one of the creators of modern developmental science was asked to address the confluence of psychoanalysis and developmental science: Piaget was asked by the American Psychoanalytic Association (Piaget, 1973) to discuss potential areas of overlap. Focusing on the fundamental psychoanalytic construct of the unconscious, Piaget contrasted the psychoanalytic mainstay as the "affective unconscious" with his own life work on the emergence of processes of thinking, which he called "the cognitive unconscious". Neither process is immediately available to introspective access and hence remains unconscious unless a higher level of organization of experiences takes place through language-mediated thinking. In psychoanalytic therapy, the individual gains introspective access to, say, repressed memories, via the interpretations offered by the analyst in the process of the therapeutic "inter-view"—that is, through acts of communication (Farr, 1984). In this sense, the psychoanalytic setting makes possible the conversion of nonconceptual affective states into narrative memories through the ongoing communicative process. For example, early unpleasant memories might be rediscovered via the dynamics of free association. Piaget argued that many forms of cognitive learning were of a similar nature. In one observation he exemplifies this process in the following way:

> When a child manages (on his own or by imitation) to use one or two fingers to send off a pingpong ball on a horizontal surface in such a way that it starts backwards by itself, he does not see that he made it turn backward from the start. He believes that first it was rolling forward and then it changed direction by itself. To explain the lacunae or the distortions in the conscious awareness, one would be tempted to resort to a seemingly obvious reason—that is, that the child simply does not "understand" what he did, and so all he can remember is that which is intelligible to him. But we believe that this interpretation is inadequate. It is not true that the child has not understood anything of his successful action (reverse rotation of the pingpong ball). He did understand the essential, but *in action*, and not by thought; that is, by sensorimotor and not representational schemas. In other words, he "knows" how to cast the pingpong ball, and he knows it as a function of a certain perceptual motor learning (and by no means innately). [Piaget, 1973, pp. 254–255]

Piaget was, therefore, very much aware of learning and meaning that occur as a result of sensorimotor experiences in the world. He quotes Binet's whimsical expression: "Thought is an unconscious activity of the mind" (p. 250). And he goes on to describe a series of examples, typically characterized by processes of automatic behaviours or overlearned skills: for example, we can all crawl if asked to, but most of us are unable to provide a narrative that correctly accounts for how we do so; or we can run down a flight of steps, or play tennis, or improvise on the piano (if we are a little musical), but these processes not only are "unconscious", they are also disrupted if we try to think about it while performing the task (thinking about each note you play on the piano may disrupt your improvisational attempt; worrying about the physical trajectory of the tennis ball may, in fact, ensure that you will miss the ball flying at you at great speed). This was his way of validating the psychoanalytic unconscious, although he was cautious to separate his cognitive one from psychoanalysts' "affective" one. The "unconscious" brought the two camps together for a moment, but it is very unlikely that his audience greeted this intellectual exercise as true rapprochement. Their unconscious was loaded with emotional meaning, conflictual motivations, and social trauma. Throwing a ping-pong ball in reverse rotation was very different from having ambivalent feelings of identification and annihilation towards one's father.

Whether it was the pressures inherent in addressing the hostile audience of the American Psychoanalytic Association or his genuine belief in processes affecting learning that were outside his "child as a little scientist" model of development, Piaget did point to forms of meaning that were generally outside the realm of conscious thinking. His focus on sensorimotor schemas is particularly enlightening, given his articulate descriptions of learning as a result of the coupling of a child's bodily sensations and actions towards the surrounding world. What he was less prepared to tackle was the possibility that we use "sensorimotor schemas" to learn more about the world than what he described in his genetic epistemology (Piaget, 1970). There may have been a father or a mother responding in some affective way to the child's actions on the ping-pong ball after all.

What Piaget omitted in his accounts, another creator of developmental science made into the pillar of his developmental theories. In Piaget's world, caregivers could be imitated, but they were otherwise non-players in the child's development. The child protagonist proceeded relentlessly in scientific pursuits of world discovery almost by himself or herself. Not so for Vygotsky (1978). In his work, and in the work of decades of Soviet developmental psychology that he generated (Wertsch, 1979), thought itself was a social phenomenon, or the inalienable result of being born immersed in social experiences. As for the American Pragmatist George Herbert Mead (1934), symbols emerged from social interaction, with its cultural relativity and complexity, but with a shared sense of regularity captured by conventional symbols such as language, which, in turn, reflected shared regularities in social experiences. The works of both Vygotsky and Mead are primarily known for their accounts of the social emergence of symbols and language (e.g., Mead's work was reduced by his students to the concept of "symbolic interactionism", or a call to the relativism of culture). Put simplistically, the contents of our thoughts reflect our social–cultural experiences or upbringing. Taken in this manner, Vygotsky's and Mead's work would have little to add to our discussion of the unconscious, except maybe the notion that we unconsciously use cultural tools that are embedded in our cultural pool. But there is nothing about the process of learning or about how cognition may result from sensorimotor actions and experiences. In other words, there is little that we can use to add the social element to Piaget's sanitized world of the infant's "learning in action" (where feelings and motivations are kept at bay by his scientific stance).

Thankfully, there is much more in Vygotsky's and Mead's work than what has crystallized as their main contributions in the literature about their writings. One of Vygotsky's (1962) important concepts in his account of the emergence of thought and language was one that he borrowed from his predecessor, William Stern (in Vygotsky, 1962).

Stern made the important distinction between the meaning of words (say, the conventional dictionary definition of a word) and the *sense* of words (or the body of vaguely defined, personalized, and individualized sensations that are associated with a given word). The former reflects some more-or-less accidental result of cumulative communications within a group of people or some cultural determinism shaped by the experiences of this community. Words are conventionalized to become the language of a given people within a well-delineated geographical environment and cultural landscape. The sense of words, however, reflects the individualized experiences of a person in the process of acquisition of that word or concept. Although the meaning of a word is community-wide and fairly static, a convention that can be enshrined in a dictionary, the sense of words is an individualized phenomenon, a cumulative body of feelings and sensations experienced by one person in relation to that word or concept. Thus while the meaning of the word "Mother" is a noun defined by descriptions such as "a female parent, a woman in authority, a caring female dedicated to the well-being of their offspring", the sense of the word "mother" is as varied as one individual's numerous experiences with a mother or mother-like figure. While the meaning of the word "mother" is by force a conscious thought, the sense of the word "mother" is an amalgam of feelings and sensations with portions that can be—but not necessarily are—brought to conscious awareness at any moment in time. And yet, they predispose us to act towards mothers in a certain way or ways. While the meaning of words may become entangled in strange associations that require free-associative narratives to become conscious thought, the words themselves are not fodder for unconscious conflicts. In contrast, the sense of words is the province of psychoanalytic thought and therapy since it reveals growths and formations of individualized meanings and experiences that hang from the fairly straightforward word definitions. In many ways, word meanings can be referred to as computer semantics (once the symbol is fully described, the computer software or the human linguistic apparatus can manipulate it to convey straightforward messages); in contrast, the sense of words can be referred to as human semantics (an almost solipsistic mapping of a person's cumulative experiences, mapped in terms of the person's unique life of feelings and predispositions associated with events involving that concept). Although Stern was as removed from Freud as Vygotsky was, they were contemporaneous thinkers, and it is impossible to discard some form of influence crossing the porous borders of the early Soviet Union.

Mead's thinking about the emergence of symbols within the realm of social interaction was much better defined and elaborated. He described the process of the emergence of mind with the precision of an eighteenth-century philosopher. A student of Darwin's writings, Mead's life's work was an attempt to trace the emergence of the human mind from the social environment not unlike Darwin's treatment of human biped locomotion. And his starting point was, in fact, Darwin's *The Expression of the Emotions in Man and Animals* (1872). Mead's ideas are as applicable in phylogenetic discussions of the emergence of mind as in ontogenetic accounts. Humans make gestures to one another. These gestures are facial (e.g., grimaces), bodily (e.g., waving away), or vocal (e.g., inflected sounds, speech-like vocalizations). A gesture becomes a symbol when the gesture-maker is capable of anticipating the response of the other to his or her gesture prior to actually making the gesture. The aspect of Mead's thinking that is most pertinent to the current discussion is that Mead defined the response of the other as the meaning of a gesture. In so doing, he was not only describing the emergence of symbolic communication (and eventually of language); he was also describing a process of learning. Within the highly charged settings of human dyads, triads, or group interaction, the individual's actions upon others become imbued with meaning as a result of the reactions of the others to those actions. These meanings are composites of feelings of pleasure, displeasure, fright, tenderness, safety and lack thereof, helplessness, panic, predispositions to approach or to flee, to hit or to caress, or, more generally, they are as complex as there are experiences resulting from the interaction of people. Thus while Mead focused a great deal of his work on what eventually becomes cultural symbols such as words, the learning mechanism that he described was a more general one.

In fact, the learning mechanism that Mead described in his philosophical writings bears great resemblance to the formation of intrapsychic dynamics between people in psychoanalytic thinking. And unlike contemporaneous cognitivist psychology, Mead's mental meanings are as real and immediate as the reactions of others were at the times of incipience or change of these constructs. They are not algorithmic ghosts, because they stand as affective and predispositional proxies to the reactions of others. To exemplify this: to a digital being like a computer, the word "terrifying" may mean something different from the word "loving" only because the words have been given, *a priori*, different definitions. The computer might hardly notice an incorrect use of these words if they are syntactically correct within a sentence.

Nor is the computer likely to frown at the text "The mummy opened its cavernous mouth in a *loving* grimace to the explorer." In a way, words have meanings only if they have definitions that can fit into a procedure (e.g., a syntactically correct answer, or a correctly spelled word). Otherwise, computers are totally neutral to semantics: words do not mean anything to them. To non-digital beings like human beings, however, it would be impossible to stay neutral to the mummy statement. There is nothing loving about mummies. The word has meaning to us in that it makes us feel in a certain way (e.g., we feel terror), and predisposes us to behave in a certain way (e.g., to run away). In some situations, words and combinations thereof can bring about overwhelming feelings and reactions in us. They can only do so because they are proxies to real experiences that left indelible traces in our senses and emotional make-up.

The combination of Piaget's, Vygotsky's, and Mead's ideas forms the starting point for the approach to the emergence of mind that we summarize in this chapter. There is a need to de-sanitize Piaget's observations by inserting people and social learning into his developmental account. While sensorimotor learning, or learning in action, works for throwing ping-pong balls in reverse rotation, they may also work in similar ways for the infant–mother dyad. If so, there is more than a "cognitive unconscious" (i.e., learning that takes place as a result of sensorimotor explorations of the physical world); there is also a "social–affective unconscious" (i.e., learning that takes place as a result of sensorimotor explorations of the social world). Had he made this point in his 1973 address to the American Psychoanalytic Association, there might have been the impetus to compile a book like the current one at the time of his historical presentation. And while Vygotsky emphasized the social nature of the emergence of conventional language (1978), he also discussed the highly individualized senses of words (i.e., the experiential foundations of language and concepts). Echoing Stern, he suggested that those experiential components of language also emerged from within the social immersion of the child. Vygotsky's famous definition of thought as internalized speech (1962), if encompassing the sense of words, would suggest that "linguistic experiences", and not only words, also become part of our internal lives. And, finally, Mead (1934), whose paradigm for symbol learning was the power to anticipate the reaction of the other to one's gesture (in other words: the meaning of one's action is the response of the other person), provides the social process for the emergence of mind as the internalization of other people and their responses. This revisionistic approach to the work of these giants of developmental theory would make them fully compatible with psychodynamic theory. There is room for a social–affective unconscious (i.e., internalized experiences of other people and their actions), and for object relations (since the meaning of others, and of oneself, is also seen as the internal consolidation of social–affective experiences emerging in social interaction).

An attempt to create such a synthesis, however, never happened. And developmental constructs that could be integrated into a more unified theory of development spun their own literatures across rigid partisan lines. It is of interest that even within the field of non-psychoanalytic child psychology, these tensions were never resolved. And, over time, there were winners and losers. For example, Mead's (1934) role-taking framework for the development of mind—and its Darwinian roots—was reinvented as the "theory of mind" framework. This was the notion that in order to ascribe mental states such as intentions, beliefs, and feelings to others, the child must have a "theory" (e.g., a problem-solving algorithm) that other people have minds (Leslie, 1987; Premack & Woodruff, 1978; Pylyshyn & Demopoulos, 1986). John Flavell, whose work became a seminal landmark for theory of mind research (Flavell, 2004), first published a study testing the validity of Mead's role-taking hypothesis regarding the emergence of children's understanding of mental states (Flavell, Botkin, Fry, Wright, & Jarvis, 1968). Research on social referencing (the child learns the meaning of an entity in the world by monitoring, and internalizing, the adult's reactions to that entity; Campos & Sternberg, 1981) with its psychodynamic roots has by and large given way to research on joint attention (the child's ability to attend to what the adult is attending to: see Tomasello, Carpenter, Call, Behne, & Moll, 2005[4]) with its cognitivist roots. While in these two instances it made sense to distil more experiment-friendly concepts from the original and more convoluted ones, it may be unfortunate that this also implied the construction of purely cognitive (and computer-like) models of the emergence of mind (e.g., Mandler, 1992), which may have stripped babies from their emotions, motivation, actions, and bodily sensations. Had this not happened, the reconciliation between psychoanalytic theory an developmental science would perhaps be a more easily attainable goal.

It is the case, however, that cognitive theories of the emergence of mind have generated a large body of experimental evidence, and this growing literature has crossed the mind–brain divide through an ever-increasing number of neurofunctional studies of social cognition (Schultz, 2005). If one is to argue for some reintegration of body and emotions into the field of mind development in children, it is incumbent upon the writer to justify the need for such an approach. The need for models of embodied (in contrast to algorithmic) minds is probably best illustrated in a brief consideration of autism—a neurodevelopmental disorder derailing the process of socialization from birth—to which we now turn.

Autism and mechanisms of socialization

Autism is a neurodevelopmental disorder impacting on a child's social, communication, and play skills (Volkmar, Paul, Klin, & Cohen, 2005). It disrupts the basic course of socialization, as children are unable to intuit other people's feelings, "read" other people's thoughts, and, more generally, to develop reciprocal relationships. There is a strong genetic component, with recurrence rates among sibships of 2–10%. Its prevalence is much higher than previously thought, with rates ranging from 2 to 5 per 1,000 individuals, if one considers the variants of the condition. There is tremendous variability in manifestation of the syndrome. Intellectual functioning ranges from profound mental retardation to gifted intelligence; many individuals are entirely nonverbal, whereas others may "talk too much"; some are extraordinarily isolated and aloof, whereas others make continuous social approaches but in awkward, inappropriate, or eccentric ways.

There are two predominant psychological theories of autism: the first, mentioned above, posits a disruption of the capacity to impart mental states to others (e.g., beliefs, desires, intentions, and feelings) or to have a "theory of mind" (ToM: see Baron-Cohen, 1995); the second posits that the universal human drive to integrate information into coherent "wholes" or to link pieces of stimuli or meaning into contextual entities is lacking in autism, and, in this sense, individuals with this condition have a cognitive apparatus marked by "weak central coherence" (WCC). While ToM focuses primarily on social cognitive deficits, the WCC is a more general theory describing cognitive deficits with implications to learning more broadly, with the social deficits being one instance only, albeit an important one. Both hypotheses share the emphasis, however, on cognitive skills required for successful social adaptation.

ToM and WCC both have strong face validity. Individuals with autism have variable but typically deficient abilities in understanding other people's behaviour in terms of mental determinants. Therefore, they may become overly focused on manifest behaviour at the expense of intentions contextualizing the meaning of that behaviour; they do not adjust their communications to other people's expectations; their play is typically devoid of representational elements or symbolic themes. In many ways, persons with autism appear to navigate the social world as if there were no minds or other people's subjectivity upholding them as an object of thought and observation. These individuals also have an extremely fragmented view of the world, often focusing on unrelated aspects of the environment rather than on ways in which different elements fit into a more integrated entity or event. They go from "parts to whole", missing the overall meaning or context of what they experience, be it in learning, in communication, or in social interaction. Their thinking often becomes entangled in leaves while missing the forests. This learning style has a disastrous impact on their social adaptation, since, for example, in order to understand what a person is communicating, there is a need to listen to her speech, to observe facial and bodily gestures as well as posture and voice inflection, and to appreciate the specific setting where the communication is delivered. If those contextual cues go unnoticed, the person is likely to respond in an overly literal manner, thus missing the true meaning of an interaction. This is particularly true in peer interaction when children say many things that they do not mean, and they mean so many things that they do not say.

Despite the strong face validity (and the considerable literature supporting its predictions, e.g., Baron-Cohen, Tager-Flusberg, & Cohen, 2000; Happé, 2005), there are some concerns that while these hypotheses are right, they may not be touching at the developmental causes of autism. In other words, they may result from disruptions in sociability that predate them both chronologically and causally—that is, ToM and WCC may be distilled results formed from more fundamental and pervasive social disruptions (Klin, Jones, Schultz, & Volkmar, 2003). In order to illustrate this contention, we present some clinical observations and experimental studies carried out at the Yale Child Study Center. Note that there is virtually no area of overlap between ToM and WCC on the one hand and psychodynamic theory, given the cognitive/affective chasm separating cognitivist and social affective views of the emergence of mind. It is, in fact, paradoxical that these prevalent theories have moved so far from Leo Kanner's (1943) original hypothesis of autism as a disorder of "affective contact".

Let us begin with a 15-month-old girl (called "Helen" for the purpose of this chapter), whose older brother had been diagnosed with autism some 20 months before her (Klin et al., 2004).

> Helen toddled into the playroom behind her father, entirely oblivious to the presence of the examiner. Attempts to engage her through exaggerated facial gestures and inflected vocalizations from a distance as close as two inches from her face did not alter her overly focused exploration of cause–effect toys. And although she could not "see" the examiner standing so close to her, she did turn around very purposely at one point, crawling quickly towards an M&M (i.e., a piece of candy) that was lying on the floor some 5 feet away from her.

As clinicians, we are also mobile laboratories of social engagement, hoping to make ourselves into malleable forms to be shaped by our child clients. In this case, the examiner had a clear sense that, in contrast to similar situations with typical children when their world changes in the presence of any adult, Helen had no internal sense of the examiner's mind, focus of attention, or desires—in other words, she does not have ToM. But the examiner's feeling was in fact much more fundamental than that. It appeared that Helen did not have much of a "theory of body" either, since she was oblivious to being the focus of the adult's intense gaze and vocalizations. Typical babies are preferentially drawn to speech sounds relative to other environmental sounds from birth or soon thereafter (Mills & Melhuish, 1974). They are more likely to look at adults looking at them (rather than looking away) from the time they are 4 days old (Farroni, Csibra, Simion, & Johnson, 2002). By the age of 7 weeks or so, they are not only looking preferentially at people, but within faces, they prefer to look at the more socially revealing elements aspects of faces, such as eyes, rather than at less expressive aspects of faces such as mouths or contours of the head (Haith, Bergman, & Moore, 1977). At 15 months, Helen, whose nonverbal cognitive functioning was not delayed, was not displaying sociability known to be present already in very young babies.

Still, this failure is even more profound than that, since humans hold no exclusive privileges over these fundamental mechanisms of socialization. When our smaller and hairier predecessors jumped from branch to branch, there was a need to process information from cospecifics' eyes, since the other animal's intentions might have been to kill or to mate. The acuity of this phenomenon pervades our own daily lives. Most of us are extraordinarily aware of being looked at since we have a clear sense that "looking at means thinking about", and being the objects of others' subjectivity is one of humans' obsessions. And this phenomenon is not only seen in the visual domain. Given the fragility and prolonged infancy period of primates, becoming estranged from caregivers means certain death. It does make sense, therefore, for baby primates, us included, to gravitate towards our caregivers' voice. Such multimodal mechanisms of socialization appear to push babies towards adults, who reciprocate in kind, creating a mutually reinforcing choreography that sets the stage for socialization and the development of social cognitive skills. In this context, Helen's lack of social engagement would place her in a developmental path disrupting every single process known to require social experiences, And since our brains not only determine what we will be but also become repositories of repeated experiences—in other words, our brains "become who we are" (LeDoux, 2002)—brain organization and specialization are also likely to be compromised.

Given these clinical observations, we questioned what the social world looks like from Helen's isolated stance and what the contents of her mind are. In other words, we wanted to image the surrounding world through her eyes and probe for mental representations of people and people's actions (Klin & Jones, submitted). In order to test whether or not Helen can think about social action, we filmed adults acting typical scenes of caregivers approaching their babies (e.g., "pat-a-cake, "peek-a-boo", "so big"). We then rendered these people's actions as point-light displays (see Figure 1.1 and Klin et al., 2003). When stationary, these point-light displays are described by children as "stars", but when they move, they may say "Oh, it's a man of stars." First pioneered by Johansson (1973), these lights capture biological movement, and, in our case, the movements of an approaching caregiver. We presented these animations in a split-screen setting. On one side, we showed the right-side-up animation. On the other side, we showed the same animation, but upside-down and played backwards (the latter was necessary in order to discourage children's looking back and forth between the two animations once they had noticed that they were mirror images). We also played back the audio of the

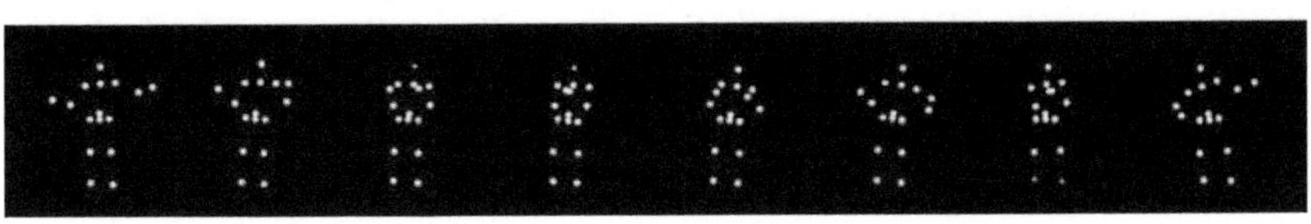

Figure 1.1: Series of static images of the human form rendered as point-light displays

situations (e.g., the nursery rhyme, or whatever sound had been used by the model caregivers when the scenes were filmed). Our assumption was that if children could "fill in the blanks between the dots", as it were, and recognize that these were people, they would then look preferentially at the right-side-up animation (rather than the upside-down one) since in their experience they would be more likely to see caregivers approach them in this way. In other words, they would match the sound effects with their mental template of that action, which was facilitated by the visual animation, whereas if they had no internal representations of human action, they would move their focus of visual attention randomly between the two displays. Similar abilities have been documented in 3-month-old human infants (Fox & McDaniel, 1982), in non-human species like monkeys (Oram & Perrett, 1994), and even in birds (Regolin, Tommasi, & Vallortigara, 2000). The recognition of motion as "biological" is a highly conserved and unique system that makes possible the recognition of movement of others in order to move towards or away from them.

Helen viewed 11 such animations. In 10 of these animations her view paths were entirely random, whereas two control children, one matched on chronological and nonverbal mental age (at 15 months) and one matched on basic understanding of language (at 7 months), had a robust preference for the right-side-up animations. However, in one of the animations, Helen showed a close to 90% viewing preference for the right side up. This was very perplexing, and therefore we revisited that animation. It depicted an adult acting the "pat-a-cake" game. A more careful look at our design led us to a serendipitous observation. Remember that our upside-down animations were played both upside-down and backwards. However, the speech accompanying the two animations was the same for both—namely forwards—since the presentation of the stimuli was simultaneous side by side. When "pat-a-cake" became point-light displays, the effect was of balls or lights hitting each at midpoint (i.e., the clapping) synchronously with the original sound of clapping. This was the only animation in which a sound was actually temporally contingent to something in the visual display. In all of the other animations, the sound effects (or speech/nursery rhymes) provided only the context for the display. An inadvertent implication from this design is that in the "pat-a-cake" animation we created a disynchrony in the upside-down display (i.e., because the animation was played backwards, there was no synchrony between the balls colliding and the clapping sound). This design problem generated the following hypothesis: Could it be that

Helen was acutely aware of this physical contingency (if something collides, it makes a synchronous sound) and was therefore looking at the right-side-up animation (and away from the upside-down one) because only in this one did the physical contingency occur correctly? In other words, although she might not have mental representations of people, she did have mental representations or expectations for physical events? Note that from our visual-preference data summary she could have been looking at any portion of the right-side-up side of the screen. But for this hypothesis to be corroborated, she would have to be looking exactly at the collision of balls or lights.

We were able to corroborate this prediction in the following way: As Helen had watched the video stimuli within an eye-tracking laboratory, we could actually map her visual attention onto the viewed scenes for the entire procedure. The eye-tracking set-up involves the utilization of two cameras—one filming the viewed scene and the other, an infrared one, focused on the child's eye to obtain two coordinates showing the exact location of the child's visual focus (or foveation). By superimposing the recording from these two cameras, it is possible to display, moment by moment, where the child is visually focusing during the video presentation. As we replayed our recording of Helen's data for the pat-a-cake animation, it was apparent that she followed very closely the point-lights' collision at midline. Therefore, despite her inability to "see" the other animations as human actions, she was exquisitely aware of a cross-modal physical contingency. In other words, she could not think about people, but she could think about things.

We then presented real-life videos of caregivers acting out typical approaches to babies (these individuals were filmed from the shoulders up). When we analysed Helen's visual fixations for some 12 caregiver clips, she spent the majority of the time looking at people's mouths, some time looking at background objects, and virtually no time looking at their eyes. Given our clinical experiences with her, the lack of fixation on eyes was to be expected. But the fixation on mouths was not. However, given her visual fixations in the experiment with the point-light displays, we can hypothesize that, possibly, she was looking at the mouth because this is where an important physical contingency takes place—namely, the lip movements match the speech sounds (in the same way as balls make a sound when they collide). If so, our conclusion would be that Helen was watching a face but was not "seeing" a person; she was, instead, seeing physical contingencies. Data for the two controls were very different. Both of them showed an overwhelming preference for the caregivers' eyes. This sad hypothesis will be pursued in the future by purposely desynchronizing lip movements and speech sounds.

The notion that a child with autism may watch someone without seeing a person has obvious implications for development—in addition to bringing up core psychodynamic concepts such as object relations. It would imply that her mind was specializing on things rather than people, and that her brain would show equally atypical specialization. Three sets of studies of adolescents and adults with autism support this prediction: (a) Can adolescents and adults with autism think about people (or are they, like Helen, more adept at thinking about things)? (b) When they are looking at people, are they drawn to socially salient features of scenes (or are they, like Helen, drawn to inanimate aspects or physical contingencies in what they see)? And (c) is the brain circuitry subserving the processing of social stimuli in typical individuals equally involved in individuals with autism (or do these neuronal systems, like the prediction resulting from the experiment with Helen, become specialized in the processing of non-social events)?

In the first set of studies, a group of normative-IQ adolescents and adults with autism were presented with the famous Heider and Simmel (1944) cartoon animation in which geometric forms move and act like humans (see Figure 1.2). Typical viewers immediately recognize the social nature of the cartoon and provide narratives that include a number of social attributions involving relationships portrayed there

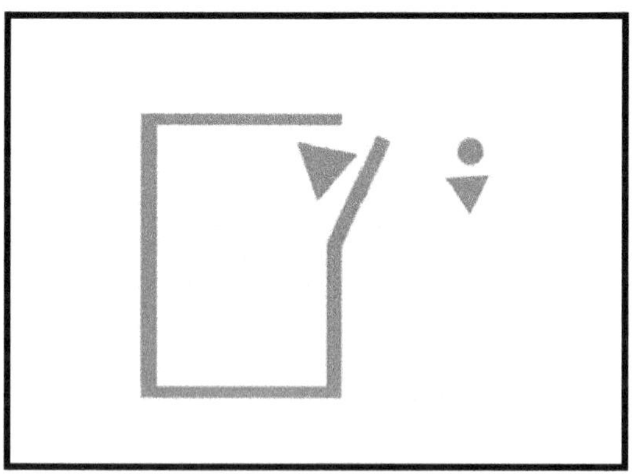

Figure 1.2: Screen shot showing cast of characters from Heider & Simmel's (1944) cartoon.

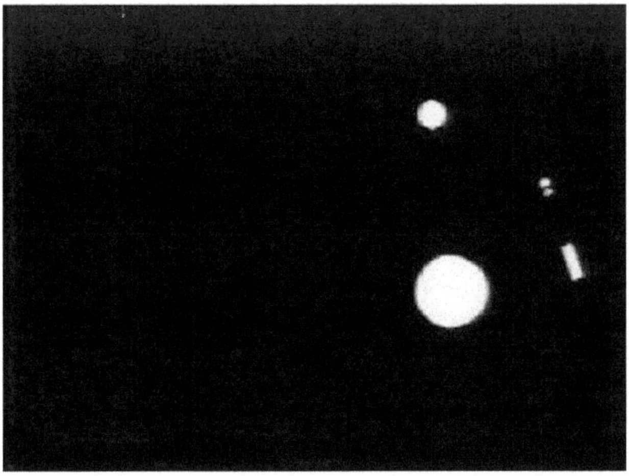

Figure 1.3: Screen shot illustrating the Physical Attribution Task (Klin & Jones, 2006).

(e.g., being a bully, being a friend), the meaning of specific actions (e.g., trapping, protecting), and attribution of mental states (e.g., being shy, thinking, being surprised). In contrast, the individuals with autism have great difficulty making these attributions (Klin, 2000). As this difficulty could be the result of "weak central coherence" (connecting the various forms and movements into a coherence social story), a similar group of individuals with autism were presented with an animation in which a physical scene (rather than a social one) was depicted with geometric forms (it portrayed the launching of a rocket into space: see Figure 1.3). We called this task a "physical attribution task" (PAT), to contrast it with the "social attribution task" (SAT) depicted above. This new group of individuals with autism had very similar difficulties with the SAT as the original group had had, showing marked deficits in their ability to think about people when viewing ambiguous visual displays of human action. Interestingly, however, they were equally able, and sometimes superior to typical controls, when making physical attributions on the PAT (Klin & Jones, 2006). This dichotomy is probably best exemplified by the narratives obtained for a 38-year-old very bright man with autism. When looking at the SAT, his attributions were entirely physical:

> "Starts when a small equilateral triangle breaks out of a square. A small sphere or circle appears and slides down the broken

> rectangle. The triangles were either equilateral or isosceles. Later the small, I think, isosceles triangle and sphere bounce around each other, maybe because of a magnetic field. . . ."

When looking at the PAT, his attributions were among the best for either experimental or control groups:

> "The rocket is being launched and is in preliminary orbit around the earth, winding around the moon at the appropriate distance so that the satellite can be released. The satellite was launched from the rocket, and it actually landed on the moon. The satellite was actually more like a lunar module. . . ."

This person showed an exquisite ability to think about physical events while being unable to attribute social meaning to a display that is recognized as social by infants (Gergely et al., 1995), and even primates (Uller & Nichols, 2000). His results, like those of others in this study, would suggest that Helen's developmental path might also move towards a specialization on things rather than people. Of interest, the results on the PAT study showed that individuals with autism are not entirely impaired in their ability to integrate information into coherent wholes, as predicted by the WCC hypothesis. They seem to be able to do so, at least in some situations such as in that particular study, but in the physical rather than the social domain.

In the second set of studies, adolescents and adults with autism watched scenes from a commercial film while we recorded their visual fixations and visual scan paths in our eye-tracking laboratory (Klin, Jones, Schultz, Volkmar, & Cohen, 2002a, 2002b). Relative to controls, the individuals with autism spent three times less time fixating on the characters' eyes, two and half times more time looking at their mouths, and almost three times more time looking at objects. Given the variability within the autism group, we examined the possibility that their visual fixation patterns might predict social adaptation in real life as well as the degree of their social disability. Our hypothesis was that, within the autism group, those who fixated more on eyes would be both more able and less disabled. However, there was no correlation between fixation on eyes and social competence. These results suggested that additional fixation on eyes did not afford greater competence in real life, which, in turn, suggested that the individuals with autism may be unable to extract information of social meaning from the eyes of others. To our surprise, however, greater fixation on mouths was strongly correlated with more social ability and less social disability among individuals with autism. These results appeared to suggest that in contrast to eyes, the mouth, or the language that comes from the mouth, is meaningful to these persons, since they can at least get the manifest theme of social scenes. Clearly, however, without attention to contextual factors such as facial and bodily gestures as well as the reactions of others to the speaker, there is the constant danger of misinterpretation (e.g., in a sarcastic remark). Those who fixated more on objects were the most disabled in the group. In a sense, while those who fixated on mouths were actually focusing on the social action (albeit via language only), the former were actually more removed from the social scenes, focusing on inanimate objects instead.

While the results of these studies are compelling, the individual illustrations might in fact be a more powerful indicator of the phenomena observed. In one scene, two of the protagonists of the film are involved in a passionate kiss in the foreground of the picture, but one viewer with autism is visually fixating on a light switch at the corner of the room (Klin et al., 2003). In another scene, a husband and wife show facial expressions of terror after a frightening action displayed by one of the protagonists. The viewer with autism moves alongside the eyes to focus on the husband's mouth, which, in contrast to the terrified eyes, is entirely expressionless. This viewer would appear to have missed the entire meaning of the scene. In another scene the husband of the same couple is interrupted by his wife who begins to tell a story that embarrasses her husband. The viewer with autism focuses on the mouth of the wife, missing the reactions of the non-speaking husband and thus failing to appreciate the fact that he is now very embarrassed. We were once presenting these studies at a public conference in which a lady with autism had previously spoken about her first-person experiences of having the condition. When we began to show our video clips with eye-tracking data, this lady interrupted us and stated: "I can't see the movie because of the door handle!" Indeed, after viewing these video clips possibly hundreds of times for eye-tracking data coding, neither of us was aware of the door handle, although this was indeed the salient feature of this movie to this lady with autism.

These pronounced social deficits make us speculate about the ways in which individuals with autism re-create in their minds the world around them. Imaging their creation from the standpoint of their eyes, they seem to populate their minds with light fixtures, moving inanimate objects, physical contingencies, and language that may not necessarily map on social experiences. Clearly, they have difficulties with mental states, as predicted by the ToM hypothesis, but this is almost stating the obvious. Their mental recreation of the world around them appears to go beyond a psyche devoid of concerns with other people's mental states; their internal world appears to be skewed in the direction of things and physical or factual entities. Our typical obsession with others is not there, and it is replaced by atypical preoccupations with non-social regularities occurring in the environment. And it is important to note that all individuals completing the various studies reported here were able to make attributions of mental states to others if the situation was explicitly and verbally given to them, like a problem-solving task. Some might speak in an articulate manner about people and their attitudes, about beliefs and intentions, and even about relationships. But they are unable to translate this knowledge into real-life competence, or experiments like the ones described here that attempt to simulate naturalistic situations and are, therefore, implicit rather than explicit. Our hypothesis for this puzzling issue is that individuals with autism with sufficient intelligence and language are capable of learning *about* the world by acquiring factual information that can be acquired as a set of explicit symbols, but they are not capable of learning *in* the world—in action, as it were—by accumulating experiences in an immersive social environment, which, in turn, leads to the emergence of social capacities such as entertaining other people's beliefs and one's own, as well as desires, intentions, and predispositions. This pattern of learning seems to lead higher-functioning individuals with autism to the successful acquisition of concepts and complex linguistic competence, and they can reason about explicit social phenomena. These are the "roof-top" of our social and communicative development. But we contend that this conceptual competence is normatively the result of a lifetime of social–affective experiences, embedded in fast-pace social interaction and rooted in survival responses demanding fast reactions and adaptation. In other words, the roof-top is built atop experiential columns. For the individuals with autism, however, their roof-top appears to be free-standing.

A final hypothesis originating from our clinical observations of Helen was that not only the formation of her mind, but the organization of her brain would be altered as a result of her extricating herself from the realm of social interactions. This prediction is supported by a series of functional neuroimaging studies led by Robert Schultz (Grelotti et al., 2005; Schultz et al., 2000). In one functional magnetic resonance imaging (fMRI) study, higher-functioning adolescents and adults with autism were presented with pictures of faces and objects and their patterns of brain activation were compared with those of controls. In contrast to controls, for whom face processing was associated with activation of the lateral fusiform gyrus (a midtemporal structure specializing on face recognition: see Kanwisher, McDermott, & Chun, 1997), face recognition in individuals with autism was associated with activation in inferior temporal gyrus structures, an activation pattern that was obtained for controls when they were processing objects. The conclusion from this study was that individuals with autism processed faces as objects. There are clear advantages in processing faces in a special way. Most of us need to know thousands of faces in order to function competently in our social lives. If we saw faces as objects, we might in fact have a much more reduced repertoire of familiar faces in our minds, just as we have a reduced number of objects in a given category in our minds. For example, we might not create too much havoc if we mistakenly pick up the wrong bag at the luggage-claim carousel in an airport, but we would certainly be doomed if we failed to recognize our mother-in-law rushing to us in the airport's waiting area. We do know that individuals with autism are able to recognize some important faces in their lives, although overall they have great face-processing deficits (e.g., Klin et al., 1999). What is more interesting, however, is that they seem to acquire the ability to recognize faces in a way that is different from their typical peers: perhaps as an object with a given configuration, but without the immediacy that comes from our repeated experiences, from birth onwards, that there is a person behind that face.

The study by Schultz and colleagues (2000), and subsequent studies that corroborated the reported findings of hypoactivation of the fusiform gyrus to face stimuli, generated some speculation that this issue could be at fault in autism and could, in fact, play a causative role in the syndrome. This would run counter to the hypothesis that the brain crystallizes the repeated experiences of the person—in this case, because we all experience, seek, run away from, recognize, contemplate so many faces in the course of our development from birth that the fusiform gyrus reflects this specialization (thus mind becomes brain). To test this hypothesis, David Grelotti and colleagues (2005) conducted an intensive study with one higher-functioning young adult with autism whose main love in life is Digimon characters: cartoon figures that appear in computer and video games, on TV shows and in films. This individual was presented with three kinds of stimuli—faces, objects, and Digimon characters—and patterns of brain activation were compared to controls. As expected, there was no fusiform activation for either faces or objects; however, there was strong activation in the fusiform and associated limbic structures to the Digimon characters. Thus, it certainly appeared to be the case that this individual's fusiform and associated circuitry were functioning well, but they had specialized to something other than faces, probably reflecting this person's repeated experiences and expertise with these figures (see also Gauthier, Tarr, Anderson, Skudlarski, & Gore, 1999).

These preliminary results evoke a number of speculations as to what might happen to Helen's brain specialization, given her preferential attention to physical contingencies over social ones in her naturalistic viewing of the world around her. Collectively, though, these various lines of study seem to call into question any notion that the fundamental derailment in socialization processes in individuals with autism can be explained without a deeper understanding of these individuals' reward systems—that is, what draws their eyes and their minds and what does not, and the neuronal circuitry associated with relative salience of things in the world to a given organism. Reward systems may involve higher-level thinking in complex situations lived by human children and adults; but fight-or-flight reactions inherent in reward systems are much more visceral in human infants and non-human species. Some of these visceral reactions remain with us for the duration of our lives, despite our complex symbolic existence. We may still turn to a frightening stimulus—or a loved one—at the blink of an eye, or respond first to someone with our predisposition and unconscious intentions prior to reining them in with our explicit thoughts.

The fact that autism has its onset in infancy suggests the need to embrace these fundamental mechanisms of socialization. As in Piaget's examples, we need to study how we learn, in action, about others. Our contention is that successful interaction with others requires fast-paced, intuitive, and overlearned reactions. In fact, we believe that social competence has more in common with a game of tennis than with computer programming. And that rather than looking for humans' phylogenetically unique cognitive accomplishments in order to understand social competence, we may have to look down at our phylogenetic cousins whose lives are still more directly guided by Darwinian principles of survival. In fact, it is our view that successful social interaction, even in technological societies, would be impossible without the infusion of these more instinctual drives and learning processes. In that, the approach to the emergence of mind that we propose has more in common with Freudian theory than with prevailing cognitive science. This approach is called "embodied cognition" or "enactive mind", to which we now turn.

"Enactive mind", or from actions to cognition

Peter Hobson opens his book on the emergence of mind (2002) with the following dilemma embedded in the current debate about the ontogeny of mental processes:

> Ever since the 17th century, when Aristotle's distinction between knowledge and desire was elaborated into a threefold division of mental activity involving cognition (thought), conation (the will, motivation) and affect (feelings), we have had a terrible time trying to piece Humpty Dumpty together again. . . . [Hobson, 2002, p. 7]

A mixture of a clinician and psychoanalyst, experimental psychologist and theorist of social development, Hobson has found the need to weave these elements of social action into a more unitary blend of Aristotle-free concepts such as Identification. This was necessary because in early childhood particularly, the academic segregation of mental domains implies the mutilation of reality as we experience as clinicians when faced with a little person. A similar effort is ongoing in cognitive neuroscience, although still at its margins. This framework for studies of cognition—the "Enactive Mind" (EM), is established by a series of stances and emphases:

1. It assumes an active mind that sets out to make sense of the social environment, changing itself as a result of this interaction (Mead, 1934). Just like experimenting with a ping-pong ball, children constantly experiment with people, "moving" them in different directions (e.g., emotionally), and learning in action how to do so (e.g., moving the mother in a downward spiral).

2. It focuses on the adaptive functions that are subserved by cognitive accomplishments rather than distilling the computational accomplishment from its nourishing home. To use a metaphor from physics (Thompson, 1942), every time we blow on a straw that has been dipped in soapy water, we will produce a round bubble. It is round because this is the inevitable solution of the equation of maximum volume in minimum surface. The roundness of the bubble is not pre-programmed; if one is to understand it, there is a need to understand the invisible outside forces operating to create it. Similarly, EM states that the nature of some results of learning is inescapably tied to the contextual processes that gave rise to that learning incident. In

other words, we cannot dissociate our social understanding from the social experiences that led to the emergence of that understanding;

3. It makes the adaptive function within which cognition operates the main process for study. To use a metaphor from developmental physiology, Anokhin (1964) described the fact that the maturation of the muscles of the hand in primates does not follow an anatomic timetable but a functional one. Some muscles (relative to adjacent ones) in the hands undergo accelerated maturation towards the end of gestation, because the animal will have to be able to grasp tightly to the mother almost immediately after birth. The animal could die otherwise. Similarly, we need to highlight the adaptive functions subserved by social cognitive accomplishments such as orienting preferentially to social stimuli, seeking social pleasure and avoiding social pain, following gaze direction, using the pointing gesture, reinforcing the caregiver's loving approach and avoiding the caregiver's ambivalent or angry approaches, inferring the other person's desires and intentions, and so forth. Fishing these out from this pool of social interaction and adaptation could render these skills unfathomable or, alternatively, one may have to simply deem them innate and genetically determined. To use the soap-bubble metaphor once again, this would be like trying to find a gene (or a Kantian or Humean ideal template) for roundness in bubbles;

4. Given the focus on an almost Darwinian adaptation (which can become quite convoluted and conflicted, yet experientially real, in Freud's version), EM highlights consideration of the mental fuel of social development—namely, affective and predispositional responses.

5. EM shifts the focus of investigation from what can be called "disembodied cognition", or insular abstractions captured by computational cognition (e.g., algorithms in a digital computer) to "embodied cognition", or cognitive traces left by the action of an organism upon an environment defined by species-specific regularities and by a species-specific topology of differential salience (i.e., some things in the environment are more important than others).

Of particular importance in the EM framework is the premise that agents (e.g., a butterfly, a human infant, a cognitive psychologist) may vary in what they are seeking in the environment, resulting in highly disparate "mental representations" of the world with which they are interacting (Clark, 1999; Varela, Thompson, & Rosch, 1991). Uexkull (1957) probably best represented this principle when attempting to "take a stroll through the world of animals and men". He showed that a typical street would be constructed very differently by a man, a fly, a butterfly, or a mollusc, because their visual systems and "motivations" are so different. To describe this work informally, the butterfly's version of the street has this complex set of stimuli simplified into no more than some blurred hot spots (flowers to feed from). Different humans would also render that street in a simplified manner. A lonely teenager would create "hot spots" around a congregation of girls and boys; someone trying to cross the street would focus on the crossing traffic. In other words, that street would be continuously recreated in the person's mind in accordance with the adaptive task to be performed.

This individualization or "bodification" of cognition is often judged as being incompatible with scientific enquiry because of the complexity that it engenders in our attempts to generalize and test a construct in groups of people. In mainstream science, we constrain experiments to simple variables in explicit designs that abstract and isolate capacities that otherwise could not be measured. The EM framework would push us in the other direction. We should take the world as is, embracing the individual's recreation of that world while making a concerted effort to develop methods that capture and quantify that complexity. In many ways, this principle is very reminiscent of psychodynamic theory. For example, in psychoanalytic therapy, the process of recreation takes place using the narrative method to shed light on predispositional forces that envelop the patient without his or her knowing. This sea of meanings blends feelings and motivations accrued over the developmental periods of mind formation. Conscious awareness, through free-associative narratives, is used as a ray of light thrown around to illuminate these meanings. Manifest thought and behaviour needs to be "dipped" into this sea if it is to be understood. More importantly still: if we do not do so, we may do what our clients with autism often do—namely to be overly literal in our interpretation of what we hear and see. From a clinical standpoint, this literalness is harmful, since dealing exclusively with manifest behaviour, thus ignoring the mental fuelling of that behaviour, might alter or alleviate little if at all any conflicted feelings that result from that behaviour. In social interaction, the EM framework conceives of a similar "sea of meanings" that engulfs two or more people engaged in social exchange. Were we to analyse the fast-paced sentences, facial expressions, postural changes, synchronous gestures, and anticipations, among a host of other phenomena making possible natural social interaction on the basis of some linear problem-solving algorithm such as sequential language or theory of mind skills, we might find ourselves in awe of how inadequate our theoretical social cognitive abstractions are to begin to account for this ballet of synchronous bodies, imaginations, beliefs, feelings, background knowledge, cultural judgements, among a host of other phenomena that populates the "sea of meanings" that surrounds people involved in the simplest act of social and communication exchange. Were we to focus only on explicit knowledge (via language, or computational cognition), interactions between people would be as clunky and comically slow as one expects from two digital robots making acquaintance through conversation (Winograd, 1975; Winograd & Flores, 1986). Unfortunately, in developmental science one cannot use the free-associative method to throw rays of consciousness onto the contextual forces determining developmental outcomes, but we can focus on the moment-by-moment process of developmental learning if we recapture the more primal nature of social interaction. The need for such an approach comes directly from an examination of what are the challenges involved in adaptive social functioning, which can be simplified here in terms of three facts: (a) the social world is an "open-domain" adaptive task; (b) it involves contextual forces or adaptive functions; and (c) it has important temporal constraints.

The social world as an "open-domain" task

In the EM approach, a fundamental difference between explicit (as in an experiment) and naturalistic (as in real life) social tasks is captured in the distinction between "closed domains" and "open domains" of operation (Winograd & Flores, 1986). Research paradigms based on computational models of the social mind often reduce the social world to a set of pre-given rules and regularities that can be symbolically represented in the mind of a young child. In other words, the social world is simplified into a "closed-domain" task in which all essential elements to be studied can be fully represented and defined. This is justified in terms of the need to reduce the complexity of the social environment into a number of easily tested problem-solving tasks. By contrast, the EM approach embraces the open-ended nature of social adaptation. This implies the need to consider a multitude of elements that are more or less important depending on the context of the situation and person's perceptions, desires, goals, and ongoing adjustment. Successful adaptation requires from a person a sense of relative salience of each element in a situation, preferential choices based on priorities learned through experience, and further moment-by-moment adjustments.

In many ways, social competence is seen like the skill of driving a car. The "driving domain" involves wheels, roads, traffic lights, and other cars. But it also involves attention to pedestrians (in an urban street but not on the highways), driving regulations (but these can be overridden by safety factors), local customs (e.g., Italy vs. US), variable weather conditions, signals from other drivers, the driver's tardiness to work, and so on. This rich texture of elements defines the "background" of knowledge necessary to solve problems in the driving domain. Similarly, the social domain consists of people with age, gender, ethnic, and individual differences, facial and bodily gestures, language and voice/prosodic cues in all of their complexity and context-dependent nature, posture, physical settings and social props, and situation-specific conventions, among a host of other factors. Successful driving, or social adaptation, would require more than knowing a set of rules—at times referred to as "knowing that". Rather, it would require "knowing how", or a learning process that is based on the accumulation of experiences in a vast number of cases that result in being able to navigate the background environment according to the relative salience of each of the multitude of elements of a situation and the moment-by-moment emerging patterns that result from the interaction of the various elements.

If a person is to function successfully in such an environment, one has to move away from any veridical representation of the social world, where every bit of information is ideally present for an action to be performed (which would be a requirement to build a robot capable of functioning successfully in a world of people). For people—and young children in particular—this task needs to be simplified and organized differently. In the EM approach, the child "enacts the social world", perceiving it selectively in terms of what is immediately essential for social action. Thus the vast complexity of the surrounding environment is greatly simplified in terms of a differential "topology of salience" that separates aspects of the environment that are irrelevant (e.g., light fixtures, door handles, a person turned away) from those that are crucially important (e.g., someone staring at you or moving in your direction). And there is no need to know what to do prior to engaging in this dynamic of interaction—for example, babies do not need to infer mental states to interact with their caregivers. Babies simply do something that is simpler than fully fledged imputing of mental states to others. But repeated social interactive experiences give rise to an ever-increasing body of mental representations of that individualized social world, which makes it possible for babies to jerry-build an ever more complex social cognitive apparatus, which, in turn, makes possible ever more complex social experiences in an iterative process of social cognitive growth. In other words, cognition refers to the mental traces left by these recursive experiences (Varela, Thompson, & Rosch, 1991). And however complex these traces become (e.g., linguistic abstractions describing mental states), they are still speech-acts or acts of communication (Searle, 1980) because they hearken back to the original experiences of adaptation, which are, in turn, embedded in feelings, bodily sensations, and predispositional responses.

No other clinical condition can best concretize the distinction between open and closed domains than does autism. For individuals with this condition, the most entrenched difficulty inherent in treatment has to do with the lack of generalization. We teach them better social competence through the use of methods relying on explicit rules and drilling. In other words, we teach them in a closed-domain environment, and then we expect them to use the skill that we taught them in the "open-domain environment, that is their daily lives".

Contextual elements of social competence

The classic computational model in cognitive science assumes that cognitive processes are rule-based manipulations of symbols representing the external environment (Newell, 1991). Similarly, computational models of the social mind build on the notion that to operate socially is to execute algorithms involving mental representations (Baron-Cohen, 1994), By contrast the EM approach raises the non-trivial question of how a representation acquires meaning to a given child, the so-called "mind–mind" problem (Jackendoff, 1987). The question is what is the relationship between computational states (e.g., manipulation of mental representations) and a person's experience of the real-life referent of the computational state? How do we progress from having a representation of a person's intention to experiencing that intention by reacting to it in a certain way? This is clearly not a problem in computer programming (as noted, the symbols mean whatever is in the mind of the programmer) or in psychoanalysis (since words there are always appendages to feelings, bodily sensations, or affective attitudes). But in developmental psychology from a cognitivist standpoint, this is a problem. How do mental representations (e.g., words and symbols related to friendship, time, mind, home) acquire meaning to a developing child?

In autism, individuals often acquire a large number of symbols and symbolic computations that are devoid of shared meaning with others—that is, the symbols do not have the meaning to them that they have to typical children. Examples are hyperlexia (reading decoding skills go unaccompanied by reading comprehension) (Grigorenko et al., 2002), echolalia and echopraxia (echoing of sounds or mimicry of movements) (Prizant & Duchan, 1981; Rogers, 1999), "metaphoric language" (e.g., neologisms, words used in idiosyncratic ways) (Lord & Paul, 1997), and prompt-dependent social gestures, routines, or scripts (e.g., waving bye-bye without eye contact, staring when requested to make eye contact), among many others. While it is difficult for one to conceive of a dissociation between knowing a symbol and acting upon it (e.g., knowing what is the meaning of the pointing gesture and spontaneously turning one's head when somebody is pointing somewhere), this actually happens in autism. We know that children with autism can learn associatively (e.g., a symbol becomes paired with a referent). This happens, for example, in vocabulary instruction using simple behavioural techniques. But one of the big challenges for these children is often to pair a symbol with the adaptive action subsumed by the symbol (Wetherby, Prizant, & Schuler, 2000).

In the EM approach, symbols, or cognition in general, have meaning to the child using them because they are "embodied actions" (Clark, 1999; Johnson, 1987), meaning that "cognition depends upon the experiences that come from having a body with various sensorimotor capacities", and that " perception and action are fundamentally inseparable in lived cognition" (Varela, Thompson, & Rosch, 1991, p. 173). An artificial separation of cognition from the other elements would render the given cognitive construct a "mental ghost" once again. This principle takes Piaget's (1973) cognitive unconscious into the realm of social cognition. That is one reason why developmental skills have been increasingly described as "perception-for-action" systems (e.g., Thelen, Schoener, Scheier, & Smith, 2001). In other words, perception and cognition on the one hand, and an act of adaptation on the other hand, are tied together into a unit of social adaptation. Humpty Dumpty is put together again. In other words, perceiving something (e.g., seeing and hearing a roaring lion) means something internally to us because this perception—and the cognition associated with it—cannot be severed from the action that it engenders (e.g., fright, fleeing). This principle is also reflected in new neuroimaging studies that are showing overlapping brain circuitry subserving action observation and action generation (e.g., Blakemore & Decety, 2001; Iacoboni, 2000).

Perception-for-action systems are particularly relevant to a discussion of social adaptation. Consider the skill of imitation—one of the major deficits in autism (Rogers, 1999). It is interesting that while children with autism have great difficulty in learning through imitation, they do exhibit a great deal of "mirroring" or "copying" behaviour, both vocally (e.g., echoing what other people say) and motorically (e.g., making the same gesture as another person), which, however, are typically devoid of the function that these behaviours serve to typical people displaying them. One hypothesis derived from the EM approach would predict that this curious discrepancy originates from the aspect of the typical person's action that is most salient in the child's perception. Whereas typical children may see a waving gesture as a motion embedded in the act of communication or emotional exchange, children with autism may dissociate the motion from the social context, focusing on the salient physical facts and thus repeating the gesture in a mechanical fashion, not unlike what a typical child might do in a game of imitating meaningless gestures or what a neonate might do when sticking its tongue out in response to seeing an adult doing so (Meltzoff & Moore, 1977). This hypothesis originates from the notion that while perception-for-action may occur in the absence of social engagement (e.g., in neonates), in typical infants sometime around the middle of their second year of life imitation is much more likely to serve social engagement and social learning than to occur outside the realm of social interaction, as in autism. Supporting this hypothesis is a series of studies in which, for example, 18-month-old infants were exposed to a human or to a mechanical device attempting to perform various actions. The children imitated the action when it was performed by the human model but not when it was performed by the mechanical device (Meltzoff, 1995).

Perception-for-action systems are also of interest in the context of survival abilities (e.g., responding to a threatening person or a lethal predator). A central example of such systems is the ability to perceive certain patterns of movement as biological motion (like Johansson's, 1973, type of displays). This system allows humans, as well as other species, to distinguish motion of biological forms from motion occurring in the inanimate environment. In the wild, an animal's survival would depend on its ability to detect approaching predators and predict their future actions. In humans, this system has been linked to the emergence of the capacity to attribute intentions to others (Frith & Frith, 1999). Remember our results for Helen, the little girl with autism, who was unable to respond to the point-light displays as social animations (or portrayals of biological movement/human action). Where she to be in the wild, she would not be aware of a predator's attack. In her nursery school, she is unaware of an approaching peer.

Temporal constraints in social adaptation

Computational models of the mind place less emphasis on the temporal unfolding of the cognitive processes involved in a task (Newell, 1991). This stance is justified when a given task is explicit and fully defined. However, in naturalistic situations there are important temporal constraints in social adaptation, as failure to detect an important but fleeting social cue, or a failure to detect temporal relationships between two social cues, may lead to partial or even misleading comprehension of the situation, which may, in turn, lead to ineffective adjustment to the situation. For example, if the viewer of a scene fails to monitor a non-speaker in a social scene who is clearly embarrassed by what another person is saying, the viewer is unlikely to correctly identify the meaning of that situation (Klin et al., 2002a).

The EM approach sees social adaptation along the same principles currently being considered in research of "embodied vision" (Churchland, Ramachandran, & Sejnowski, 1994). This view holds that the task of the visual system is not to generate exhaustive mental models of a veridical surrounding environment but to use visual information to perform real-time, real-life adaptive reactions. Rather than creating an inner mirror of the outside world to formulate problems and then to solve them ahead of acting upon them, vision is seen as the active retrieval of useful information as it is needed from the constantly present and complex visual environment. From the organism's adaptive perspective, the topology of salience of this visual tapestry—from light reflections to carpet patterning, to furniture and clothing, to mouths and eyes—is far from flat. We would be overwhelmed and paralysed by its richness if we were to start from a position of equal salience to every aspect of what is available to be visually inspected. Rather, we actively retrieve aspects of the visual environment that are essential for quick adaptive actions by foveating on sequential locations where we expect to find them. These "expectations" are generated by a brain system dedicated to salience (a lion entering the room is more important than the light switch next to the door) and an ever more complex (going from infancy to adulthood) understanding of the context of the situation, the so-called "top-down" approach to vision (Engel, Fries, & Singer, 2001).

A pertinent example of this view of vision is Clark's description of a baseball game in which an outfielder positions himself or herself to catch a fly ball:

> It used to be thought that this problem required complex calculations of the arc, acceleration and distance of the ball. More recent work, however, suggests a computationally simpler strategy (McBeath et al., 1995). Put simply, the fielder continually adjusts his or her run so that the ball never seems to curve towards the ground, but instead appears to move in a straight line in his or her visual field. By maintaining this strategy, the fielder should be guaranteed to arrive in the right place at the right time to catch the ball [Clark, 1999, p. 346).

We had previously discussed similar examples from tennis playing and sending ping-pong balls in reverse rotation (Piaget, 1973), but a whole host of similar examples are available in intersubjective adaptation (Zajonc, 1980). To generalize, therefore, the EM approach sees the "social game" to be not unlike the outfielder's effort described by Clark (1999). A typical toddler entering a playroom pursues a sequence of social adaptive reactions to split-second environmental demands with moment-by-moment disregard of the vast majority of the available visual stimulation. Such a child is ready to play the social game. For individuals with autism, however, the topology of salience, defined as the "foveal elicitation" of socially relevant stimuli (as exemplified in our eye-tracking illustrations and in studies of preferential attention to social vs. non-social entities described briefly in previous sections) is much flatter. In the case of Helen, the examiner was hardly a "hot spot" in her Uexkullian inner world, which instead had representations for the faraway M&M.

Social cognition as social action: a call for embodied psychoanalysis

The radical assumption made in the EM approach is that mental representations as described in computational models of the mind are proxies for the actions that generated them and for which they stand

(Lakoff & Johnson, 1999; Thelen & Smith, 1994; Varela, Thompson, & Rosch, 1991). This counterintuitive view can be traced back to Mead's (1934) account of the social origins of mind, as discussed before. Mead saw the emergence of mind as the capacity of an individual to make a "gesture" (e.g., bodily sign, vocal sound) that means the same to the other person seeing or hearing it as for the person making it. The meaning of the gesture, however, is in the reaction of the other. A gesture used in this way becomes a symbol—that is, something that stands for the predicted reaction of the other person. Once a child has such a symbolic gesture, she can then uphold it as a representation for the reaction of the social partner, thus being able to take a step back from the immediate experience and then to contemplate alternatives of action using such symbols as proxies for real actions. In the EM approach, the fact that the emergence and evolution of a symbol is tied to actions of adaptation, which in turn are immersed in a context of somatosensory experiences, salience, and perceptually guided actions, makes the symbol a proxy for these elements of the action. When we uphold and manipulate symbols in our mind, therefore, we are also evoking a network of experiences resulting from a life history of actions associated with that symbol.

It is of interest that our sensorimotor apparatus (as per Piaget, 1973) fits well in this scenario. These systems typically act in pairs or in self-referential ways—for example, we talk and we hear, we touch and we feel, we move and we balance. The visual system is odd in this regard because it is unidirectional. In other words, in natural environments we see but we do not see ourselves (this might have been adaptive at one point; witness what happened to Narcissus). There is a need for a natural mirror surface if vision is also to become self-referential. Nature has placed other people's eyes as our natural mirrors, and their agency and subjectivity imbue their eyes with visceral proprioception to us. In this sense, other people become our natural mirrors. And from the EM perspective, we use this visual proprioception to adjust our actions to the ongoing social demands, not unlike tripping over something would be followed by correcting one's balance when walking.

In psychoanalysis this process is dramatized by the fact that different subjectivities do not always mesh well, not even in our infantile states. And in the same way that we internalize symbols *à la* Vygotsky and Mead, so we also identify with others who begin to populate our internal worlds, sometimes de-identified in our unconscious, sometimes identified in psychoanalytic therapy. Just as our symbols are embodied pieces of cognition, so are these products of identification, who become embodied psychodynamic products pushing and pulling our psyche in—sometimes—conflicted directions. Thus they share the process of embodiment, vestiges of sensations, and predispositions that make our elusive unconscious a clinical reality.

Commentary

Peter Fonagy

Klin and Jones's beautiful chapter offers an exceptionally helpful suggestion for a mutually beneficial integration of a developmental psychology dominated by cognition and an adultomorphic psychoanalysis that has traditionally considered emotion its home base.

The chapter maps out a domain at the crossroads between developmental psychology and psychoanalysis and links this with the newfound concern with embedded cognition. Criticisms of classical cognitive psychology are, of course, almost as old as the subject itself. Jerome Bruner (1990), one of the most important cognitive scientists of our time, had always maintained that the essential concern of cognitive psychology with understanding meaning was coming to be obscured by a study of mental mechanisms—a formalist, functionalist model of mind. The heuristic devices that cognitive scientists have adopted from general systems theory and computer science to study thinking and reasoning have always been alien to psychoanalysts. Cognitive scientists borrowed the notion of hypothetical processes, each with its own input and output, which together could be seen as providing a metaphor for a mental activity.

The incompatibility between the cognitive science and psychoanalytic approaches is partly one of content. The cognitivist models turned out to be helpful ways to describe phenomena that were of little interest to psychoanalysts. There have been distinguished historical attempts at bringing general systems theory models to psychoanalysis (Horowitz, 1988; Horowitz, Fridhandler, & Stinson, 1991; Peterfreund, 1971, 1975, 1980; Rosenblatt & Thickstun, 1994, 1977). None of these had a significant impact on either discipline. Each failed the first test of psychoanalytic theorization: they have little heuristic value for the clinician.

Klin and Jones claim that the polarization of the mind between the software of mental processes and the hardware of brain mechanisms was rejected by Freud and other psychoanalysts, who saw mental function as driven by bodily energy, creating a bridge between the two worlds. The ego is first and foremost a body ego. This is only partially true; as Klin and Jones point out, the Freudian unconscious is ultimately neo-Cartesian. Even if concerned with the body in content, it remains an isolated container of abstractions and exists separately from the body and the social world.

Klin and Jones offer the contribution of three key developmentalists to illustrate the choices made by developmental cognitive science that led it on a path away from psychoanalysis. Piaget missed an opportunity when he focused on sensorimotor learning as a foundation of cognitive abstraction and ignored the sensorimotor learning in action that occurs in the infant–mother dyad. Vygotsky could have gone beyond his emphasis on the social nature of language and missed the opportunity to fully explore the experiential components of language that emerged from the social world. George Herbert Mead, whose work on symbolic interactionism was used as the basis for cultural relativism, was also clear that the meaning of gesture and action arose out of the reaction of the other. Taking these aspects of the work of these giants of psychology together, Klin and Jones have identified a space for a social-affective unconscious that consists of internalized experiences of other people and their actions. It also incorporates object relations, since the internal consolidation of social affective experiences in the context of social interactions amounts to a matrix of meanings for self and other. The computer-like models of cognitive science "stripped babies of their emotions, motivations, actions and bodily sensations".

Klin and Jones politely refrain from mentioning this, but one of my intellectual heroes, John Bowlby, may also be to blame. Bowlby, particularly in the last volume of his trilogy (Bowlby, 1980), explicitly linked his motivational theory to a specific, then predominant position in cognitive science rooted in the computer metaphor. A schema-oriented general systems model of the internal world, the internal working model of attachment relationships, remains at the core of the attachment theory model. This general information theory model was the promising bridge to science that Bowlby chose in his mission to rescue psychoanalysis, but it was perhaps appropriately seen by many analysts as in many ways dehumanizing, clinically irrelevant, and incompatible with some fundamental psychoanalytic ideas.

The evidence upon which Klin and Jones draw heavily comes from research on the neuro-developmental disorder of autism. In a remarkably elegant series of studies the Yale Group demonstrated that children with autism failed to evidence an ability to link pieces of stimuli, or, more generally, meaning, with their contextual entities. The weak central coherence (WCC) hypothesis might have great explanatory potential. Being insensitive to the social context leads them to respond in an over-literal manner to social interactions. Autistic infants show a general lack of social interest, reduced levels of social engagement and social–communicative exchanges, limited eye contact, and less visual attention to social stimuli (Klin et al., 2003). Perhaps they never acquire a "theory of mind". At a time when most infants begin more fully to integrate object exploration with social interaction to become more intentional, infants with autism seem to be less interested in people (Klin & Jones, submitted). But Klin and Jones's theoretical ambitions take them beyond currently dominant formulations.

An impressive accumulation of data from a programmatic series of investigations provides support for their formulation. In the chapter it is reported in the context of a "psychoanalysis-friendly" single case study of a 15-month-old autistic girl. Helen fails to do what very young babies already do, orient towards the eyes of adults. She also fails to recognize human body movements in the movement of animated dogs. She orients towards physical contingencies, so when watching people speaking, she looks at their mouth rather than their eyes, as this where the physical contingencies between sound and movement take place. Her brain has come to be specialized in understanding physical, non-social events. In studies autistic individuals fail to attribute social meaning to cartoons that are seen as having meaning even by infants. Watching films, they fixate on the mouth of characters and on physical objects. Those individuals who fixated on physical objects while watching a social interaction were the most disabled. But even when watching someone they may be looking at the "display" without seeing the person. It is not that they are impaired in their ability to integrate information into coherent wholes, as the WCC hypothesis might predict, but that this integration occurs in the physical rather than the social domain.

Children with autism may not be able to translate either implicit or explicit knowledge about people into real-life competence. They are able to learn *about* the world but are not capable of learning *in* the world from an immersive social environment. This incapacity is what underpins their failure to be able to entertain other people's beliefs or desires. It turns out that is not the brain tissue normally underpinning the processing of face stimuli (the fusiform gyrus) that is dysfunctional. It seems more likely that the areas normally specializing in social stimuli come to mediate the processing of the movement of physical objects in which individuals with autism have greater interest. While for most children human interaction is inherently rewarding, for children with autism physical aspects of the world are of greater interest. By linking the inherent experience of pleasure in an activity to the nature of a cognitive deficit, Klin and Jones begin to move towards an integration of Freudian theory with developmental science. They find this integration in the biological predispositions that the human mind, through a process of selection, has evolved to bring to social interaction.

In identifying the common ground between developmental science and psychoanalysis, they point to the understanding of modern-day cognitivists of mind as embedded in the physical experiences that have created it and that continue to closely link cognition and affect. The "Enactive Mind" (EM) is embedded in social interaction and changes itself in response to this interaction. Consistencies in development may not be usefully interpreted as the consequence of a specific computational process but, rather, as the inevitable consequence of the contextual processes that gave rise to a particular experience of learning. It is the adaptive function of cognition in its social context that shapes the emergence of cognition, and affect and predispositional responses that are its mental fuel. In place of the insular abstractions of computational cognition, the focus is moved to cognition as the residue of the actions of an organism upon the environment.

The EM framework implies a number of profound epistemological changes that move developmental science closer to psychoanalysis. Psychoanalysis was never comfortable with the closed domains of computational models, in which elements to be studied can be fully represented and defined. The EM approach, by contrast, is respectful of the open-ended nature of social adaptation. The domain must remain open because the context of the situation, the active desires and goals of the individual, define what is relatively salient, and successful adaptation requires moment-by-moment adjustments to these. In common with the psychoanalytic emphasis, a world created out of desire (Winnicott), the EM approach moves away from an insistence on the veridical representation of the social world to a stance of enactment based on what is perceived by the child to be essential. The social world becomes individualized, unique to each of us, through recursive experiences that we have with our objects that leave behind the process of thought and cognition (Varela, Thompson, & Rosch,

1991). Thus, cognition at its most complex—language—is still an "act of communication" because it reaches back to the language of gestures that remain embedded in feelings, bodily sensations, and biologically predisposed responses (Fónagy, 2000). In an as yet unpublished paper, we have tried to elaborate the significance, for psychoanalytic theory and practice, of looking at attachment and language with the EM approach and suggested that the gulf that has existed between attachment theory and psychoanalysis could perhaps in part be bridged by conceptualizing attachment within this frame (Fonagy & Target, in press).

In their answer to the question of how children acquire meaning, Klin and Jones once again move closer to psychoanalytic ideas. The EM approach assumes that cognitions have meaning because they are embodied actions (Clark, 1999). Meaning arises out of the origin of cognitions within the body, with its various sensorimotor capacities. Recent neuroscientific work, tying together the action with the perception of action by the mediation of a single set of brain structures, supports this set of contentions (Ferrari, Gallese, Rizzolatti, & Fogassi, 2003; Rizzolatti & Craighero, 2004). Similarly, George Gergely's recent study of imitation, showing that the child's imitation was highly selective and dependent on the assumption the 18-month-old baby made about the context of the actions of the model, illustrates that social learning occurs within the realm of social interaction (Gergely, Bekkering, & Király, 2002).

Finally, Klin and Jones move closer to psychoanalysis in their model of how children adjust to social situations. A computational model would assume a complex series of mental operations quite incompatible with psychoanalytic ideas of impulsive, affect- and drive-driven actions, rapid, intricate elaborations associated with unconscious processes. The EM approach resolves the problem, insurmountable for computational models, of the speed with which complex social adaptation is made in real-world social interactions by assuming a highly selective process that is adapted to extract a very narrow range of salient information, disregarding the vast majority of available cues. Klin and Jones suggest that we may assume that children are influenced by unconscious wishes and beliefs by an analogous highly selective process.

In conclusion, the radical proposal in this chapter is based on the idea that all mental representations are proxies for the actions that generated them and for which they stand. Thus, mind emerges out of gesture, but the *meaning* of mind is rooted in the reaction of the other to the child. It becomes a symbol in the mind of the actor, as the reaction is internalized. Interestingly, we have suggested a psychoanalytic model of this sort in our theory of the emergence of affect regulation through an internalization of contingent, marked mirroring of actions that emerge as second-order representations of the child's constitutional self-state (Fonagy, Gergely, Jurist, & Target, 2002; Gergely & Watson, 1996). Placing this model into the emerging context of the EM approach, or embodied cognition (Lakoff & Johnson, 1999; Thelen & Smith, 1994; Varela, Thompson, & Rosch, 1991), creates a valuable bridge to modern developmental theory—the bridge that Klin and colleagues have created, and which, we hope, will be increasingly used by psychoanalysts. Klin and Jones have made a major theoretical contribution in their chapter. It is rich and thought-provoking and, in my view, a landmark contribution to which I, along with many other readers, will return as a source of understanding and inspiration.

CHAPTER TWO

The social construction of the subjective self: the role of affect-mirroring, markedness, and ostensive communication in self-development

György Gergely

Introduction: the multiplicity of subjective self-experiences

We tend to take for granted the existence of our subjective awareness of the continuous flow of affective experiences during our everyday life. In fact, it is quite easy for us to intuitively assume that this is just the way our human psyche is built, and so the continuity, coherence, relative intensity, and characteristic affective quality of our dynamically changing emotional experiences are basically similar to the subjective emotional lives of our fellow human beings. As it happens, this naive psychological belief in the universality and interpersonally shared nature of our subjective self-experience is likely to play an important functional role as a useful idealization or background working assumption of our intuitive "theory of mind" that facilitates our attempts to infer other people's intentional mental states and subjective emotional experiences when trying to predict or interpret their behaviour.

The general validity of this assumption, however, is seriously challenged by our clinical experience with patients suffering from severe self-pathologies whose reports during psychotherapy about their subjective emotional experiences suggest radical differences in their affective self-organization and functioning as well as in their subjective awareness of their emotional self states. Individuals with borderline, narcissistic, or dissociative personality disorders, for example, describe their subjective experience of their internal affective world as being variably characterized by fragmentation, discontinuity and incoherence, feelings of flat affect or emptiness, chaotic emotional experiences involving undifferentiated mixtures of affects, a prevalence of periods of intense, intolerable, and uncontrollable negative emotional states, or feelings of being "absent", detached, "switched off", or even dead. Our clinical experience with such self-pathologies also highlights the fact that the subjective awareness of one's emotional self states has a number of crucial organizational and control functions in the everyday management of one's social life and intimate attachment relationships, these being the domains of adaptive functioning in which patients with self-pathologies exhibit serious deficits. Many of these dysfunctions seem clearly related to the qualitative differences in these patients' subjective experiences of their affective self states. We can differentiate at least four functional aspects of subjective self-experience that are often severely undermined in such self-pathologies:

1. *Self-perception and self-attribution of dispositional emotion states: anticipating emotion-based action-tendencies and the possibility of self-control.* The ability to introspectively monitor and correctly perceive one's dynamically changing emotion states makes it possible to attribute to the self—and consequently to represent the self in terms of—its current dispositional states. This requires introspective monitoring of internal self-states on the one hand, and representing one's emotion states in a cognitively accessible format, on the other. The ensuing self-state attributions and the consequent subjective awareness of one's dispositional self-states are cognitive prerequisites for the ability to foresee and evaluate the probable external consequences of one's anticipated actions that the self's currently active emotional states are likely to automatically induce. This ability for subjective self-perception of emotion states and for the consequent anticipation of one's likely affect-induced actions are therefore crucial prerequisites for one's capacity to inhibit dysfunctional action-tendencies and to exercise affective self-control over one's emotion-driven actions and public emotion displays in the interpersonal sphere (Gergely & Watson, 1996).

2. *Social self-presentation and interpersonal reality testing: mentalizing about others' mind states in relation to the self.* Being subjectively aware of the emotional states one is in or that one is publicly displaying is

also a prerequisite for succeeding in one's attempts to predict, evaluate or manipulate the perceptions, reactions, and attitudes of interactive social partners and attachment figures towards oneself. Erroneous evaluation of the consequences of one's self-presentation and communicative emotion displays can have disastrous consequences for one's ability to adaptively function in everyday interpersonal and intimate attachment relationships.

3. *Internal self-evaluative attitudes, self-referential feelings, and self-directed actions: the affective regulation of the self's inner emotional life.* Distorted self-perceptions, unrealistically harsh negative self-image, disastrous self-evaluative emotional attitudes, intense feelings of guilt, shame, embarrassment, or self-hatred are highly characteristic dysfunctions of the affective self-experience of patients with self-pathologies. Such distorted and dysfunctional self-perceptions and evaluations often lead to tormenting negative self-referential feelings and attitudes that generate unbearable emotional pain and lead to self-punitive tendencies that can take the form of self-debasement, self-harm and even suicide.

4. *Differentiating subjective emotions from reality: the "psychic equivalence" mode of mental functioning.* A further dysfunctional aspect of the subjective experience of one's affect states that is characteristic of pathologies of the self has to do with the weakness or lack of ability to differentiate intense emotional states of the self and their related action-fantasies from reality—what we have termed elsewhere the "psychic equivalence" mode of mental functioning (Fonagy, Gergely, Jurist, & Target, 2002; Fonagy & Target, 1995, 1997; Fonagy, Target, & Gergely, 2000). This is, then, a further source of unbearable fear, insecurity, and suffering that stem from subjectively experiencing the self's emotional states as being part of external and objective reality or as threatening to easily turn into reality. This confusion between subjective affective states and objective reality also underlies the tendency for uncontrolled acting out that is often characteristic of patients with certain self-pathological conditions.

* * *

It seems clear, therefore, that such clinical observations suggest a more complicated view of the internal organization of the affective sense of self than the intuitive notion of a universal and interpersonally shared sense of affective subjectivity that our everyday psychology (or naive "theory of mind") seems to presuppose. To account for the existence of significant individual differences in subjective self-experience and the severe functional pathologies stemming from certain types of maladaptive affective self-organizations, it seems necessary to consider the affective self as a representationally complex and multi-layered developmental construct, the ontogenetic unfolding and variable developmental pathways (both normal and pathological) of which are likely to be a function of complex interactions between genetic, temperamental, and social environmental factors during early development. This raises the central question I aim to address here: what are the developmental and social–environmental origins of our subjective sense of affective self states?

The Cartesian view of the nature of the subjective sense of self

It is noteworthy that—in spite of the arguments summarized above—a historically as well as currently popular answer to this question has been the Cartesian one which upholds the basic assumptions of the universality and interpersonally shared nature of the sense of subjective self-experiences across individuals and through development (see Dennett, 1991). This Cartesian view assumes an innate, prewired organization of our mind that ensures "primary introspective access" to our internal mental states providing us with "first person authority" over the contents of our internal and private subjective mental life (for a critical discussion of this general view, see Fonagy, Gergely, et al., 2002; Gergely, 2002; Gopnik, 1993; Wegner & Wheatley, 1999). The Cartesian approach is often coupled (in so-called "simulationist" models of mind-reading; e.g., Gallese & Goldman, 1998; Gallese, Keysers, & Rizzolatti, 2004; Goldman, 1993; Gordon, 1995; Harris, 1991, 1992) with the idea that the way we come to understand (or, in a sense, to internally directly "perceive") *other* people's subjective mental states is by (automatically) "putting ourselves in their shoes" using (in our imagination) our self as a mental model of the other. Through this process of internally "simulating" the other person's goals and particular situation one comes to infer and represent the other's mental states as well as anticipating the actions these intentional mind states are likely to cause. This involves mentally inducing the internal subjective states of the other in our selves through some psychological process that generates the mental simulation of the other by imagining our self in her situation (by imitation, imagination, identification, or lately, through "neuronal resonance" evoked by the automatic activation of our brain's "mirror neuron system" during the observation of the other person's behaviour: see Gallese, Keysers, & Rizzolatti, 2004). Once such a mental model has been set up, all one has to do is to introspectively access its contents and "read off" from this "off-line self-simulation of the other" what the other must be feeling, intending, or believing in the given situation. In other words, by accessing the intentional and emotional mental self-states that oneself would have in the other's—internally represented—situation, one can attribute (by analogy) these simulated subjective states (as belonging) to the other person's mind. Note that this simulationist account of understanding other minds relies on the assumption that the basic set of subjective mental states of different individuals are identical and "interchangeable" and that similar situations generate the same causal mental states and consequent action-tendencies in all of us.

The Cartesian infant: The myth of primary "intersubjectivity" in current-day infancy research

This Cartesian approach to the self (a) presupposes as a given the availability of direct introspective access to subjective intentional and emotional mind states, and (b) implies strong innatist and universalist assumptions about the existence of prewired, universal—and subjectively equally accessible—intentional and emotional self states that are constitutionally shared by all human individuals. Furthermore, this view offers little room for developmental change induced by social environmental factors as potential causal sources of individual variability in the quality and content of subjective self-experience of affective and mental states across different persons. To the degree that individual differences and variability exist in the variety and kinds of internal mental and emotional states, in their relative degree of subjective accessibility, or in the ability to use them to simulate the contents of other minds, these phenotypical variations are best explained as a result of genetic differences, maturational dysfunctions, or brain injury.

In spite of the fact that the Cartesian view of the mind and the self has been seriously challenged and criticized on a number of grounds in current philosophy of mind, cognitive neuroscience, social psychology, developmental psychology, and clinical theory (Csibra & Gergely, 2006; Damasio, 1994; Dennett, 1991; Fonagy, Gergely, et al., 2002; Gergely, 2002, 2004; Gopnik, 1993; Wegner & Wheatley, 1999), it has nevertheless continued to be rather influential in numerous recent theories of early socio-emotional development and attachment. These developmental theories share a common emphasis on the centrality of what has come to be termed primary "*intersubjectivity*" that is assumed to characterize the mental experience of infants during infant–caregiver interactions from the earliest phases of life (Braten, 1988, 1992; Gianino & Tronick, 1988; Hobson, 1993; Meltzoff & Gopnik, 1993; Meltzoff & Moore, 1977, 1998; Stern, 1985; Trevarthen, 1979, 1993; Trevarthen & Aitken, 2001). The concept of primary "intersubjectivity" involves a "rich" mentalistic interpretation of the nature of the young baby's subjective experience of her own as well as of the caregiver's mind states during the organized patterns of mother–infant interactions basically from the start.

However—as we have argued in greater detail elsewhere (Csibra & Gergely, 2006; Fonagy, Gergely, et al., 2002; Gergely, 2002, 2004)—theories of primary "intersubjectivity" make a number of strong innatist assumptions that seem neither necessary nor empirically warranted about the initial availability and introspective accessibility of differentiated mental states in the young infant as well as about the early availability of inferential mechanisms through which the baby can identify and attribute similar subjective mind states to its interactive partners. This "strong intersubjectivist" view assumes (a) that human infants are born with innate perceptual and inferential mechanisms to identify and attribute a rich set of subjective mental states—such as intentions, desires, goals, and feelings—to the other's mind during early contingent social interactions; (b) that from the beginning of life there is a relatively rich set of differentiated mental states of the self—such as emotions, intentions, motives, and goals—that are introspectively accessible to the infant, resulting in subjective awareness of them; (c) that these subjectively experienced mental states of the self can be recognized as being similar or identical to the corresponding subjective mental states displayed by the caregiver's behavioural expressions during turn-taking interactions, and, as a result, (d) the infant experiences these subjective self states as "being shared" with the attachment figure (e.g., Braten, 1988, 1992; Stern, 1995; Trevarthen, 1979, 1993; Trevarthen & Aitken, 2001; for a collection of papers on "intersubjectivity", see Braten, 1998).

For example, Trevarthen (1993) proposes that infants are born with a "dialogic mind", with an innate sense of "the virtual other" (see also Braten, 1988, 1992) and can interpret the other's affectively attuned interactions in terms of a rich set of underlying motives, feelings, intentions, and goals. Stern (1995) also suggests that "from a very early age, the infant perceives intentions in the self and the other, that he or she 'sees past' the specific overt behaviors in order to read in them the intentions that organize these behaviors" (p. 420). Meltzoff and his colleagues (see Meltzoff & Gopnik, 1993; Meltzoff & Moore, 1997, 1998) proposed a specific innate mechanism that underlies intersubjective attributions of intentional and feeling states to the other during early imitative interactions. In their "active intermodal mapping" model (Meltzoff & Moore, 1997), the affective/intentional behavioural acts of the other are mapped onto a "supramodal body scheme" that allows the infant to recognize the other person as "just-like-me". Furthermore, it is assumed that by imitating such acts, infants generate the corresponding internal subjective intentional and/or feeling states of the other in themselves (Meltzoff & Gopnik, 1993). A similar assumption is made by proponents of differential emotions theory (Izard & Malatesta, 1987; Malatesta & Izard, 1984), who suggest that "there is an innate expression-to-feeling concordance in the young infant" (Malatesta, Culver, Tesman, & Shepard, 1989, p. 6). In Meltzoff's view, the intentional and feeling states generated by imitating the other are introspectively accessed by the infant and then attributed to the other by inference. Thus, Meltzoff and Gopnik (1993) argue that "imitation of behavior provides the bridge that allows the internal mental state of another to 'cross over' to and become one's own experienced state" (p. 358).

A central characteristic of these models of primary "intersubjectivity" is a shared emphasis on the *continuity from infancy to adulthood* of the qualitative nature of subjective *emotional experience*, of the kinds of *intersubjective states of interpersonal relatedness* and of the *identity of basic human motives* that are supposed to drive the bidirectional coordination and mutual affect regulation and attunement that are assumed to characterize dyadic human interactions from the beginning of life. Such theories often assume—either explicitly or implicitly—a basic human-specific drive to "*share psychological states*" with others: "a species-unique motivation to share emotions, experience, and activities with other persons" (e.g., Tomasello et al., 2005, p. 675). This is often seen as the ultimate and intersubjectively shared basic goal that is inherent in and determines the structure of human interactions from the beginning of life.

From the point of view of recent dynamically oriented psychotherapeutic approaches to adult self-pathologies, it is interesting to note that the empirical viability of such developmental models advocating primary "intersubjectivity" of early interactive experience is often simply taken for granted and directly relied on by many of the current "intersubjectivist" and relational psychoanalytic theories. These psychotherapeutic approaches tend to embrace theories of primary "intersubjectivity" as their natural developmental cousins when looking for the ontogenetic origins of the complex intersubjective experiences of minds that are generated and explored during the therapeutic relationship. (For a review of psychoanalytic attempts to directly relate to or derive intersubjective phenomena in adult treatment from the assumed initial states of primary "intersubjectivity" in infancy, see the special issues, in 2003 and 2004, of the journal *Psychoanalytic Dialogues*, edited by Beatrice Beebe, that are fully devoted to this topic.)

In fact, there is very little empirical evidence to support the rich mentalistic innatist assumptions of the proponents of early "intersubjectivity", and the evidence referred to is in most cases subject to alternative interpretations (for a review, see Csibra & Gergely, 2006; Gergely, 2002, 2004). In fact, there are many researchers of early emotional development (often of rather different theoretical persuasions) who share the view that differentiation of discrete emotions and/or their conscious access are not yet present during the first few months, but are either the consequences of early self-organizing dynamic systems processes (Fogel et al., 1992; Lewis & Granic, 2000) or, alternatively, of cognitive developmental processes leading to the early socialization of, and sensitization to, differential internal emotion states during affect-regulative caregiver–infant interactions (Gergely & Watson, 1996, 1999; Sroufe, 1979, 1995). Lewis and Michalson (1983) also argue that during the earliest phases of infancy internal states and expressive behaviours are not yet coordinated. In their view, conscious feeling states that are linked to discrete expressive displays emerge only later due to the influence of socialization and cognitive growth (see also Barrett & Campos, 1987; Kagan, 1992; Lewis & Brooks, 1978).

In fact, many infancy researchers (e. g., Csibra & Gergely, 2006; Fonagy, Gergely, et al., 2002; Gergely, 2002, 2004; Gergely & Watson, 1996, 1999; Thompson, 1998; Tomasello, 1999) hold that the basic evidence marshalled in favour of primary "intersubjectivity", such as the intricate organization of the early bidirectional affective and imitative interaction sequences and their characteristic contingent "protoconversational" turn-taking structure (Beebe, Jaffe, Feldstein, Mays, & Alson, 1985; Brazelton, Koslowski, & Main, 1974; Brazelton & Tronick, 1980; Stern, 1985; Tomasello et al., 2005; Trevarthen, 1979; Tronick, 1989), can be parsimoniously explained without attributing intersubjective mentalistic understanding to the young infant. Examples of such early social competences include the innate attentiveness and preference for the pattern of the human face, a prewired interest in eye contact, and early propensity to follow gaze shift (Csibra & Gergely, 2006; Fantz, 1963; Farroni, Massaccesi, Pividori, Simion, & Johnson, 2004; Morton & Johnson, 1991), the innate inclination to imitate certain human facial gestures (Meltzoff & Moore, 1977, 1989), or the early sensitivity and motivation to explore and analyse the causal contingency structure of interactive behavioural exchanges (Gergely & Watson, 1999; Lewis, Allessandri, & Sullivan, 1990; Watson, 1972, 1994, 2001).

Critics of primary "intersubjectivity" also argue that there are plausible alternatives to the central functionalist and motivational interpretations proposed by the intersubjectivist school as the primary organizational factors behind the rich contingent protoconversational turn-taking structure of early affective caregiver–infant interactions. Such primary intersubjectivist functional explanations include the postulation of a basic human-specific drive for "sharing psychological states" with other humans, achieving "affect attunement", "mutual and bidirectional affect regulation", establishing and maintaining interpersonal "reciprocity", or "identification with the other" by recognizing, sharing, and maintaining identical emotional and intentional states between the interactive partners. In contrast, there exist a number of well-documented innate cognitive and perceptual capacities of the human infant that can account for the early turn-taking structural organization of affective interactions without invoking mentalization or attribution of intersubjective emotional states to the other (Csibra & Gergely, 2006; Gergely & Watson, 1996, 1999; Watson, 1994).

For example, there is clear evidence of innate *sensitivity to and preference for contingent reactivity* to the infant's responses (e.g., sucking, or leg kicks) that is *not restricted to humans or even to animate objects,* as these effects are also evoked by inanimate sources of external stimulation—for example, by a mobile, geometric shapes, or sound stimuli (e. g., Floccia, Christophe, & Bertoncini, 1997; Lewis, Allessandri, & Sullivan, 1990; Watson, 1972, 1994). Similarly, infants seem to be innately equipped with a sophisticated contingency-detection module (Gergely & Watson, 1999; Watson, 1979, 1994) that analyses the causal contingency and conditional probability structure of response–stimulus events irrespective of the social or non-social nature of the stimuli over which the infant exerts different degrees of contingent control. Furthermore, infants show positive emotional reactions when discovering their causal influence over an external event and exhibit frustration when their contingent control is lost (Lewis, Allessandri, & Sullivan, 1990; Watson, 1972, 1994). Such emotional reactions to self-induced contingent reactivity—or to its loss—is also equally present irrespective of the human or inanimate nature of the external event (Lewis, Allessandri, & Sullivan, 1990; Watson, 1972, 1979). Therefore, the intrinsic motivation driving the infant's active engagement of such external contingencies does not seem to be primarily tied to the social domain: rather, it may represent a domain-general drive to discover the degree of contingent control that the infant's specific responses can exert over different aspects of the external stimulus world (Gergely, 2002; Gergely & Watson, 1999; Lewis, Allessandri, & Sullivan, 1990; Watson, 1972, 1979, 1994). Similarly, contingent reactivity (e.g., beeping or light effects evoked by infant vocalization) by physical objects lacking any human features triggers in the infant visual following of a directional movement cue in the object's frontal orientation (Johnson, Slaughter, & Carey, 1998; Movellan & Watson, 2002). Infants also seem to actively test (by periodically increasing the rate of their leg-kicking followed by periods of inhibiting their response emission) whether or not a non-human external stimulus exhibits a turn-taking structure of contingent reactivity (Watson, 1985, 1994).

In short, infants seem innately motivated to engage and discover the contingent reactivity of the stimulus environment as well as their own degree of causal efficacy in controlling aspects of the external world around them. At the same time, there is no indication that this innate interest in causal contingencies would be restricted to human conspecifics or even to self-propelled animate agents only. One plausible explanation (e.g., Watson, 1994) for the existence of the infant's innate contingency detection device and the intrinsic biological function it serves (that would clearly be adaptive for the infant's survival in its environment) is to consider its primary function to be the discovery and representation of the degree of causal power that different responses of the infant exercise over different aspects of the external world, be it human or non-human in nature. Note that this account is not only plausible on its own right, but it is also sufficient to account for the infant's active engagement in and emotional reactivity to bidirectional social interactions with the caregiver that exhibit a characteristic turn-taking structure of contingent reactivity.

Similarly, there seems to be no evidence to suggest that the infants' positive or negative emotional reactions evoked by such contingencies—or by their loss—would result in attributing similar emotional reactions to the external stimuli that show contingent reactivity to them. In general, the intersubjectivist proposal that infants' emotional reactions during engaging turn-taking contingencies is driven by a motivation to "share" their emotion states with those of the reactive object, or, indeed, that they attribute specific emotions (or other intentional mental states) to the contingently reactive other is not based on any strong evidence either.

1. These claims presuppose that young infants experience the same type of discrete emotion states that they observe expressed in their mother's emotion displays during early affective interactions. Even though proponents of differential emotions theory (Izard, 1991; Malatesta & Izard, 1984) claim that expressions of discrete emotions such as fear, anger, or sadness can be objectively demonstrated in early infancy, using the MAX (Izard, 1979) or the AFFEX (Izard, Dougherty, & Hembree, 1983) coding systems, others—using a different coding system, the Baby–FACS (see Oster, Hegley, & Nagel, 1992)—dispute this claim and argue that young babies' negative expressions show only undifferentiated distress at first. Camras (1992, 2000) reviews several further empirical phenomena that are problematic for the view that in early infancy basic emotion expressions are linked to similar internal feeling states and are evoked by similar stimulus conditions as in adulthood.

2. If early emotional interactions were indeed driven by a primary motivation for "sharing" affective states, then one would expect that (a) the majority of emotional exchanges between infant and caregiver would involve the expressions of identical emotion states, and (b) that one would observe the full variety of emotions that are expressed by the interactive partners to be "shared" (i.e., exhibited simultaneously or sequentially) more or less equally often. But, as several researchers have observed (e.g., Gianino & Tronick, 1988, Sroufe, 1995; Tronick, 1989), matched emotional states during early interactions make up less than 30% of all affective interactive episodes, and they mostly involve shared positive affects only. Thus, the majority of sequential (turn-taking) exchanges of emotion expressions tend to involve emotions that are different in content, being complementary rather than identical. It is arguable therefore that such emotional interactions primarily serve the need for the baby to be affectively regulated through the affect-modulating influence of the parent's complementary emotion displays (as well as gentle physical contact by the caregiver), rather than serving the assumed primary function of "sharing" internal psychological states with each other (Fonagy, Gergely, et al., 2002; Gergely, 2002, 2004).

Furthermore, the claim that newborn or a-few-weeks-old infants can differentiate among a set of discrete basic emotion expressions (Field, Woodson, Cohen, Garcia, & Greenberg, 1983; Haviland & Lelwicka, 1987; Izard & Malatesta, 1987) such as happiness, surprise, or sadness has been strongly called into doubt by more recent findings. Nelson (1987) has questioned whether the basis for such early perceptual differentiations is indeed the truly emotion-specific expressive patterns of basic emotion displays or, rather, some other, non-emotion-specific salient perceptual features. For example, Caron, Caron, and Myers (1985) demonstrated that 4- to 7-month-olds could differentiate between toothy and non-toothy emotion expressions, but could not differentiate between angry and happy expressions if both of them showed teeth. Caron, Caron, and MacLean (1988) also showed that 4-month-olds could not discriminate between happy and sad dynamic facial/vocal expressions, and 5-month-olds failed to do so with happy and angry displays. Such findings suggest that even if one accepts the notion of basic emotions theory (Ekman, 1992; Ekman, Friesen, & Ellsworth, 1972) or differential emotions theory (Izard, 1991; Malatesta & Izard, 1984) that there is a set of universal, prewired, discrete facial emotion expressions, there seems to be no compelling evidence to suggest that infants would be able to discriminate such emotion-expressive facial patterns in others before 5–6 months of age.

Csibra and Gergely (2006) have recently provided a detailed critical analysis of the flaws inherent in the standard functional explanations currently widely accepted in the developmental literature for many of those early infant social competencies that together constitute much of the evidential basis to which proponents of the primary "intersubjectivity" theory refer. They argue that these early social interactional phenomena are better and more coherently explained in an entirely different theoretical framework as being the manifestations of a human specific adaptation for "pedagogy" (discussed in greater detail below). Pedagogy is hypothesized to be a primary cognitive system of mutual design that has evolved to facilitate the fast and efficient transmission of relevant cultural information from knowledgeable conspecifics to ignorant, but specifically receptive, human infants (Csibra & Gergely, 2006; Gergely & Csibra, 2006). In this theoretical framework the phenomenon of early turn-taking protoconversational interactions, for example, is interpreted as manifesting the infant's innate sensitivity to and preference for stimuli exhibiting "contingent reactivity". This innate propensity to engage in turn-taking contingencies (Floccia, Christophe, & Bertoncini, 1997), together with the infant's innate preference for eye contact (Farroni et al., 2002; Farroni et al., 2004) and for the characteristic intonation pattern of infant-directed speech or "motherese" (Cooper & Aslin, 1990; Fernald, 1985), belong to the set of cues of "ostensive communication" that function to identify a potential communicative agent for the infant. As we shall see, such ostensive cues are hypothesized to be interpreted as signalling the presence of a communicative intention in the other that is "addressed" to the infant. Ostensive cues trigger a specific receptive attentional and interpretive attitude (the "pedagogical stance") in the infant and an active expectation for further cues of referent identification and communicative manifestation of new and relevant knowledge about the referent. Thus, early turn-taking—together with other early social communicative phenomena, such as joint attention, "proto-declarative" pointing, social referencing (Egyed, Király, & Gergely, 2004), or imitative learning (Gergely, Bekkering, & Király, 2002; Gergely & Csibra, 2006; Király, Csibra, & Gergely, 2004), are interpreted as examples of pedagogical communication whose primary function is the efficient transfer of relevant cultural information rather than that of intersubjective "sharing" of internal psychological states. Below I argue that "marked" affect-mirroring interactions can also be interpreted as a special case of pedagogical communication that functions to "teach" infants about the presence and dispositional content of their primary emotions through mediating the establishment of cognitively accessible second-order representations for such—initially non-conscious—procedural automatisms.

The social construction of the subjective sense of affective self states

In contrast to developmental theories of primary "intersubjectivity", we have proposed an alternative model of early self-development (Fonagy, Gergely, et al., 2002; Gergely & Watson, 1996, 1999) within the framework of contingency detection theory and attachment theory (Watson, 1985, 2001), according to which the infant's subjective sense of affective self has important social interactional origins. We find it important to emphasize from the point of view of clinical theory and therapeutic practice that in our alternative approach *"intersubjectivity" is viewed as a developmental achievement and the capacity for intersubjective experience as an emergent subjective property of the self* rather than it being an initial and universal starting state of the human infant's mental life. We propose that the subjective sense of differential self states (e.g., awareness of being "angry", rather than just experiencing some undifferentiated negative state of tension) is established as a result of the infant's repeated experience with the pattern of contingent reactions and social "mirroring" feedback that her automatic expressions of—initially non-conscious—affective self states evoke from her attachment environment. Our model is based on two central assumptions:

The "constitutional" or introspectively "invisible self". We assume (together with numerous others) that the infant's innate "constitutional self"—that we could equally refer to as the "biological", "temperamental", or the "true" self (see Winnicott, 1971)—has a richly structured internal organization from the beginning. Though the constitutional self is likely to be characterized by significant genetically based individual temperamental differences, it contains a basic set of pre-wired universal categorical emotions that are primary biological adaptations (Ekman, 1992; Ekman, Friesen, & Ellsworth, 1972). These basic emotions can be best conceived of as prewired, stimulus-driven, procedural behavioural automatisms that are not accessible to conscious awareness and over which the baby has no voluntary control at first. Affect regulation at the earliest stages is carried out mainly by the attachment environment as the caregiver, reading the infant's automatic behavioural emotion expressions, reacts to them with appropriate affect-modulating interactions and emotion displays (Gergely, 2002, 2004; Gergely & Watson, 1996). Thus, while infants may be sensitive to the general (positive vs. negative) hedonic quality of affective experience, we assume that babies at the beginning of their lives have no subjective awareness of their discrete basic emotion states as differentiated subjective categories of internal self-experience (for empirical arguments to support this presupposition, see Gergely & Watson, 1996). It is in this sense that we consider the initial constitutional self to be introspectively "invisible": while it contains discrete and categorically differentiable emotional states, these pre-wired automatisms are at first not accessible to introspective awareness, and so they do not present themselves as subjectively experienced differential internal states of the self.

We further hypothesize (contrary to classical approaches, such as Bruner, Olver, & Greenfield, 1966; Mahler, Pine &, Bergman, 1975) that at the beginning of life the human infant exhibits a primary built-in bias towards actively attending to and learning about external events (that is, a primary sensitivity bias towards exteroceptive stimulation), while showing little active introspective attentional orientation towards internal self states to start with (Fonagy, Gergely, et al., 2002; Gergely & Watson, 1996, 1999).

The social construction of subjectivity or the emergence of the introspectively "visible self". We assume that for the categorically differentiable affective states of the primary constitutional self (which includes the universal set of basic emotions) to become introspectively "visible" and subjectively experienced, two basic conditions need to be established developmentally. On the one hand, the primary and procedural affective states of the constitutional self (that are prewired initially non-conscious automatisms) need to become associated with *second-order representations* that, when activated, are cognitively accessible to introspectively oriented attention and monitoring processes. In other words, we suggest that the initially non-conscious primary emotion states become introspectively "visible" differentiated self states of subjective awareness through the activation of their associated second-order representations only. For this to happen, it is also necessary that the primary bias towards external attentional orientation of the newborn should become modified so that *the direction of the infant's attention could be turned towards the self's internal states* to a sufficient degree to allow for the active introspective monitoring and perception of the second-order representations of the primary procedural self states. This can then lead to the introspective self-perception of "being in" a particular differentiated emotion state giving rise to the discrete subjective awareness of that state.

The cognitively accessible and introspectively monitored second-order representations of the primary emotion states can then provide the basis for the establishment of a—continuously updated—representation of the dynamically changing affective self. This allows for the possibility of internally generating self-predictions of one's likely actions by anticipating the dispositional action-tendencies associated with the emotion states that the self is currently in. The ability to become subjectively aware of the current dispositional states of the self before the automatic activation of the emotion-based action-tendencies would take effect is a major precondition for the possibility of exercising affective self-control (Gergely & Watson, 1996). This is so because by foreseeing and then internally evaluating the likely external consequences of the self's anticipated actions one can decide to inhibit or modify them in an adaptive manner rather than being automatically induced to act out one's emotion-based action-tendencies.

Our central developmental proposal is that both of the above preconditions for the construction of the introspectively "visible" subjective self become established as a result of, and to the degree to which, the social attachment environment of the infant provides *systematic contingent feedback reactions* to the automatic expressions—or inferred presence—of the initially non-conscious dynamic affect states of the constitutional self. In other words, it is the experience of one's current internal states being externally "mirrored" or "reflected" back through the infant-attuned contingent social reactions of the attachment environment that makes it possible to develop a subjective sense and awareness of one's primary affective self states.

Of course, no amount of contingent social "mirroring" could result in the establishment of these two (representational and attentional) preconditions unless infants were equipped with an appropriately structured perceptual information-processing mechanism that could efficiently detect the contingent relatedness between their automatic state expressive behavioural displays on the one hand, and the corresponding external mirroring reactions of the social environment on the other. Furthermore, some further mechanism is needed to internalize the representation of the external "mirroring" feedback signal and to establish an association between this second-order representation and the primary self states that has contingently evoked the external "mirroring" reaction in question.

In previous work on the *social biofeedback theory* of parental affect-mirroring (Gergely & Watson, 1996, 1999), we have proposed and structurally characterized the workings of such a perceptual and representation-building mechanism in the form of an innate "*contingency detection module*". Briefly, this prewired contingency perception device (Watson, 1985, 1994) automatically monitors and assesses over time the degree of contingent relatedness between the infant's responses and events in the external (social) stimulus environment. By monitoring three different aspects of contingent relatedness in parallel (the degree of temporal contingency, spatial similarity, and correspondence of relative intensity), the contingency detection device can identify those stimulus aspects of the social environment that are under (some specific degree of) *causal control* of the infant's state expressions and behavioural displays. One important consequence of this perceptual contingency analysis is that to the degree that the social environment exhibits systematic and differential contingent reactivity to the baby's particular types of responses, the consequent discovery of being in contingent control over the social environment generates an experience of causal efficacy and self-agency in the infant.[1]

The role of "markedness" of affect-mirroring expressions in the internalization of second-order representations of affective self states

A most probably species-specific characteristic of the human attachment system is the inclination of sensitive, infant-attuned caregivers to repeatedly present their infants during affect-regulative interactions with empathic emotion displays that imitatively "mirror" their baby's momentary affect-expressions (including the empathic mirroring of negative affect displays as well).[2] In our earlier works on this topic (Fonagy, Gergely, et al., 2002; Gergely & Watson, 1996, 1999) we have emphasized the functional importance of the fact that in the case of sensitive, infant-attuned caregivers such empathic affect-mirroring displays tend to be executed in a saliently *"marked"* manner that makes them perceptually clearly distinguishable from the caregiver's corresponding realistic emotion expressions for the infant. Such "marked" affect-reflecting displays are *saliently transformed versions* of the normative display patterns of the corresponding realistic emotion expressions of the caregiver.[3] Some of the typical features of "markedness" involve (a) *exaggerated, slowed-down execution* of the spatial–temporal display pattern of the realistic, normative emotion expression; (b) *schematic, sometimes abbreviated or only partial execution* of the normative display pattern; (c) the "mirroring" display being *sometimes mixed with*—simultaneous or quickly alternating—*components of other emotion* displays; and (d) it being typically introduced or accompanied by *ostensive communicative "framing" cues* such as raised eyebrows, slightly tilted head, widely opened eyes, and so on.

Our earlier interpretation of the function of "marking" parental affect expressions (Gergely & Watson, 1996) emphasized its importance as a cue signalling to the infant that the emotion display "is not for real", its expressed emotional content should be "decoupled" from the caregiver, or, in other words, that its attribution to her as her real emotion state should be inhibited. This was considered especially important in cases when the caregiver was mirroring a *negative* emotion display of the infant. When salient "marking" of the mirroring display is absent in such cases, the infant could easily confuse it with the corresponding normative emotion expression of the parent. This would lead to the attribution of the expressed emotion to the caregiver as her actual, realistic negative affect state. The consequent perception of the parent being in—and expressing towards the infant—a realistic negative emotion state could then induce traumatic escalation—rather than soothing—of the baby's negative emotion state.

In what follows, I elaborate further the functional characterization of "markedness" by generalizing it in two ways:

1. I shall place the construct within a larger theoretical framework identifying "marked" emotional mirroring displays as a particular instance of the general class of communicative "teaching" acts that are marked by *cues of ostensive communication* that human caregivers seem instinctively inclined to produce when, being in the "*pedagogical mode*" of communication (Csibra & Gergely, 2006; Gergely & Csibra, 2006), they referentially manifest new and relevant cultural information and behavioural skills for their infants to learn. This provides a more principled and generalized explanatory account of *why "marked" mirroring displays are interpreted self-referentially by the infant,* leading to their referential "anchoring" (in the form of internalized second-order representations) to those primary procedural emotion states that the mirroring displays contingently reflect. This new interpretation of "marked" mirroring displays as a form of "pedagogical" communication that functions to "teach" the infant about the presence and dispositional kind of her primary emotion state will also provide us with an improved account of *why the perception of ostensive communicative cues involving "markedness" of mirroring expressions (together with cues of referent identification) help to establish an introspective orientation of the infant's—initially externally biased—attentional processes.* Considering "marked" mirroring as a case of pedagogical communication referencing the infant's self states will also shed further explanatory light on the consequent *increase in sensitivity to subjective self states and their contingent effects on the external social environment.*

2. I review briefly some examples of new empirical research that our theoretical conceptualization of the developmental functions of "mirroring" and "markedness" has recently inspired and the preliminary results of which provide initial support for the hypothesized functional significance of "marked" contingent social mirroring on the development of attachment security, internal sensitivity to self states, and representational competence for pretence during later stages of self development.

Human "pedagogy": The functions of cues of "ostensive communication" and "referential knowledge manifestation" in communicative knowledge transfer

Pedagogy is hypothesized to be a human-specific adaptation of mutual design the evolutionary function of which is the facilitation of fast and efficient intergenerational transfer of relevant cultural information from knowledgeable conspecifics to ignorant juveniles (Csibra & Gergely, 2006; Gergely & Csibra, 2006).[4] The natural initial domain in which such pedagogical communications first occur are the early infant–caregiver interactions that take place within the human attachment system. The types of new and relevant cultural knowledge that are typically transmitted through pedagogical communication include new words, gestural symbols, artefact functions, and the stereotypic use of artefacts, valence information about object kinds, culturally habitual manners of actions, culture-specific emotion display rules, and so on. Here I argue that this list should be extended to include relevant *knowledge about the existence and culturally shared dispositional contents of specific categorical emotion states of the infant's constitutional self* that are initially made accessible to the infant through the caregiver's pedagogical communicative interactions involving ostensively "marked" contingent mirroring displays.

The hypothesis that the primary cognitive adaptation of human pedagogy has a built-in *mutual design* implies specific biological preparedness on the part of both the adult and the infant for providing and receiving cultural information that is new and relevant for the infant. On the "teacher's" part, knowledgeable caregivers, when taking a pedagogical attitude towards the infant, show a natural inclination to exhibit *ostensive communicative cues* and specially *"marked" forms of referential knowledge manifestations*. These pedagogical cues are hypothesized to trigger in the infant a specific type of attentional orientation and interpretive attitude to be applied to the "referential knowledge manifestation" produced by the "teacher". (a) They identify for the infant that the other has an overt communicative intent that is "addressed" to them (cf. Sperber & Wilson, 1986). (b) They evoke an expectation that the other is going to manifest new and relevant information about a referent that the infant needs to infer from the communicative cues contained in the manner in which the "teacher" manifests the new knowledge for the infant. (c) The ostensive communicative cues put the infant into a receptive learning mode supporting fast mapping of the manifested information to its referent. There are *two types of pedagogical communicative cues* produced by adults for which infants show specific receptivity: *cues of "ostensive communication"* and *cues of "referential knowledge manifestation"*.

"Ostensive cues" of communication have two major functions: (a) they inform the infant that the adult has an *overt "communicative intent"* (cf. Sperber & Wilson, 1986) towards the addressee, and (b) they function as *"addressing cues"*, signalling to the infant that the upcoming communication is specifically addressed to her. Ostensive cues involve the establishment of *eye-contact* typically marked by further ostensive gestures such as "knowingly" *raising one's eyebrows* (the "eyebrow flash"), momentarily *widening (or shrinking) one's eyes,* and *tilting one's head slightly forward* towards the addressee. These are often accompanied by verbally *addressing the infant by name* using the salient and specific type of "marked" speech intonation pattern of "*motherese*".

An important semantic feature of such ostensive cues that differentiates them from the "marked" forms of "referential knowledge manifestations"—which they introduce or accompany—is that they do not encode or convey specific informational content about the relevant knowledge to be transmitted to the infant. Instead, the referential meaning that these ostensive cues express is simply—and only—the fact that the person producing them has an "overt communicative intent" that is specifically directed to the addressee.

As we have argued, the perception of "ostensive" communicative gestures triggers in the infant an active expectation that new and relevant knowledge will be manifested about some referent. Therefore, the infant will need to identify the intended referent of the communication in order to map the manifested new information onto it. This will induce a search for the intended referent entity by the infant. This referent identification process is based on—and is directed by—the adult's presentation of *referential orienting cues* such as *eye-direction*, *gaze-shift*, or a *pointing gesture* indicating the intended referent about which new knowledge is going to be manifested. For example, such referential orienting cues will lead the infant to identify the new object the name of which is going to be demonstrated by the adult, as in fast mapping word-learning situations (Tomasello, 1999), to single out the referent object about which valence information is going to be provided by the object-directed emotional attitude manifestations by the adult, as in social referencing situations (Baldwin & Moses, 1996), or to specify the referent object about whose new functional affordance properties the adult's goal-directed action manifestation is going to provide relevant information, as in situations of ostensively induced imitative learning about artefact functions (Gergely, Bekkering, & Király, 2002; Király, Csibra, & Gergely, 2004).

The *second type of pedagogical communicative cues* is provided by the *specific "marked" manner* in which the action demonstrations, serving as *"referential knowledge manifestations"*, are executed by the adult. The function of "referential knowledge manifestations" is to convey to the infant the content of the adult's "referential intention" (cf. Sperber & Wilson, 1986)—that is, to communicate *the content of the new and relevant knowledge about the intended referent* that the infant should infer and map onto the representation of the referent.

"Marked" manifestations involve a *modified and saliently transformed version* of motor execution of the primary procedural motor scheme that is activated and forms the basis of the action display serving as "referential knowledge manifestation". The *cues of "markedness"* correspond to this special form of *saliently exaggerated, slowed down, schematic, and sometimes only partially executed version* of the habitual procedural motor pattern. "Marked" forms of knowledge manifestations serve several functions in pedagogical knowledge transfer. First, they cue the infant about the fact that the "marked" behavioural display is produced to achieve the *communicative and referential goal* of manifesting the knowledge content to—and for—the infant, rather than simply using the procedural motor routine in its everyday habitual manner to achieve its normative, primary function. Take the example of demonstrating to an infant how to eat with a spoon with the pedagogical intention of teaching him about this curious—culturally habitual and shared—human manner of food intake. Clearly, you don't simply start to eat your soup, as you normally do, in front of the infant, passively letting her watch your smooth and efficient functional use of the spoon. Rather, after having established "ostensive communicative contact" with the infant through the production of the kind of ostensive addressing cues discussed earlier, you produce a saliently "marked", modified, schematized, exaggerated, and transformed version of the primary motor scheme of eating with a spoon. Apart from cueing the infant about your referential communicative teaching intent, a further function that is served by performing the saliently "marked" form of the motor display is to cue the infant to take the "pedagogical stance" towards your behavioural manifestation and to infer from it what is the new and relevant knowledge to be learned.

Furthermore, it should be noted that the "marked" form of referential knowledge manifestation is characterized by a *"recipient design"* that also serves several functions in human pedagogy. (a) By taking into consideration the current state of knowledge and mobilizable inferential capacities of the infant, the adult can produce a "marked" modified transform of the primary motor scheme that foregrounds and saliently exaggerates those particular aspects of knowledge that are new and relevant for the infant. In this way, the demonstrator facilitates, constrains, and directs the infant's inferential processing of the referential knowledge manifestation by directing her attention to those aspects of the demonstrated action that convey new and relevant information for her. (b) By producing a "recipient-tailored" version of the motor manifestation emphasizing certain aspects of the procedural scheme over others, the adult can help the infant who is imitating or practicing the new skill by correcting her or directing her attention to those relevant functional aspects of the procedure that the infant has not yet fully understood.

Finally, this evolutionary "mutual design" involves built-in assumptions of the infant's "pedagogical stance" whereby she conceives of the "teacher" as a repository of relevant cultural knowledge that can be expected to exhibit cooperative benevolence in communicating only new and relevant information to the baby. Therefore, the infant can faithfully and quickly learn the content of the ostensively communicated knowledge or skill without any further need for testing its relevance by herself or even for understanding why and how (exactly) what she has acquired actually works to fulfil its relevant function. Note that these tacit assumptions built into the infant's "pedagogical stance"—about the communicator as a repository of relevant cultural knowledge and as having a communicative attitude of cooperative benevolence—are crucial for making possible the efficient and fast intergenerational transfer of *arbitrary* and *conventional*—and sometimes not transparently (or not at all) functional—forms of knowledge the existence of which is specifically characteristic of human culture. Through human pedagogy, such—ostensively communicated—arbitrary aspects of cultural knowledge can become acquired and used (thereby also causally contributing to the stabilization of such forms of knowledge in human culture: see Sperber, 1996, 2006), *even when* the nature of their causal or functional efficacy—or whatever other property it is that justifies their existence in human culture—remains cognitively "opaque" to the infant.

The role of cues of "ostension" and "markedness" in inducing the self-referential interpretation of "marked" affect-mirroring displays

If one looks at the characteristic formal features of empathic "marked" affect-mirroring displays and the ostensive affective interactions in which they appear, it becomes apparent that both types of pedagogical cues described above are centrally involved in the affect-mirroring communicative acts performed by sensitive, infant-attuned caregivers. The manner of execution of "marked" emotion expressions shares the characteristic features of other types of ostensively communicated referential knowledge manifestations in that "marked" affect displays are themselves salient and schematically executed transformations of the corresponding normative, realistic emotion expressions. Also, "marked" emotion displays are typically accompanied by such ostensive cues of communicative intent as "raised eyebrows", "slightly tilted head" or gestural "widening (or shrinking) the eyes". As we have argued elsewhere (Fonagy, Gergely, et al., 2002; Gergely & Watson, 1996, 1999), one of the consequences of the presence of these cues of "markedness" is that the infant will inhibit the attribution of the emotion to the caregiver as her "real" feeling, referentially "decoupling" the emotion display from her. In other words, the infant is cued by the "marked" form of display execution and the other ostensive cues accompanying it that the emotion display is not performed in its primary function as expressing the caregiver's actual emotion state. At the same time, the joint presence of cues of ostension and "marked" forms of emotion manifestation in the caregiver's affect-mirroring display will, by hypothesis, induce the referential interpretive attitude of the "pedagogical stance" in the infant. In other words, they will activate a search for the intended referent of the caregiver's "marked" behavioural manifestation and will lead to setting up a referential interpretation for the "marked" affect display ("anchoring" it to a referent state *other* than the caregiver's actual emotion state). In trying to establish the referent entity that the—"decoupled"—"marked" emotion display is about, the infant will rely on the cues of referent identification (such as eye-gaze direction) of the caregiver that accompany her communicative emotion display. Since the caregiver is looking at and being oriented towards the infant while producing such infant-directed "marked" emotion mirroring displays, *the infant's attention will be directed towards her own face and body, i.e., her own physical self as the spatial locus of the referent entity* that the caregiver's attention orienting referent identification cues indicate and to which the "marked"—and "decoupled"—affect display should be *referentially "anchored"*. This indicated spatial locus of the intended referent coincides with the spatial locus from which those automatic state-expressive behavioural—and proprioceptive—cues emanate that exercise a high degree of contingent control over the caregiver's mirroring responses, as this is signalled to the infant by the output of the automatic contingency analysis that her contingency detection device performs (Gergely & Watson, 1996). These two sources of converging information then *identify the referent of the "marked" mirroring display as being located in the infant's own self*: the intended referent being the infant's dispositional emotional self-state the expressive behavioural components of which exert high contingent control over the caregiver's "marked" empathic mirroring response. As a result, the infant will referentially "anchor"—and associate—the "marked" mirroring display as referring to her own primary emotion state and will internalize its representation as a second-order representation for that—inferred—primary self state.

It is in this way, then, that by activating the infant's pedagogical stance, repeated experience with ostensive "marked" affect-mirroring feedback reactions from infant-attuned caregivers in the baby's early attachment environment can (a) "teach" the infant about the existence of her internal subjective emotion states, (b) lead to the internalization of the caregiver's "marked" mirroring displays as second-order representations associated with the infant's—inferred—primary self states, and (c) introspectively sensitize the infant's attentional system to the presence of internal referents in the self. This process (together with the sensitization effects of the contingency-based social biofeedback mechanism described by Gergely & Watson, 1996) also leads to a heightened awareness of the internal proprioceptive cues of emotional self-expressions and the potential instrumental effects of contingent control that these internal state cues of the self exert over the reactivity of the social environment.

This is, then, in short, the manner in which an infant-attuned social mirroring-environment contributes to the construction of the introspectively "visible" subjective self, populating it with second-order internal state representations that form the basis of a subjective sense of awareness of internal self states.

The cognitive "costs" involved in ostensive communication, "marked" communicative manifestations, contingent affect-mirroring, and their significance for an infant-minded caregiving attitude and secure attachment

Above it was argued that—apart from their role in the direct interactive regulation of the infant's affective states within the attachment system (see Gergely & Watson, 1996)—contingent empathic "mirroring" reactions and "marked" ostensive forms of communicative parental displays also serve the further "pedagogical" function of "teaching" the infant about the existence and referential content of her internal subjective self states. As we have seen, this process of social construction of an introspectively "visible" subjective sense of self involves the internalization of contingent and "marked" mirroring displays by the infant as second-order representations of her primary affective self states. These second-order structures are cognitively accessible, they are subject to introspective awareness, and they can "stand for"—or signal the activation of—the primary and non-conscious procedural emotion states of the constitutional self to which they have become referentially "anchored".

This proposal has been based on the realization that "marked" affect-mirroring displays involve the very same infant-directed cues of "ostensive communication" and "referential knowledge manifestation" that play a key role in the hypothesized species-specific cognitive adaptation for human pedagogy, a dedicated system of mutual design selected for the fast and efficient intergenerational transmission of cultural knowledge in humans (Csibra & Gergely, 2006; Gergely & Csibra, 2006).

It should be pointed out that the human-specific ability to produce these types of pedagogical communicative cues in a functional manner is not at all a trivial matter, as it necessitates special—and probably human-specific—cognitive capacities the application of which involves significant cognitive processing "costs" for the caregiver. On the one hand, in order to generate "marked" forms of referential knowledge manifestations (a specific instance of which are the infant-directed "marked" affect-mirroring displays), the caregiver needs to apply specialized cognitive resources. This is so because in order to produce such "marked" knowledge manifestations the caregiver needs to have *metacognitive access* to the internal structural organization of her own primary automatic procedural knowledge representations the contents of which she manifests for the infant (rather than simply using them in the habitual manner to fulfil their primary function). Furthermore, the caregiver must also possess the cognitive capacity for *motor re-planning and voluntary control over the manner of execution* of such habitual action schemes to produce modified versions of them in a goal-directed manner. This is needed to allow her to transform these habitual and primary motor execution patterns into the kind of "marked, schematized, exaggerated, slowed down, only partially executed, and saliently transformed display versions" that are used in pedagogical communications in which knowledge is not simply used but is, rather, demonstrated. On the other hand, metacognitive access and voluntary modification of stereotypic motor execution patterns are also crucial for generating referential knowledge manifestations with a functional "recipient design" being individually "tailored" to fit the level of cognitive needs of the particular infant to whom they are communicated. Apart from cueing the infant—through ostensive cues and the salient "markedness" of the display—to take the "pedagogical stance" and interpret the knowledge demonstration referentially, the manifestation must include—or needs to exaggerate—only those aspects of procedural information that will enable the infant to infer from it the new and relevant information that she should represent and retain in memory. This involves additional cognitive "costs" for the caregiver who—in order to create such a "recipient-tailored" and "marked" version of knowledge manifestation—must be able and willing to actively *monitor and diagnose the infant's actual state of knowledge* and mobilizable inferential capacities.

In sum, to produce the right cues of ostensive communication at the right time and to generate pedagogically functional "recipient-tailored" "marked" forms of knowledge, manifestations represent high cognitive and computational "costs" and, as such, involve significant evolutionary investment in the infant on the part of the caregiver. From the point of view of the *development of attachment security*, this observation has important predictive significance. Caregivers differ greatly in their available cognitive capacity, mobilizable attentional resources, and attachment motivation that they can invest into actively monitoring their infant's knowledge and affective states. However, as argued above, these are the necessary preconditions for generating successful pedagogical communications with a functional "recipient design" that can facilitate and direct the extraction of relevant new knowledge by the infant.

This leads to the prediction that "infant-minded" caregivers, who are high pedagogical "investors" in the evolutionary sense, will be more likely to frequently exhibit such "costly", appropriately "marked", infant-attuned, and infant-directed contingent "mirroring" displays as well as appropriate and well-timed ostensive communicative "addressing cues" during their communicative interactions. Therefore, the relatively high rate of producing adequate ostensive communicative cues and "marked" forms of contingent "mirroring" reactions observable during infant–caregiver interactions can be expected to function as diagnostic signs or behavioural "fingerprints" indicating a highly infant-attuned and infant-minded attitude of the caregiver.[5]

Such caregivers will, in general, tend to be more vigilant and perceptive than others in relation to their infant's internal self states, which they are more likely to actively monitor. As a result, they will be better in correctly identifying their infants' signals when those indicate emerging attachment needs as well. They will, therefore, be more able to mobilize their resources quickly and efficiently to establish proximity and to successfully regulate their baby's disequilibrated affective states, thus fostering the development of attachment security. Also, there are several other ways in which the frequency of ostensive communications involving contingent "mirroring" and "marked" parental referential displays are likely to contribute to the development of secure attachment in the infant. Attachment figures who produce these behavioural indicators adequately and with relatively high frequency are clearly more ready to invest "costly" cognitive resources into benevolently monitoring as well as appropriately and efficiently enriching the subjective sense of the infant's self through their "marked" mirroring feedback of the infant's primary self states. Such a richly responsive contingent "mirroring" environment also contributes to the development of a sense of causal self-efficacy and agency as the infant—through the workings of the contingency detection device (Gergely & Watson, 1996)—detects and becomes sensitized to the degree of causal control that her automatic affective self-expressions exercise over the contingent reactivity of her attachment environment.

Recent research on the developmental consequences of early contingent "mirroring" and "markedness" of communicative parental displays on the development of the subjective self

The aim of this final section is to briefly and informally illustrate some new and—and often still preliminary—research findings that our approach to the social origins of the subjective sense of self and, in particular, our theoretical analysis of the functional role of early contingent "mirroring" and "markedness" of emotion displays have given rise to in recent years. It should be clear that the few selected examples briefly discussed below do not represent a systematic review of the existing body of evidence that is relevant for our theory of self development. Rather, they simply serve to illustrate some of the interesting and promising new directions of research that have grown out of our specific theoretical proposals.[6]

1. *Mirroring, markedness, attachment security, and the development of pretence competence.* We have already referred to the remarkable similarity between the formal features of "markedness" of infant-directed parental emotion displays and other forms of "marked" referential knowledge manifestations, on the one hand, and the characteristic "marked" manner of emotion expressions, actions, and verbal utterances produced in pretend play, on the other (see Fonagy, Gergely, et al., 2002; Gergely & Watson, 1996). By the end of the second year (Harris & Kavanaugh, 1993; Leslie, 1987), normally developing children start to spontaneously produce and understand pretend play—both solitary and social—in which the execution of habitual motor schemes is modified, transformed, exaggerated, abbreviated, schematically or only partially realized in ways that seem very closely related to the manner in which "marked" forms of parental mirroring displays and other types of infant-directed referential knowledge manifestations are produced. Pretend play is also characterized by the production of ostensive cues and "marked" forms of intonation contour and elevated pitch that are typical features of the infant-directed speech pattern of motherese. Furthermore, pretend play and "marked" parental knowledge manifestations certainly seem to require the very same cognitive mechanisms allowing for metacognitive access and voluntary transformation of procedural knowledge representations for their production. (It is also noteworthy that just as these metacognitive abilities, so the propensity to spontaneously engage in pretend play seems also a species-unique characteristic of humans.) We have argued that the cue of "markedness" in caregiver–infant communicative interactions fulfils two important interpretive functions: (a) it triggers referential "decoupling" of the content of the manifested display from its primary referent, and (b) it triggers the referential "anchoring" of the display content to a new referent entity. As first pointed out by Alan Leslie (1987) in his seminal paper on the metarepresentational structure of pretend play, the very same representational operations and interpretive referential functions of "markedness" are also cru-

cial cognitive requirements for producing and understanding pretence (see Gergely & Watson, 1996, pp. 1196–1200). On these grounds, Gergely and Watson (1996) have specifically hypothesized that repeated experience with "marked" parental mirroring interactions—and their consequent internalization as second-order representations of primary self states—may play an important causal role in the establishment of "a generalised communicative code of 'marked' expressions characterized by the representational functions of referential decoupling, anchoring, and suspension of realistic consequences" (p. 1200).

As part of a larger longitudinal study, we could recently examine the developmental relation between contingent maternal mirroring and the "markedness" of contingent maternal reactions in a group of 12-month-old infants, on the one hand, and different aspects of pretence competence of the same children at 2.5 years of age, on the other (Futó, Bátki, Koós, Fonagy, & Gergely, 2004). Maternal mirroring and contingent "markedness" was measured at 12 months in the so-called three-phase Mirror Interaction Situation (MIS) (see Koós & Gergely, 2001) that is a modified version of the standard Still-Face paradigm (Tronick, Als, Adamson, Wise, & Brazelton, 1978). We designed this procedure to induce contingent mother–infant interactions in an affect-regulative situation that involved the induction of mild stress in the infant. Mother and infant were seated next to each other in front of a—one-way—mirror. They were separated by an occlusion screen that prevented them from physically contacting each other: however, they were free to interact facially and vocally with each others' mirror image. (We videotaped these sessions from the other side of the one-way mirror for later off-line analysis.) After a first phase of free interaction, the mother was instructed to put on a motionless, neutral "still-face", looking at but not reacting to her infant. This "interaction deprivation" period was followed by a third phase during which the mother was again free to interact with her baby. Since the temporary deprivation of maternal reactivity during the second—still-face—phase induces mild stress in the infant (Koós & Gergely, 2001; Tronick et al., 1978), the mother could attempt to regulate her baby's affectively disequilibrated state through vocal and facial interactions during the third phase (without the possibility, however, of soothing her baby by direct physical contact). The video-taped, synchronized, and time coded "split-screen" record of mother–infant interactive behaviours was coded later in a micro-analytic manner for the relative frequency and duration of a number of interactive and state-expressive behavioural variables. The category of "contingent maternal reactivity" ("mirroring") involved facial and/or vocal imitative maternal reflections of the infant's behaviours as well as temporally contingent verbal "acknowledgements" by the mother that made reference to the infant's behavioural, attentional, intentional, or emotional state. We have separately coded those contingent verbal reactions of the mother that involved a saliently "marked", exaggerated form of expression.

We followed up a sub-sample of these infants and at between 2 and 3 years of age we administered in the child's home a modified and enriched version of the battery of pretence tasks originally developed by Harris and Kavanaugh (1993) to measure representational aspects of pretence competence along the lines of Leslie's (1987) analysis of the metarepresentational structure and representational operations implied by understanding and producing pretend play. We also developed further coding categories to specifically measure those aspects of spontaneous elaborative and creative use of pretence that went beyond the representational task requirements of the Harris–Kavanaugh tasks such as elaborations, modifications, creative extensions, and role-reversals. We considered these aspects of pretence competence to be particularly important in the functional use of pretence play for affect-regulative purposes (such as re-enacting traumatic episodes by adaptively modifying their contents by changing the role of passive recipient to active agent or by modifying or extending the episode to include a happy ending, etc.: see Freud, 1920g). We also included open-ended pretence scenarios that involved separation or physical injury and invited the children to spontaneously complete them. These extensions of the set of pretence tasks and modifications of the coding categories allowed us to measure the children's ability to use pretend play creatively for affect-regulative purposes. The sessions were videotaped for later off-line coding. Our complex coding system allowed us to characterize each child's overall *representational pretence competence* on the one hand, and level of *spontaneous, creative, and elaborative use of pretence* that is involved in the functional use of pretend play for affect-regulative purposes, on the other.

For *"markedness"*, our preliminary findings (Futó et al., 2004) indicate that a high degree of "markedness" of contingent maternal references to infant state (during the first and third phases of the MIS) at 12 months significantly predicted both higher overall representational pretence competence scores and higher scores on spontaneous, adequate, and creative extensions in the use of pretence at 2.5 years of age. For *"mirroring"*, we found that high contingent maternal reactivity ("mirroring") at 12 months (during the first and third phases of the

MIS) predicted high scores on spontaneous, adequate, and creative extensions of pretence performance at 2.5 years. (Interestingly, we also found that low tolerance to loss of maternal contingency during the still-face period of the MIS at 12 months predicted low pretence performance in open-ended pretence situations involving separation or physical injury at 2.5 years of age.)

Since at 12 months we had also measured the infants' attachment security using the standard Ainsworth Strange Situation procedure (Ainsworth, Blehar, Waters, & Wall, 1978), we could also look for developmental correlations between security of attachment at 1 year and later pretence competence at 2.5 years of age. We found that secure attachment at 12 months predicted significantly higher overall representational pretence competence scores at 2.5 years than did insecure attachment.

In sum, these preliminary results clearly support our hypotheses that (a) *high contingent maternal responsivity ("mirroring")* and (b) *high degree of "markedness" of contingent maternal references* to infants' state-expressive behaviours during the first year *facilitate the development of representational pretence competence* in general, and the capacity for *rich creative and spontaneous use of pretence* associated with affect-regulative use, in particular. In the previous section we argued that the same features of maternal interactions—that is, contingent reactivity and "marked" forms of mirroring reactions—are likely to facilitate the development of attachment security in infants. Our finding of a significant positive correlation between security of infant attachment at 1 year and high levels of representational pretence competence at 2.5 years of age is clearly in line with this argument.

2. *Contingent maternal reactivity, markedness, attachment security, and the emergence of introspective sensitization to subjective self states and their contingent effects on the external world.* Finally, I shall briefly summarize some recent results that are relevant for testing a further central prediction of our theory about the developmental consequences of the caregiver's "marked" forms of infant-directed emotion displays and contingent "mirroring" reactions for the establishment of the infant's emerging subjective awareness of her internal self states. Above it was hypothesized that the perception of "markedness" of contingent parental mirroring displays helps to establish *an introspective orientation of the infant's—initially externally biased—attentional processes.* In particular, it was proposed that repeated experience with "marked" mirroring reactions of sensitive, infant-attuned caregivers will result

in a *heightened sensitivity* (a) *to the internal proprioceptive stimulus cues* that are activated by the emotional state expressions of the self, and, consequently, (b) *to their potential instrumental effects of contingent control* that—through their behavioural expressions—these internal state cues exert over the reactivity of the external (social) environment.

A recent study reported by Stanley, Murray, and Stein (2004) provides evidence that is directly relevant for the above predictions. These researchers measured contingent maternal reactivity to infant behaviours during face-to-face interactions at 2 months (in a sample of infants with post-natally depressed mothers and non-depressed controls). Months later these infants participated in an Instrumental Learning Task in which they had to learn that their spontaneously emitted responses exerted contingent causal control over an external event (inducing the contingent movements of a mobile). Stanley and colleagues reported that high contingent maternal reactivity at 2 months predicted faster instrumental learning in infants (irrespective of maternal status with regard to depression). This finding is in line with our hypothesis that maternal contingent reactivity to the infant's state expressions increases the introspective accessibility of internal proprioceptive cues that accompany the infant's state expressive behaviours. This increased sensitivity to and accessibility of proprioceptive cues may have allowed for the faster discovery, registration, and learning of the instrumental contingent control that the infant's spontaneous responses exerted over the mobile's movements, leading to the more efficient learning performance of infants with highly contingently reactive mothers. The finding also indicates that the experience of causal agency and self-efficacy gained by those infants whose responses evoked high degrees of contingent maternal reactivity may have resulted in a generalized interest in attending to—and active testing of—the causal potency of their actions in controlling different aspects of the external world around them.

In closing, I wish to describe some preliminary findings (Gergely, Fonagy, & Watson, in preparation) from our own social instrumental learning task that we have designed to test infants' relative degree of sensitivity to internal (proprioceptive) cues produced by their own facial emotion expressions versus their sensitivity to the external—visual—stimulus equivalents that they perceive when the same facial expression is displayed by a face that the infants are looking at. In our paradigm, 12-month-olds were seated in front of a large monitor showing a schematic female face in the centre looking and smiling at the infant (without her lips being separated). The screen also showed two identical black magician's hats in an upside-down orientation, one appearing in the upper left corner, the other in the upper right corner. During the experiment, the external face opened her mouth from time to time. Similar mouth-opening behaviour was also spontaneously produced from time to time by the infant herself, whose facial behaviour was being videotaped through a hidden camera placed above the monitor. An experimenter (watching the live image of the infant's face on a monitor in another room) pressed a key on the keyboard whenever the baby opened her mouth.

This was the basic set-up for our discriminative learning task in which there were three conditions.

1. In the "Other" (exteroceptive cue only) condition, the discriminative stimulus was the mouth-opening action of the female face on the screen: whenever she opened her mouth, for the next 5 seconds a "reward" became available for the infant (a rabbit with a carrot in its mouth came out of one of the black hats while a pleasant musical tune was heard). For the reward to become activated, however, the infant had to look up at the hat (discriminative response) within the 5-second time-window of reward availability that started at—and was signalled by—the onset of the mouth-opening action of the female face. So the infant needed to learn the signal value of the external visual stimulus of the female face's mouth-opening action as indicating reward availability. Instrumental learning was measured as the increase in frequency of the infant successfully harnessing the reward within the 5-second reward availability window following the external mouth-opening event by looking up at the right corner, thereby activating the reward event.

2. In the "Self" (interoceptive cue only) condition, the only difference was that it was the infant's *own* mouth-opening action that served as the discriminative stimulus the onset of which signalled the availability of the reward. (Note that in this condition, the external face opened her mouth with equal frequency across subjects—in a "yoked control" design—as in the "Other" condition, but without signalling reward availability.) So for instrumental learning to occur in the "Self" condition, the infant had to discover the predictive power of his own mouth-opening gesture which required sensitivity to and monitoring of the internal (proprioceptive) cues produced by her facial response.

3. In the "Self–Other" ("mirroring") condition we arranged for the mouth-opening action of the external face to be contingent upon the infant's own mouth-opening responses. In other words, the external face contingently and imitatively reacted to the spontaneous

mouth-opening responses of the infant, effectively "mirroring" them whenever they occurred. Note that in this "Self–Other" condition *both* the internal (proprioceptive) cues generated by the infant's *own* mouth-opening gestures and the contingent external (exteroceptive) cues of the imitative mouth-opening acts of the female face acted as potential discriminative stimuli: in other words, the internal and the external cues had equal predictive power in signalling the availability of the reward. So to achieve instrumental learning, the infant could rely equally on either the internal self-cues or the external other-cues (or both).

Looking at the relative difficulty of instrumental learning across the three conditions, we found a significant difference between securely versus insecurely attached infants. Interestingly, insecure infants performed significantly better in the "Other" (exteroceptive cue only) condition than did the secure babies, whereas in both the "Self" (interoceptive cue only) and the "Self–Other" ("mirroring") conditions the opposite pattern was obtained: securely attached infants tended to produce better instrumental learning scores in both of these conditions than did insecurely attached infants.

This intriguing pattern of results can be interpreted as indicating that while the direction of attentional processes of insecure infants remains dominantly externally oriented, by 1 year of age securely attached infants have already learned—as a result of their experiences with the "marked" contingent mirroring reactions of their sensitive, infant-attuned caregivers—to direct at least part of their available attentional resources in an introspective direction, actively monitoring the dynamic changes of their internal self states as well as the proprioceptive cues produced by their own emotion-expressive behaviours. For example, it may be that secure infants are switching their available attentional resources dynamically back and forth between monitoring either the external or the internal world for relevant emotion-expressive cues that allow the anticipation of both the self's and others' affectively driven action dispositions. This, in fact, is likely to be a highly adaptive and desirable strategy for optimal coping and social reality testing in the interpersonal domain.

In terms of relative efficacy of instrumental learning in the "Other" (exteroceptive cues only) condition, however, such a style of "division of attentional labour" between internal and external monitoring can actually result in a relative disadvantage for securely attached infants who can allocate proportionally less attention to monitor and learn about external cues than do insecure infants who direct the bulk of their attentional resources externally. This would explain their superior learning performance in the "Other" condition where successful learning depends solely on learning about the predictive power of external cues and nothing is gained by attending to the world of internal cues. In the other two conditions, however, where the internal cues are also informative and can be relied on for instrumental learning, the performance of securely attached infants has markedly improved, and they outperformed the insecure infants in both of these conditions. This relative improvement can be interpreted to be the result of their hypothesized ability to partially allocate their attentional resources in an introspective direction where they could pick up useful task-relevant information about the predictive power of the internal (proprioceptive) cues of their own facial behaviour. In contrast, the dominantly externally oriented insecure infants remain relatively introspectively "blind" to such internal cues and, accordingly, cannot exploit their informational value in the instrumental learning task.

An intriguing further aspect of these findings is that the learning performance of insecure infants, when compared to their level of learning efficiency in the Other (exteroceptive-cue-only) condition, has actually decreased in the Self–Other (mirroring) condition and did so to a similar degree as in the Self (proprioceptive-cue-only) condition. This was so in spite of the fact that the external stimulus cues of the other's face provided equally useful predictive information about reward availability in the Self–Other (mirroring) condition as in the Other (exteroceptive-cue-only) condition. It seems that the detection of contingent control that their own self's facial action exerted over the other's facial mirroring reaction must have negatively interfered with the insecure infants' ability to attend to and learn about the predictive value of the exteroceptive cue of the other's facial action. One possible interpretation of this finding is based on the possibility that due to their habitual affective experiences induced by the characteristic interaction patterns of their insecure attachment environments, by 1 year of age insecure infants have learned to associate the contingent reactions of others to their emotion-expressive behaviours with negative affective consequences. Therefore, the detection of their contingent influence on the reactivity of the external face may have induced negative arousal in the insecurely attached infants which could have interfered with and consequently decreased their learning performance. The fact that the negative emotional expressions of insecure–avoidant infants typically evoke systematic negative parental reactions (that can actually result in the characteristic inhibition of avoidant infants' negative affect expressions during separation episodes in the Strange Situation) seems to be in line with this hypothesis. On the other hand, in the case of insecure–resistant infants who are affectively under-regulated (Sroufe, 1995), one can argue that their emotional expressivity typically results in negatively escalating affective states and increased disequilibration due to their caregivers' typical emotional (often anxious) overreactions and contagious unmarked "mirroring" reactions to their infant's emotional signals (Gergely & Watson, 1996). Again, it can be argued that the habitual negative affective consequences of such contingent parental reactions have become associated in anxiously resistant insecurely attached infants with their perceived agentive influence on the emotional reactions of their social environment. This could explain, then, the negative interference that both groups of insecure infants showed in the Self–Other ("mirroring") condition that involves the detection of the self's contingent influence over the emotional facial behaviour of the external female face.

Conclusions

I have here contrasted two different developmental approaches to the ontogenetic origins of the subjective self and to the nature and developmental roots of the "intersubjectivity" of interpersonal experience from the points of view of developmental psychopathology of disorders of the self on the one hand, and social cognitive theories of normal self development on the other. First the Cartesian view of the subjective self and the group of related current-day developmental theories of *primary "intersubjectivity"* have been described and critically examined on both empirical and clinical grounds. These developmental theories advocate a rich mentalistic interpretation of the subjective experience that young infants may have during early turn-taking protoconversational affective interactions about the emotional and intentional psychological states of both their own self and the caregiver's mind. A number of non-trivial conceptual and empirical problems that these currently popular theories of primary "intersubjectivity" have to face have been identified, and several alternative developmental approaches that avoid these problems have been outlined. Then I summarized our alternative social constructivist approach (Fonagy, Gergely, et al., 2002; Gergely & Watson, 1996) to the early development of the subjective self that emphasizes the important causal role that habitual patterns of contingent responsivity of the infant's attachment environment may play in the emergence of a subjective sense of affective self-experience. I described the specific mechanisms and psychological processes postulated by our contingency-based "social biofeedback model of affect-mirroring" that mediate the *internalization of second-order representations* for the primary—and initially non-conscious—procedural emotional states of the "constitutional self" that are at first introspectively "invisible" and cognitively inaccessible. Our model emphasizes the central developmental role of *contingent affect-mirroring* interactions involving *"marked" forms of emotion displays* in the formation of the representational and attentional preconditions for the emergence of a subjective sense of emotional self-experience and the intersubjective mental understanding of interpersonal interactions with others. The representation-building role of "marked" forms of affect-mirroring interactions and the functional nature of the "ostensive communicative cues" that accompany them were then reconceptualized within the new theoretical framework of human "pedagogy", a primary species-unique adaptation dedicated for the efficient transmission of new and relevant cultural knowledge in humans (Csibra & Gergely, 2006; Gergely & Csibra, 2006). It was argued that the "marked" affect-mirroring interactions of infant-attuned sensitive caregivers can be conceived of as a specific form of ostensive pedagogical communications through which the caregiver "teaches" the infant about the existence and dispositional content of her primary, non-conscious, and automatic emotion states by establishing cognitively accessible second-order representations for them. This process is argued to induce a self-referential interpretation of the caregiver's ostensive "marked" affect-mirroring displays by the infant that also leads to the modification of initially externally biased attentional processes towards introspective self-monitoring, further contributing to the establishment of subjective self-awareness and control. In the final section new evidence from recent empirical studies is briefly summarized that specifically examines the role of contingent affect-mirroring and ostensive cues of "markedness" in the later development of aspects of the subjective self such as pretend play, introspective sensitivity to internal self states, and their contingent influence on the social environment.

NOTES

1. For further details and supporting empirical evidence for the workings of the contingency detection device the reader should consult Fonagy, Gergely, et al., 2002; Gergely & Watson, 1996, 1999; Watson, 1979, 1994.

2. In Gergely & Watson (1996) and Fonagy, Gergely, et al. (2002) we provide a review of the developmental and psychoanalytic literature that both demonstrates

and emphasizes the centrality of parental empathic affect-mirroring during early affect-regulative mother–infant interactions.

3. It is noteworthy (see later) that the manner in which such "marked" emotion displays transform the normative display patterns of realistic emotion expressions shares a great deal of formal similarity with the marked "as if" manner of executing "real" expressive and goal-directed action schemes in pretend play, on the one hand (Fónagy & Fonagy, 1995; Fonagy, Gergely, et al., 2002; Gergely & Watson, 1996), and to the manner in which infant-directed speech or "motherese" transforms adult communicative speech patterns, on the other (Fernald, 1992: see Gergely & Watson, 1996, p. 1198, fn. 8).

4. Reviews of the relevant infant literature supporting the postulation of such a human-specific cognitive adaptation as well as arguments for its probable evolutionary origins can be found in Csibra & Gergely, 2006, and Gergely & Csibra, 2006.

5. Karpf (2004), in an unpublished Ph.D. dissertation that has specifically examined the developmental effects of early "marked" maternal mirroring on later measures of attachment security and social cognitive development, reports findings that are generally in line with the above hypotheses. A further finding that is also relevant to the hypothesized developmental link between level of contingent reactivity of the caregiver and the development of attachment security comes from Ann Bigelow's research (Bigelow, 2001; Chisholm, Bigelow, Gillis, & Myatt, 2001). She reported that the level of maternal vocal contingency to the infant's vocalizations at 4–5 months predicted security of attachment at 2.5 years (as measured by Crittenden's preschool attachment scale).

6. A more comprehensive review can be found in our recent book (Fonagy, Gergely, et al., 2002) that includes relevant case illustrations as well both from child and adult patients.

Commentary

James F. Leckman

György Gergely leads us here through his internal world of thought, evolving theory, and empirical data documenting his search for the essential "Whats", "Whys", and "Hows" of severe "self" pathologies.

- *What* is the most fruitful perspective to consider the difficulties of individuals identified as having borderline, narcissistic, or dissociative personality disorders? Gergely introduces us to his theoretical landscape and indicates that these individuals have a "radically" different type of affective "self-organization".
- In asking the question *why* these pathologies exist, Gergely states that it is because of chronic problematic interactions with early attachment figures dating from the very beginning of their lives.
- *How* these problematic interactions transform and distort the individual's "affective self-organization" is at the heart of this chapter. Here we are treated to a mix of spirited disputation (the classical Cartesian approach to the self is flawed, or at least incomplete), the careful presentation of specific assumptions (we are all endowed with a richly structured internal organization that equips us with the "basic emotions" *à la* Paul Ekman, which, in turn, needs to be associated with second-order representations that then become accessible to introspectively oriented attention), to the presentation of an evolving "contingency detection theory". This theory proposes that we are fundamentally endowed with a "contingency detection module" and that the individual's development of their subjective sense of self is dependent upon and begins with the systematic contingent feedback reactions by the infant's social attachment environment. He next turns to a microscopic examination of the contingent

interactions ("mirroring" responses *vs.* ostensively cued "marked" parental responses) and how these interactions serve to teach the infant what is important *vis-à-vis* emotional states. Gergely then provides evidence that the presence of these features are "diagnostic and predictive" of the later development of a "secure" attachment style. In closing, Gergely shares his current passion—his view of *how* an infant establishes an introspective orientation through the repeated experience of "marked", ostensive communications by a sensitive care giver.

Point of view

Categories, the legacy of words, distort reality and ease communication by fragmenting the bewildering whole. Diagnostic categories provide an apt example. They are useful for communication and for insurance reimbursement but are probably not an all-or-none phenomenon. Nor are they an end in themselves: rather, they define a conceptual space within continuous distributions that reflect a small part of the complexity of how we experience ourselves within our unique social landscape. Diagnostic categories simply provide one perspective on the suffering of others. From this perspective, the idea of a disease entity is not a goal to be reached but, rather, our most fruitful perspective on the lives of these individuals. From this vantage point Gergely offers us an attractive landscape of thought that provides insight—and testable hypotheses—concerning certain forms of psychopathology. It also has the potential to illuminate aspects of how we become who we are within our own internal worlds and how that sense of self is always a work in progress—one that began with a nascent self: an assembly of reflections of how we were first seen in the eyes of those who cared for us at the beginning of our lives.

Following a reprise of Gergely's main points and a statement of a point of view, this brief discussion digresses to the wonders of intersubjectivity (and some tantalizing findings from a MRI study of a Clint Eastwood movie). It then moves on to what Donald Winnicott would have said (or actually did say), before returning to modern neuroscience and wondering whether we can ever witness the intersubjectivity and synchrony of parent–infant dyads and wondering at how that information might inform the care of individuals with severe "self" pathology.

The wonders of intersubjectivity

Attempting to define, diagnose, and treat psychopathology in humans is a particularly difficult enterprise as our profession operates on the border of observer-dependent and observer-independent reality (Searle, 2004). Other branches of medicine can rely on a predictable world that exists, to a great extent, independent of our social constructions and subjective states. Psychiatry and psychoanalysis cannot do so, as subjective states and social constructions are at core of the problems we seek to address and redress. While I agree with Thomas Nagel (1974) that the mind–body problem is likely to be intractable and imagine (despite periodic bouts of reductionist euphoria) that we may never be in a position to even have an accurate conception of what an explanation of the physical nature of a mental phenomenon would be, I am a psychiatrist and psychoanalyst, and I think, speak, and act as if intersubjectivity is a reality. I know that subjective states, if accurately reflected by the clinician, form the basis of our diagnoses and therapeutic alliances and that patients who feel accurately understood are more likely to remain in treatment and to have successful outcomes.

It is consciousness that makes the mind–body problem intractable. But that said, it is within consciousness that we experience rational (and irrational) thought, the ability to anticipate the future in the intentions and actions of others, play out scenarios of trial action, and take actions that reflect a sense of self and of moral responsibility. Our consciousness in the midst of a supportive family and friends is our best cushion against life's adversity, but it can turn into our greatest tormentor. Combined with language and our perceptual systems, our consciousness and our pragmatic and systematic assumption that others perceive the world, others, and themselves along similar dimensions are at the heart of who we are. Without such systematic assumptions, such things as empathy, poetry, as well as literary and cinematographic fictions would be impossible.

This brings me to one of the most interesting *in vivo* imaging studies of the last several years. Hasson, Nir, Levy, Fuhrmann, and Malach (2004) applied an unbiased analysis in which spatiotemporal activity patterns in one individual's brain were used to "model" activity in the brains of four other individuals. The investigators decided to use a 30-minute uninterrupted segment taken from *The Good, the Bad, and the Ugly,* starring Clint Eastwood. They found a striking level of voxel-by-voxel synchronization between individuals, not only in primary and secondary visual and auditory areas but also in some association cortices. The results revealed a tendency of individual brains to "tick collectively" at certain points during this film. These moments of inter-subject synchronization typically correlated with emotionally arousing scenes (the fusiform gyrus consistently activated at the same points in time that included an emotionally expressive face). Other stimuli that evoked such synchronization included scenes with other clearly discernable features, such as views of buildings (collateral sulcus) or delicate hand movements about to begin to perform some motor task (post central sulcus, in the vicinity of Brodmann area 5). These data suggest that large regions of the human cortex are stereotypically responsive to particular naturalistic audiovisual stimuli. These inter-subject correlations were found to extend well beyond the visual and auditory cortices into high-order multimodal association areas that have not been previously associated with sensory processing. This observation of inter-subject synchronization may provide a new quantifiable measure of the involvement of cortical areas associated with external sensory stimuli. And if it works for Clint Eastwood movies, how much more can we expect from the day-to-day drama of parent infant dyads.

What would Donald Winnicott have said?

Infants acquire knowledge about their caretakers and social world with remarkable speed, but exactly how they do it remains mostly a mystery. Among the unknowns are how infants acquire the skill to communicate their needs and anticipate the responses of their caregivers. This is a practical matter, but how do these developmental events initiate and shape the child's self-perceptions? As early as the 1960s, Winnicott offered a few thoughts:

> The good-enough mother meets the omnipotence of the infant and to some extent makes sense of it. She does this repeatedly. A True Self begins to have life through the strength given to the infant's weak ego . . . it is an essential part of my theory that the True Self does not become a living reality except as a result of the mother's repeated success in meeting the infant's spontaneous gesture . . . the infant begins to believe in external reality which appears and behaves as by magic . . . and which acts in a way that does not clash with the infant's omnipotence. The True Self has spontaneity, and this has been joined up with the world's events. The infant can now begin to enjoy the *illusion* of omnipotent creating and controlling, and then

> can come to recognize the illusory element, the fact of playing and imagining. [Winnicott, 1960]

Following Gergely (2003) and Winnicott—and Arnold Gesell before them—we can begin to imagine that scientists will be able to track a "universal" timeline of self-perception and self-development much in the same way that Patricia Kuhl (2004) and others have charted the "universal language timeline of speech-perception and speech-production". Just as Kuhl indicates the child's inborn capacity to discriminate phonetic contrasts in all languages and produce non-speech sounds (abilities that precede their amazing capacity to perform statistical learning of distributional frequencies and transitional probabilities and engage in "canonical babbling"), Gergely and others will chart the initial evidence for the infant's use of the "contingency detection module" to perform statistical learning of contingent interactions ("mirroring" responses as well as the ostensively cued "marked" parental responses). It is likely that this experience during face-to-face interactions beginning around the second month of life provides the basis for children's social and moral development, empathy, as well as their emerging sense of self (Fonagy, Gergely, et al., 2002). Maternal gaze matching, facial expressions, vocalizations, and regulation of arousal states during face-to-face play provide critical environmental inputs during the sensitive period of maturation of the visual cortex. Furthermore, by synchronizing with infant arousal state, mothers entrain the infant's biological rhythms and in all likelihood provide a "resonance" of internal and external experience, self and other, brain and behaviour (Lester, Hoffman, & Brazelton, 1985; Trevarthen, 1993). In addition, by entering into a synchronous affective communication with the infant, the caregiver provides an external support for the infant's developing bioregulatory abilities and in all probability conveys a measure of resilience to stress throughout life.

Can we ever witness the intersubjectivity and synchrony of parent–infant dyads?

Good-enough parenting depends on a caretaker's contingent responses to emerging subjectivity of the infant. There is a mutually reinforcing choreography that sets the stage for these two developing worlds—of the parent and of the child—which intersect in ways that push forward the development of both. It is also where the child's tools of thought and predispositional responses to the world first take shape. This choreography is in all probability reflected in electrical activity of parental and infant hearts and brains. How is it that parents synchronize with infant arousal states, entrain the infant's biological rhythms, and provide a source of "resonance" between internal and external experience, between self and other, and between brain and behaviour? Although we have relatively little understanding of how patterns of neuronal activity are transmitted and transformed, they are likely to be fundamentally important with regard to the emergence of goal-directed behaviour and the formation of habits associated with parent–infant interactions. As with respiration and the sleep–wake cycle, goal-directed behaviour and expression of habits are likely to depend upon the quasi-random oscillatory activity of groups of neurons. Their synchronization with phase-locking and frequency stabilization can be seen as a resonance phenomenon of the brain. Selectively distributed oscillatory systems of the brain exist as resonant communication networks through large populations of neurons, which work in parallel and are interwoven with sensory, motor, cognitive-, and emotional functions (Buzsáki & Draguhn, 2004; Llinás, Ribary, Contreras, & Pedroarena, 1998). For example, the "mirror neuron system" is a unique network that involves the inferior frontal cortex with superior temporal cortices that are linked via the insula to limbic structures as well as with parietal structures. It appears likely that this network underlies the understanding of the intentions of others as well as providing a neural basis for empathy and self-recognition (Carr, Iacoboni, Dubeau, Mazziotta, & Lenzi, 2003; Uddin, Kaplan, Molnar-Szakacs, Zaidel, & Iacoboni, 2005).

In closing

To close the circle and return to severe self pathologies, we would also speculate that the activity and oscillation of the mirror neuron system will be aberrant in borderline personality disorder (BPD) and related conditions. We would also predict that functional alterations in this network of cells would also be seen in individuals with disorganization of attachment (Fonagy, Gergely, et al., 2000). Although structural and functional brain imaging studies of BPD are still in their infancy, the available studies provide support for dysfunction in inferolateral prefrontal-limbic circuits (Herpertz et al., 2001; McCloskey, Phan, & Coccaro, 2005). It would also be expected that efficacious treatment of BPD would also lead to detectable changes in circuit (Bateman & Fonagy, 2004a).

CHAPTER THREE

Primary parental preoccupation: revisited

James F. Leckman, Ruth Feldman, James E. Swain, & Linda C. Mayes

> I do not believe it is possible to understand the functioning of the mother at the very beginning of the infant's life without seeing that she must be able to reach this state of heightened sensitivity . . . *almost an illness* . . . and recover from it.
>
> Donald W. Winnicott (1956)

> Part of what is introjected is the image of the child as seen, felt, smelled, heard and touched by the mother. What happens is not wholly a process of introjection. The bodily handling and concern with the child, manner in which the child is fed, touched, cleaned, looked at, talked to, called by name, recognized and re-recognized . . . shape and mould him . . .
>
> Hans Loewald (1960)

> What fascinated me most was how intimate relationships and the desire for being with the other precede the rest of cognitive development, and that this social motivation moves these other achievements forward, including meta-representation and theories about other minds. This intuitive, deeply encoded social orientation is first expressed in the mother's arms and then forms the basis for all future I–Thou relationships.
>
> Donald J. Cohen (2001)

Primary maternal preoccupation is a term coined by Winnicott (1956) to describe the mother's special mental state during the time surrounding the birth of a new infant. He described this state of mind as "almost an illness" that a mother must experience and recover from in order to create and sustain the environment that can meet the physical and psychological needs of her child. Winnicott speculated that this special state began towards the end of the pregnancy and continued through the first weeks of the infant's life. This concept, which has been incorporated into clinical formulations of disordered mother–infant relationship, has received relatively little attention, especially in the study of the normative processes of parenting (Feldman et al., 1999; Fraiberg, Adelson, & Shapiro, 1975; Kreisler, Fain, & Soulé, 1974; Leckman et al., 1999; Stern, 1997a; Zeanah, Benoit, Hirshberg, Barton, & Regan, 1994).

In this chapter we take a close look at the content of these preoccupations and the caretaking behaviours they complement and engender. Next, we consider recent research on the genetic, epigenetic, and neurobiological substrates of maternal behaviour in mammalian species and their potential relevance for understanding human risk and resiliency. Here we utilize an evolutionary point of view concerning some forms of developmental psychopathology. This viewpoint begins with the recognition that individuals vary with regard to adaptive skills and problem-solving abilities and that these individual variations may lead to differential reproductive success. The selection of a mate, bearing of viable offspring, and the formation of parental commitments that will sustain an infant through a lengthy period of dependency are just a few of the interdependent processes needed for an individual to survive. Although most of our biological and behavioural potentialities are likely to be called upon at one point or another in the service of these goals, there must be highly conserved brain-based systems that are specifically activated at developmentally appropriate moments to achieve and sustain these processes. We hypothesize that a thorough understanding of these normative processes will also lead to deeper insights into our vulnerability to develop a range of psychopathological outcomes (Leckman & Mayes, 1998).

An additional theoretical perspective adapted in this chapter is Winnicott's (1956) formulations on the "holding environment", the non-specific environment (in terms of the attachment relationship) the special provisions of which support the infant's physical and emotional growth. During the first months of life infants go through stages that

Winnicott termed "holding", "handling", and "object relating", each representing a stage in the growing specificity of the mother–infant relatedness. In line with the works of Spitz (1946), Mahler, Pine, and Bergman (1975), and Loewald (1960), the role of the early maternal environment is thought of as the provision of a core sense of safety prior to the formation of a specific object or attachment relationship. Recent research in animal models and human infants have helped specify the neurological and behavioural components of the "holding environment" by which the maternal physical presence and evolutionarily conserved set of maternal behaviours in the first post-partum period promotes the sense of safety. This early maternal environment functions to modulate the infant's stress reactivity, promote attention and self-regulatory capacities, and provide the foundation for the infant's capacities to form meaningful relationships throughout life (Feldman, 2004; Francis, Diorio, Plotsky, & Meaney, 2002).

Early parental love

For the most part, empirical studies of the early parent–child relationship have been child-centred. Most of the available empirical studies have focused on the development of attachment behaviours in the child and on the moment-to-moment observable, behavioural functioning of the parent–infant dyad. These points of focus have revealed the highly contingent nature of parental verbal and non-verbal behaviours with very young infants; the importance of early synchrony, reciprocity, and direct physical contact in parent–child interactions; and the critical impact of early experiences on the child's subsequent attachment behaviours towards the parent—and later in other intimate relationships (Bornstein, 1995; Dunn, 1977; Feldman, Weller, Sirota, & Eidelman, 2003; Stern, 1974; Trevarthan, 1979). Developmental researchers have underscored the potential negative impact of early parental deprivation and neglect on the development of social skills (Carlson et al., 1989; Egeland & Sroufe, 1981; Heinicke, 1995; Rogosch et al., 1995). The major theoretical perspectives—psychoanalysis and attachment theory—emphasize the link between the nature of early parent–infant relationship and adaptation across the lifespan as well as the interconnectedness of the physiological, behavioural, and representational components of parent–infant attachment. However, little information is available on the parents' thoughts regarding their roles as parents and the place of the infant in their inner lives, the relationship of these thoughts to their behaviours with the infant, and the impact of these thoughts on the infant's subsequent development.

Winnicott described an altered mental state that characterizes the first weeks of a mother's relationship with the infant. Suggesting that such a state of heightened sensitivity develops towards the end of pregnancy and lasts for the first few post-natal weeks, he likened it to a withdrawn or dissociated state that in the absence of pregnancy and a newborn would resemble a mental illness of acute onset. In this period, mothers are deeply focused on the infant, to the near exclusion of all else. This preoccupation heightens their ability to anticipate the infant's needs, learn his/her unique signals, and over time to develop a sense of the infant as an individual. Winnicott emphasizes the crucial importance of such a stage for the infant's self-development and the developmental consequences for infants when mothers are unable to tolerate such a level of intense preoccupation.

In a prospective longitudinal study of 82 parents, we have documented the course of early preoccupations and found that they peak at around the time of delivery (Leckman et al., 1999). Although fathers and mothers displayed a similar time course, the degree of preoccupation was significantly less for the fathers in our study. For example, at two weeks after delivery, mothers of normal infants, on average, reported spending nearly 14 hours a day focused exclusively on the infant, while fathers reported spending approximately half that amount of time.

The mental content of these preoccupations includes thoughts of reciprocity and unity with the infant, as well as thoughts about the perfection of the infant. For example, we found that 73% of the mothers and 66% of the fathers reported having the thought that their baby was "perfect" at three months of age. These idealizing thoughts may be especially important in the establishment of resiliency and the perception of self-efficacy. In a second study of 60 mothers and fathers observed in the first post-partum months and again three months later, parents similarly reported the perception of their infant as perfect and pointed to the birth of their child as a moment of transformation in their lives, associated with an alteration in the salience of career, hobbies, and other commitments and a stronger sense of spirituality. These shifts in hedonic focus were greater for mothers than for fathers and were associated with lower depression and anxiety, pointing to the importance of the parents' special mental states—the primary parental preoccupations—in buffering against post-partum depression, a condition affecting approximately 10–12% of post-partum women (Burt & Stein, 2002).

Results from studies of at-risk infants confirm the centrality of the mother's positive perceptions in shaping the mother–infant relationship. Mothers of premature infants who reported positive feelings towards their infants expressed confidence in their ability to parent and perceived their infant as not very different from an "ideal" baby were more sensitive to their infants' signals during interactions, provided more affectionate touch, and the infants were more socially alert and involved during play (Keren, Feldman, Eidelman, Sirota, & Lester, 2003).

These parental preoccupations also include anxious intrusive thoughts about the infant. In a longitudinal study of 120 couples during their first pregnancy and in the six months after birth, women reported increasing levels of worry towards the end of their pregnancy, and 25 to 30% described being preoccupied with worries about caring for the infant post-partum (Entwisle & Doering, 1981). Immediately before and after birth, this figure may be substantially higher. In our studies, we found that anxious intrusive thoughts and harm-avoidant behaviours peaked at around the time of birth. The content and timing of these thoughts and actions varied from parent to parent. After delivery and on returning home, the most frequently cited concerns were one's adequacy as a new parent, concerns about feeding the baby, about the baby's crying, and thoughts about the infant's well-being. Conditions such as these are especially commonly reported among parents of very sick preterm infants, infants with serious congenital disorders or malformations, or infants with serious birth complications (Feldman, Weller, Leckman, Kvint, & Eidelman, 1999). Less commonly, intrusive thoughts of injuring the child may beset the new mother (or father) and can in turn lead to post-partum obsessive-compulsive disorder or depression or both (Winter, 1970). In our recent study (Swain et al., 2004), mothers and fathers reported high levels of anxious and intrusive thoughts as part of their daily experience. The level of intrusive thoughts was related to the degree of responsibility the parent felt for the infant. The amount of anxious thoughts correlated to the degree of transformation the parent experienced and with the developing parental attachment with the child, in terms of both endearing mental representation of the infant (e.g., calling the infant by a special name) and the formation of special, ritualized parental behaviour (e.g., singing to the child a special song during bedtime in a special way). These highly anxious thoughts, which often have an obsessive-like intrusive quality to them, may thus be important indicators for the process of the parental attachment to the infant.

Interestingly, when the mother's preoccupation is turned to herself rather than the infant, this is a negative indicator of the emerging relationship. Mothers who reported preoccupations with their own delivery pain two days after birth, ruminated about the painful experience, and tended to magnify their discomfort reported higher levels of anxiety and depression and showed lower levels of synchronous parenting at six weeks post-partum (Ferber & Feldman, 2005).

Nursing, feeding, kissing, and affectionate touch—actions that parallel the licking and grooming behaviours seen in other mammalian species—are the parental behaviours that are perhaps most associated with a new infant. Women describe breastfeeding as a uniquely close, at times sensual, experience and one that can be associated with a timeless sense of "oneness" between the mother and infant (Bretherton, 1987). Breastfeeding contributes to the mother's caregiving behaviour, and breastfeeding mothers were shown to be more sensitive to their infants' cues during a feeding session, pointing to the importance of maternal–infant intimacy in shaping maternal behaviour (Brandt, Andrews, & Kvale, 1998). Recent studies of direct skin-to-skin contact between premature newborns and their parents (kangaroo care) also emphasize the beneficial effects of physical touch in facilitating more sensitive and affectionate interactions as the child grows older (Feldman, Weller, Sirota, & Eidelman, 2003). The physical intimacy afforded by the kangaroo experience increases nursing volume (Hurst, Valentine, & Renfro, 1997) and contributes to infant resiliency, arousal modulation, stress reactivity, and cognitive competencies across infancy (Feldman, Eidelman, Sirota, & Weller, 2002; Feldman, Weller, Sirota, & Eidelman, 2002). At five years of age, children who received kangaroo care in infancy showed better emotion regulation capacities and better executive functioning and inhibitory control, pointing to the lasting effects of early contact on the development of prefrontal cortex functioning and the child's patterns of response to stressful situations (Feldman, 2004).

Even before the child is born, most parents busy themselves with creating a safe, clean, and secure environment for the infant. Major cleaning and renovation projects are commonplace as the human nest comes into being. After birth, proximity, unimpeded access, and safety are among the parents' uppermost concerns. Safety issues include the cleanliness of the infant and the infant's immediate environment, taking extra care not to drop the infant, as well as protection from potential external threats. This sense of heightened responsibility leads parents to maintain proximity and check the infant's status compulsively, even when they know the baby is fine (Leckman et al., 1999).

For one's genes to self-replicate, sexual intimacy must occur and the progeny of such unions must survive. Pregnancy and the early years of an infant's life are fraught with mortal dangers. Indeed, it has only been during the past century that infant mortality rates have fallen from over 100/1,000 live births in 1900 to about 10/1,000 in 1984 (Corsini & Viazzo, 1997). Little wonder then that a specific state of heightened sensitivity on the part of new parents would be evolutionarily conserved.

It is also worth noting that becoming a new parent often comes at high physiological and mental cost. For nursing mothers there is the need to increase their caloric intake as well as to remain well hydrated. There is also a revaluing and reordering of what is important in life. Caregiving is just one of several competing motivational systems for parents. Parents must also consider the needs of the other children in the family, their occupational duties, the needs of the marital relationship and the demands of the larger social group, so that the advent of a new infant involves an adjustment in the parents' hedonic homeostasis as they establish lasting reciprocal social bonds and make room in their inner lives for a new family member (Clutton-Brock, 1991).

Finally, too much or too little primary parental preoccupation may be problematic. Too much can lead to obsessive-compulsive-like states (Maina, Albert, Bogetto, Vaschetto, & Ravizza, 1999), and too little may set the stage for abuse or neglect in vulnerable, high-risk families (Eckenrode et al., 2000). One condition that has been repeatedly associated with disrupted mother–infant attachment and poses a risk factor for children's development across life is maternal post-partum depression (Field, 1992; Goodman & Gotlib, 1999). In terms of the primary parental preoccupations, depressed mothers reported lower levels of preoccupations, particularly the aspect relating to the building of a meaningful relationship with the infant, such as interacting with the infant in a special way, calling him/her by a nickname, imagining the infant's future, or idealizing the child (Feldman, Weller, et al., 1999). These data suggest that the function impaired by depression is the behavioural and mental investment in forming a relationship with the new infant. On the other hand, physical intimacy with the infant—in terms of kangaroo care and breastfeeding—were found to be effective in reducing maternal depression, increasing the mother's investment in the relationship, and improving the mother's attachment behaviours towards the infant (Feldman & Eidelman, 2003; Feldman, Eidelman, et al., 2002).

Neural circuitry of maternal behaviour

Although the central nervous system events that accompany parental care and characteristic parental mental states in humans are largely unknown, it is likely that there is a substantial degree of conservation across mammalian species (Fleming, Steiner, & Corter, 1997; Leckman et al., 2006). Classical lesion studies done in rodent model systems (rats, mice, and voles) have implicated the ventral tegmental area (VTA) in the midbrain, the medial preoptic area (MPOA) of the hypothalamus, the paraventricular nucleus (PVN) of the hypothalamus, the ventral part of the bed nucleus of the stria terminalis (BNST), the nucleus accumbens, and the lateral septum (LS) as regions pivotal for regulation of pup-directed maternal behaviour (Insel & Harbaugh, 1989; Li & Fleming, 2003; Numan, 1994; Numan & Sheehan, 1997). Similarly, in rodent models repeated pup exposure also leads to the activation of many of these structures, including the MPOA, BNST, and the cingulate cortex (Stack & Numan, 2000). Subsequently, once the animal has engaged in maternal behaviour, the MPOA and parietal cortices show heightened c-fos expression in the presence of pup-associated cues.

Oestrogen, prolactin, and oxytocin can act on the MPOA to promote maternal behaviour (Bridges, Numan, Ronsheim, Mann, & Lupini, 1990; Numan, Rosenblatt, & Kiminsaruk, 1997; Pedersen & Prange, 1979). Oxytocin is primarily synthesized in the magnocellular secretory neurons of two hypothalamic nuclei, the PVN and the supraoptic nuclei (SON). The PVN and SON project to the posterior pituitary gland. Pituitary release of oxytocin into the bloodstream results in milk ejection during nursing and uterine contraction during labour. It has also been shown that oxytocin fibres, which arise from parvocellular neurons in the PVN, project to areas of the midbrain such as the VTA as well as the limbic system including the amygdala, nucleus accumbens, BNST, and LS (Sofroniew & Weindl, 1981).

There are several reports that oxytocin facilitates maternal behaviour (sensitization) in oestrogen-primed nulliparous female rats. Intracerebroventricular (ICV) administration of oxytocin in virgin female rats induces full maternal behaviour within minutes (Pedersen & Prange, 1979). Conversely, central injection of an oxytocin antagonist, or a lesion of oxytocin-producing cells in the PVN, suppresses the onset of maternal behaviour in post-partum female rats (Van Leengoed, Kerker, & Swanson, 1987). However, these manipulations have no effect on maternal behaviour in animals permitted several days of post-partum mothering. This result suggests that oxytocin plays an important role in facilitating the onset, rather than the maintenance, of maternal attachment to pups (Pedersen, 1997).

Data on the role of oxytocin in maternal behaviour in humans is scarce. Mother–infant touch and contact have been shown to stimulate oxytocin release. Newborn infants placed on the mother's chest stimulate oxytocin release by hand movement and suckling (Matthiesen, Ransjo-Arvidson, Nissen, & Uvnas-Moberg, 2001), and mother–infant skin-to-skin contact immediately after birth elevates maternal oxytocin levels (Nissen, Lilja, Widstrom, & Uvnas-Moberg, 1995). Breast pumping and breastfeeding are related to a comparable increase in oxytocin levels (Zinaman, Hughes, Queenan, Labobok, & Albertson, 1992) and thus measuring exact amounts of expressed milk may serve as an accurate proxy of oxytocin levels. Mothers of premature infants who expressed higher quantities of breast milk showed more optimal maternal behaviour, in terms of higher sensitivity and more affectionate touch during interactions. The amount of breast milk also predicted the infant's cognitive and motor development and negatively correlated with maternal depression (Feldman & Eidelman, 2003). Since oxytocin functions as an antidepressant agent, reducing anxiety and elevating social activity in humans (Carter, 1998; Uvnas-Moberg, 1998), and is increased with touch and contact, it is likely to play a role in the general complex of behaviour and mental representations related to maternal caregiving.

A recent study examined plasma oxytocin and cortisol level in a group of 64 mothers at three time-points: in the second month of pregnancy, in the third trimester, and at two weeks post-partum (Levine, Feldman, & Weller, 2004). Oxytocin was highly stable across measurement points, and oxytocin levels at two weeks post-partum were associated with more relationship-building maternal behaviours towards the infant (e.g., singing to the child in a special way) and the third trimester with the mother's report of anxious and intrusive thoughts.

Ascending dopaminergic and noradrenergic systems associated with reward pathways also appear to play a crucial role in facilitating maternal behaviour (Koob & Le Moal, 1997). For example, rat dams given microinfusions of the neurotoxin 6-hydroxydopamine (6-OHDA) in the VTA to destroy catecholaminergic neurons during lactation showed a persistent deficit in pup retrieval but were not impaired with respect to nursing, nest building, or maternal aggression (Hansen, Harthon, Wallin, Lofberg, & Svensson, 1991). There also appears to be an important interaction between dopaminergic neurons and oxytocin pathways. Specifically, pup retrieval and assuming a nursing posture over pups were blocked in parturient dams by infusions of an oxytocin antagonist into either the VTA or the MPOA (Pedersen, Caldwell, Walker, Ayers, & Mason, 1994). Recent studies have also emphasized the role of dopamine release in the nucleus accumbens in facilitating licking and grooming behaviours in rats (Champagne et al., 2004).

Brain areas that may inhibit maternal behaviour in rats have been identified (Fleming, Vaccarino, & Luebke, 1980; Sheehan, Cirrito, Numan, & Numan, 2000). Specifically, lesions of the anterior hypothalamic nuclei, the ventral medial nuclei, and the medial nuclei of the amygdala (MA), facilitate maternal behaviour. The MA in particular appears to be a crucial way station in conveying olfactory cues to the hypothalamic and limbic structures (Sheehan, Paul, Amaral, Numan, & Numan, 2001).

In summary, the initiation and maintenance of maternal behaviour involves a specific set of neural circuits. With pregnancy or with repeated exposure to pups, structural and molecular changes occur, most of which are not yet completely understood, in specific limbic, hypothalamic, and midbrain regions that reflect, in part, an adaptation to the various homeostatic demands associated with maternal care. Many of the same cell groups implicated in the control of maternal behaviour have been implicated in the processing of sensory information, the control of ingestive (eating and drinking) behaviour, thermoregulation (energy homeostasis), stress response, social (defensive and sexual) behaviours, as well as general exploratory or foraging and appetitive behaviours.

While information about these circuits in humans and other primate species is sparse, the availability of *in vivo* neuroimaging techniques is transforming this area of investigation. The available data are consistent with the same circuitry being involved in humans as is seen in other mammalian species (Fleming, O'Day, & Kraemer, 1999; Lorberbaum et al., 2002). For example, Fleming and colleagues have found that first-time mothers with high levels of circulating cortisol were better able to identify their own infant's odours. In these same primiparous mothers, the level of affectionate contact with the infant (affectionate burping, stroking, poking, and hugging) by the mother was associated with higher levels of salivary cortisol (Fleming, Steiner, & Corter, 1997). Likewise, Lorberbaum and colleagues (2002) found increased levels of activity in the cingulate cortex as well as the midbrain, hypothalamus, dorsal and ventral striatum, and the lateral septal region in response to listening to infant cry stimuli. Each of these findings supports the hypothesis that our stress response and reward pathways are adaptively activated during the period of heightened maternal sensitivity surrounding the birth of a new infant.

Using "own-baby" cry stimuli compared with "other-baby cry", we have recently reported regions of relative activation in a group of first time mothers at 2–4 weeks post-partum which included right amygdala and insula (Swain et al., 2004). Given the same stimuli at 3–4 months post-partum, amygdalar and insular activations were not observed; instead, midbrain, and hypothalamic activations were seen. It will be interesting to see how repeated measures of parental preoccupations relate to changes in brain activity. For example, does the decreased activation in the amygdala reflect a reduction in the level of anxious intrusive thoughts, or does the increased activation in the midbrain, in the area of the VTA, and in the hypothalamus relate to the increasing idealization and positive appraisal of the infant over this same interval of time?

In addition to baby cry stimuli, several research groups have used photographic images or videos of one's own infant (or child) versus other unfamiliar infants (or children) as stimuli in fMRI studies of new parents. Typically, areas within the anterior cingulate (or paracingulate regions), insula, striatum and midbrain show increased activation in response to photographic images (Bartels & Zeki, 2004; Leibenluft, Gobbini, Harrison, & Haxby, 2004; Ranote et al., 2004). In another study, Nitschke and colleagues (2004) reported bilateral orbitofrontal cortex activations, which were correlated with the mothers' ratings of a pleasant mood state while viewing photographs of their infant. These data point to the orbitofrontal cortex as well as areas in the midbrain and hypothalamus as being important nodes in the neural circuits underlying some of the rewarding and reinforcing aspects of maternal behaviour.

Longitudinal studies are needed in normal and high-risk mothers and fathers to gain a clearer picture of the time course of the patterns of brain activity that are associated with the conserved behaviours and mental states that characterize this period of life and how various forms of psychopathology, such as post-partum depression, impact on this circuitry.

Genetic determinants of maternal behaviour

Gene knockout technology has provided new insights into the molecular basis of maternal behaviour that are congruent with the existing neurobiological literature. At least ten genes have been identified as being necessary for the expression of one or more aspects of maternal behaviour (Leckman & Herman, 2002). These genes encode for three transcription factors: three enzymes, including dopamine beta hydroxylase and neuronal nitric oxide synthase; two receptors, including the prolactin and the oestrogen α receptor; and one neuropeptide, oxytocin (Leckman & Herman, 2002). By way of illustration, we briefly review one of these genes, *Dopamine beta hydroxylase* (*Dbh*).

Noradrenergic neurons in the brain project from brainstem nuclei and innervate virtually all areas of the brain and spinal cord. The enzyme Dbh synthesizes the adrenergic receptor ligands norepinephrine (NE) and epinephrine. Thomas and colleagues disrupted the *Dbh* gene in mice. Mice homozygous for the *Dbh* mutation (*Dbh* –/–) died *in utero*, of apparent cardiovascular failure (Thomas, Matsumoto, & Palmiter, 1995). *Dbh* –/– mice could be rescued at birth by provision of adrenergic agonists or a synthetic precursor of NE, L-threo-3, 4-dihydroxyphenylserine (DOPS), in the maternal drinking water from embryonic day 9.5 until birth. The majority of these rescued animals became viable adults.

In a subsequent study, Thomas and Palmiter (1997) demonstrated impaired maternal behaviour across virtually all domains evaluated. Pups were observed scattered within the bedding around the nest. Often pups were not cleaned, and their placentas remained attached. Milk was not detected in the stomachs of most pups born to *Dbh* –/– females, which suggests that the pups were not nursing despite the presence of normal mammary-gland tissue. Cross-fostering experiments revealed that almost all litters in which *Dbh* –/– dams were paired with experienced wild-type pups were raised to weaning. This observation demonstrates that the *Dbh* –/– dams can nurse and that lactation is not impaired.

The impairment in maternal behaviour in the *Dbh* –/– animals could reflect a developmental deficit caused by NE deficiency, or it could represent a physiological deficit. To distinguish between these possibilities, DOPS was used to restore NE transiently to the mutant females. When mutant females were injected with DOPS on the morning after birth, maternal behaviour was not restored, and all pups subsequently died. However, when mutant females were injected with

DOPS on the evening prior to birth, over half of the litters survived. Even more pups survived when DOPS was injected both the evening before and on the morning after birth.

These findings suggest that NE may play a key role in initiating a realignment of the dam's sense of what is salient and important in the environment. Interestingly, in 85% of the mutant females, the rescue of maternal behaviour by DOPS extended to the mother's subsequent pregnancies even in the absence of DOPS injections. However, DOPS injections did not significantly enhance pup retrieval by mutant virgin females.

In sum, gene-targeting studies have demonstrated that at least ten specific genes, including *Dbh,* are necessary for the development of maternal behaviour. We conclude that the basic microcircuitry responsible for mediating maternal behaviour is, at least in part, genetically determined. Indeed, the limbic-hypothalamic-midbrain circuit implicated by the gene knockout studies is the circuit identified by the classical lesion studies. Strikingly, some of the genetically mediated deficits in maternal behaviour can be restored through early environmental manipulations.

Non-genomic influences on maternal behaviour

Thus far, several experimental interventions have been shown to have effects on aspects of maternal behaviour, including licking and grooming, high-arched-backed nursing, and aggression towards an intruder. Other rodent maternal behaviours have also been systematically evaluated (Pryce, Bettschen, & Feldon, 2001). In general, these findings suggest that the intrauterine environment (Francis., Szegda, Campbell, Martin, & Insel, 2003) and maternal experience and behaviour in the days following birth serve to "program" the subsequent maternal behaviour of the adult offspring as well as establishing the pups' level of hypothalamic-pituitary-adrenal responsiveness to stress (Denenberg, Rosenberg, Paschke, & Zarrow, 1969; Francis, Diorio, Liu, & Meaney, 1999; Francis, Diorio, et al., 2002; Levine, 1975). This complex programming also appears to influence aspects of learning and memory. Furthermore, many of the brain regions implicated in these experimental interventions are the same as those identified in the knockout gene and earlier lesioning studies. Investigations of social primates also highlight the importance of early mothering in determining how the daughters will mother (Harlow, 1963; Suomi & Ripp, 1983). It is also clear that the effects of early maternal deprivation in primates may be difficult to reverse, as many maternally deprived monkeys are able, as adults, to function normally under usual conditions but are unable to cope with psychosocial stressors (Suomi., Delizio, & Harlow, 1976). Alternatively, in rodent models environmental enrichment in the peripubertal period appears to compensate for the effects of early maternal separation (Francis, Diorio, et al., 2002).

Embryonic transfer. Francis and colleagues (2003) recently investigated the effects of prenatal (embryo transfer) and post-natal (cross-fostering) environments in two strains of inbred mice with profound and reliable differences in behaviour. They found that some robust strain-related behavioural differences including fearfulness in novel environments may result from environmental factors during development rather than genetic differences between the offspring.

Post-natal cross-fostering studies. It has been observed that rodent mothers display naturally occurring variations in maternal licking/grooming and arched-back nursing (Francis, Diorio, et al., 1999). Since the licking/grooming behaviour occurs most frequently before or during arched-back nursing, the frequencies of these two behaviours are closely correlated among mothers. In a subsequent cross-fostering study, investigators determined that the amount of licking and grooming that a female pup receives in infancy is associated with how much licking and grooming she provides to her offspring as a new mother. They reported that the low-licking and -grooming dams could be transformed into high-licking and -grooming dams by handling. Most impressively, they also found that this change was passed on to the next generation—that is, that the female offspring of the low-licking and -grooming dams became high-licking and -grooming mothers if they were either cross-fostered by high-licking and -grooming dams or if they were handled. The converse was also true—namely, that the female offspring of the high-licking and -grooming dams became low-licking and -grooming mothers if they were cross-fostered by low-licking and -grooming dams.

These naturally occurring variations in licking, grooming, and arched-back nursing have also been associated with the development of individual differences in behavioural responses to novelty in adult offspring. Adult offspring of the low-licking, -grooming, and arched-back nursing mothers show increased startle responses, decreased open-field exploration, and longer latencies to eat food provided in a novel environment.

Oxytocin receptor binding levels have also been found to differ between the brains of rat dams depending on whether or not they are high or low "lickers and groomers" (Francis, Champagne, & Meaney, 2000). Specifically, examination of the MPOA and the intermediate and ventral regions of the lateral septum disclosed that oxytocin receptor levels were significantly higher in lactating females compared with non-lactating females. Lactation-induced increases in oxytocin receptor binding were greater in high- compared with low-licking, -grooming, and arched-back nursing females in the BNST and ventral region of the septum. Francis and colleagues suggest, therefore, that variations in maternal behaviour in the rat may be reflected in, and influenced by, differences in oxytocin receptor levels in the brain.

The adult offspring of high-licking, -grooming, and arched-back nursing dams showed, as well, increased expression of NMDA receptor subunit and brain-derived neurotrophic factor mRNA, and increased cholinergic innervation of the hippocampus. In the amygdala there are increased central benzodiazepine receptor levels in the central and basolateral nuclei. There is decreased CRF mRNA in the PVN. These adult pups also show a number of changes in receptor density in the locus coeruleus, including increased alpha2 adrenoreceptors, reduced GABA A receptors, and decreased CRF receptors (Caldji et al., 1998; 2000).

Furthermore, Francis and colleagues demonstrated that the influence of maternal care on the development of stress reactivity was mediated by changes in gene expression in regions of the brain that regulate stress responses. For example, adult offspring of high-licking, -grooming, and arched-back nursing dams showed increased hippocampal glucocorticoid receptor mRNA expression. A further exploration of this phenomenon has led to deeper understanding of the epigenetic modification of the promoter region of the glucocorticoid receptor gene within hippocampal cells that appears to be responsible for some of these enduring effects on stress response and maternal behaviour (Weaver et al., 2004). It seems that despite genetic constraints, the nature of early caregiving experiences can have enduring consequences on individual differences in subsequent maternal behaviour, anxiety regulation, and patterns of stress response.

In sum, data from animal studies indicate that the interval surrounding the birth of the rat pup or the rhesus infant is a critical period in the life of the animal that has in all likelihood enduring neurobiological and behavioural consequences. Despite genetic constraints, the nature of early caregiving experiences can have enduring consequences on individual differences in subsequent maternal behaviour, anxiety regulation, and patterns of stress response.

In the final section of this chapter we consider whether there is any evidence in human studies of similar effects.

Early life experience, risk, and resiliency

Increasing clinical and epidemiological data support the view that exposure to early adverse environments underlies vulnerability to altered physiological responses to stress and the later expression of mood and anxiety disorders (Ambelas, 1990; Brown, Bifulco, & Harris, 1987; Kendler, Kessler, Neale, Heath, & Eaves, 1993). Among the most important early environmental influences is the interaction between the primary caregiver and the infant. Building on the early theoretical work of Bowlby (1969) and colleagues, efforts to characterize this reciprocal interaction between caregiver and infant following periods of separation and to assess its impact have provided a powerful theoretical and empirical framework in the fields of social and emotional development (Cassidy & Shaver, 1999). Over the past 30 years, clear evidence has emerged that significant disturbances in the early parent–child relationship (reflected in such things as child abuse and neglect or insecure attachments) contribute to an increased risk for developing both internalizing and externalizing disorders (Sroufe, Carlson, Levy, & Egeland, 1999). While early adversity and insecure attachment may not be a proximal cause of later psychopathology, it seems to confer risk. Conversely, longitudinal studies of high-risk infants suggest that the formation of a special relationship with a caring adult in the perinatal period confers a degree of resiliency and protection against the development of psychopathology later in life (Werner, 1997; Werner & Smith, 2001).

Similarly to the findings observed in rodents (Ladd et al., 2000; Liu et al., 1997, 2000; Plotsky & Meaney, 1993), a growing body of evidence also indicates that human caregivers' levels of responsivity to their children can be traced in part to the caregivers' own childhood histories and attachment-related experiences (Miller, Kramer, Warner, Wickramaratne, & Weissman, 1997). Caregivers' attachment-related experiences are hypothesized to be encoded as "internal working models" of self and others that establish styles of emotional communication that either buffer the individual in times of stress or contribute to maladaptive patterns of affect regulation and behaviour (Bretherton & Munholland, 1999).

Of particular interest in this context is recent theoretical and empirical work on the role of a secure attachment relationship in shaping the experience and expectancies of the infant (Fonagy, Gergely, et al., 2002). By entering into a synchronous affective communication with the infant, the caregiver provides an external support for the infant's emerging bioregulatory abilities and thus conveys resilience to stress-coping capacities throughout life. The experience of caregiver and child's micro-level matching of affective states and level of arousal during face-to-face interactions emerging around the second month of life provides the basis for children's social development, empathy, and moral internalization (Feldman, Weller, et al., 1999). Maternal gaze matching, facial expressions, vocalizations, and regulation of arousal states during face-to-face play provide critical environmental inputs during the sensitive period of maturation of the visual cortex. Furthermore, by synchronizing with infant arousal state, mothers entrain the infant's biological rhythms (Feldman, 2003; Lester, Hoffman, & Brazelton, 1985), providing a "resonance" (Trevarthen, 1993) of internal and external experience, self and other, brain and behaviour. Disorganized attachment, on the other hand, is viewed as a model for the effects of relational trauma on affect dysregulation, propensity for PTSD, and reduced stress management (Lyons-Ruth & Jacobvitz, 1999).

In the next section, we review the results of early intervention programmes with high-risk families. The focus is primarily on interventions initiated in the pre- or perinatal period that included random assignment to either the experimental intervention group or to a comparison group.

Early interventions to increase parental sensitivity and child attachment security

Attachment security is a resiliency factor across the lifespan. In a recent meta-analysis of 88 intervention studies, Bakermans-Kranenburg, van IJzendoorn, and Juffer (2003) found that, overall, interventions were effective in enhancing parental sensitivity and child attachment security. Interventions focused on parenting skills, social supports, or maternal well-being were significantly more successful. So were interventions that included both mother and father. Thus, the body of research on early interventions underscores the importance of devising clear-cut short-term behavioural interventions for a variety of at-risk populations. One caveat of this important study is that the time since the termination of treatment was not systematically evaluated.

It is thus impossible to determine whether the improvement observed immediately after treatment was short-lived or had a long-term impact on risk and resiliency to later psychopathology.

Early interventions to improve child behavioural adjustment. Thus far there have been at least three selective intervention studies with random assignment, prenatal initiation, and at least one-year duration focused on child behavioural adjustment. The first set of studies was based on an intervention model that included home visits, parent meetings, and medical care (Brooks-Gunn, Klebanov, Liaw, & Spiker, 1993; McCarton et al., 1997). It showed early effects at 2 and 3 years of age that attenuated by 5 years of age. A second intervention that also included home visits by nurses, parent meetings, and medical care showed less of an effect early on, at 4 years of age, which became significant at 5 and 6 years of age (Gutelius, Kirsch, MacDonald, Brooks, McErlean, 1977; Gutelius et al., 1972). Finally, a third set of studies that included home visits by nurses that began prenatally and continued for 30 months has shown a remarkable number of positive outcomes as late as at 15 years of age (Kitzman et al., 2000; Olds et al., 1997, 1998, 1999, 2002). For example, the Nurse Home Visitation Program developed by Olds and colleagues reduced the number of subsequent pregnancies, the use of welfare, child abuse and neglect, and criminal behaviour on the part of low-income unmarried mothers for up to 15 years after the birth of the first child. These studies by Olds and colleagues provide some of the strongest evidence to date that early intervention can make a difference in the lives of high-risk children. Although the mechanism by which these effects are achieved remains in doubt, Olds and colleagues have argued that one key element is the length of time between the first and second pregnancies by the mothers participating in the home visitation programme. On average, the time to the second pregnancy was more than 60 months in the experimental group that participated in the home visitation programme and less than 40 months in the comparison group. This suggests that there was a greater maternal investment in the children who were in the Nurse Home Visitation Program compared to the children born to the comparison mothers.

In a recent study based in Denver women visited by nurses had fewer subsequent pregnancies (29% vs 41%) and births (12% vs 19%); they delayed subsequent pregnancies for longer intervals; and during the second year after the birth of their first child, they worked more than did women in the control group (6.83 vs 5.65 months). Nurse-visited mother–child pairs interacted with one another more responsively than did those in the control group. At 6 months of age, nurse-visited infants were less likely to exhibit emotional vulnerability in response to fearful stimuli (16% vs 25). At 21 months, nurse-visited children born to women with low psychological resources were less likely to exhibit language delays (7% vs 18%); and at 24 months, they exhibited mental development superior to that of their control-group counterparts. Of interest for most outcomes on which either visitor produced significant effects, the paraprofessionals typically had effects that were about half the size of those produced by nurses.

Recently, centres for the diagnosis and treatment of infants and toddlers aged 0 to 3 have been established across the world, and a diagnostic system for classifying disorders of infancy (DC 0–3) has been validated (Guedeney et al., 2003; Keren, Feldman, & Tyano, 2001; Thomas & Guskin, 2001). Treatment methods such as dyadic psychotherapy or interaction guidance (McDonough, 2000) were found useful for the treatment of children and their parents. Furthermore, psychoanalytically informed psychotherapy for mothers and infants, which combines insight into the mother's representational world and observations of mother–infant interactions, has been found useful in increasing the infant's behaviour adaptation, promoting the mother–infant relationship and the maternal interactive behaviour and improving the mother's mental representation of the infant and the parenting process as measured by narrative instruments (Feldman & Keren, 2004).

In sum, data from selective early-intervention programmes indicate that the interval surrounding the birth of the infant is a critical period in the life of the infant that is likely to have enduring behavioural consequences. Thus far, the most compelling data suggest that these early intervention programmes reduce a variety of maladaptive outcomes such as early involvement in the juvenile justice system. Less clear is the impact of these early interventions on the later rates of depression and anxiety disorders as the children reach maturity. Nor is it clear what effect these early intervention programmes have on an individual's stress responsivity, susceptibility to drug abuse, or capacity as a parental caregiver. It is also worth noting that none of these selective early intervention programmes has monitored maternal preoccupations as a possible proximal predictor of individual differences in outcome.

Conclusions

Behavioural, neurobiological, and genetic and neurobiological studies in model mammalian systems have the potential to inform clinical practice, particularly early intervention programmes for high-risk expectant parents. "Good-enough" genes, combined with "good enough" parental care, are needed to ensure positive outcomes in childhood and beyond. Among these positive outcomes is a resiliency to subsequent adversities in life and the capacity to be a good-enough parent for the next generation. Consequently, it is possible that effective early-intervention programmes may have consequences for generations. Measures of "primary parental preoccupations" may be useful in future early-intervention programmes as an index of change within a key domain of functioning.

Close collaborations between clinicians and the designers of model intervention programmes have been long-standing. These collaborations are now beginning to include neuroimagers, developmental neurobiologists, and geneticists. Our capacity to study genes and the development of the brain has never been stronger. Future studies should permit the examination of how successful early intervention programmes influence brain development, problem-solving abilities, stress response, as well as vulnerability to later psychopathology.

NOTE

This research has been supported by grants from The Institute for Research on Unlimited Love (JFL and JES); the Harris Programs in Perinatal Mental Health (LCM); Israel Science Foundation (RF), the Bi-National Science Foundation (RF), and the Ricklis Foundation (RF), and grants from the National Institutes of Health MH49351, HD03008, MH30929, DA06025, DA00222 (LCM), and RR06022.

Commentary

David R. Shanks

In the space of a few years the scale and range of explanations we are able to offer for important aspects of human behaviour such as psychopathology, intelligence, the capacity for language, and—the subject of this chapter—maternal caregiving have grown beyond recognition. Only a short while ago it seemed a far-distant prospect that we might one day be in a position to sketch out the determinants of one of these kinds of behaviour at every level from genes to physiology to cognition to social interaction, yet this is no longer a prospect but a reality. It has been made possible by many converging events: the human genome project and our ability to identify and manipulate genes thought to be connected to specific behaviours, technologies for imaging the brain while it is directed towards a behaviour, improved lesion techniques and drug interventions, and an infinitely greater understanding of how neural events cause behaviour and instantiate mental processes. This chapter, by James Leckman, Ruth Feldman, James Swain, and Linda Mayes, elegantly illustrates how a story about maternal caregiving at all these levels is beginning to be sketched out, which, while of course incomplete and missing many critical details, seems to have surmounted most of the *conceptual* difficulties that confronted us only a brief time ago such as how even to begin to determine the influence of specific genes on behaviour.

With such dramatic changes taking place around us, it becomes important to reflect continually on the fundamental questions that have driven psychology since its earliest days. One of these is the nature/nurture debate, and in this commentary I consider how discoveries such as those described here might incline us to rethink long-held views. I will also consider one aspect of the emerging story about genes, brain, and behaviour where we are not at present fully exploiting the tools available to us: this is the important contribution that computational modelling can play in theory development.

Nature and nurture

To what extent are behaviours such a maternal caregiving programmed by genes or acquired though learning and interaction with the environment? As our understanding of genetics and psychological mechanisms has accelerated, it has become clear that it is misguided to expect an either/or answer to this question. Instead, genes and the environment contribute in a complex interactive way to probably every behaviour we might care to study. While genetic influence on a vast range of behaviours and cognition has been amply demonstrated in classic twin studies (Bouchard & McGue, 2003), environmental influences are equally easy to demonstrate. The striking studies of Francis and her colleagues (2003) on mouse behaviour show, for instance, that emotional behaviour (e.g., fearfulness) can be radically altered by environmental interventions, such as transferring a mouse's prenatal embryo early in its development. Perhaps even more compelling is the finding that such changes in behaviour can, once environmentally induced, be transmitted across generations. Thus a mouse that, given its genetic strain, might be expected not to lick or groom its offspring very much can be induced to do so by cross-fostering to an environment where it receives a high level of licking and grooming as a pup.

But it is not just that genes and environment make separable contributions to behaviour: they interact. In the realm of psychopathology, a study by Caspi and his colleagues (Caspi et al., 2003) shows this very clearly: in a large longitudinal sample in New Zealand, they found that childhood mistreatment was a risk factor for subsequent susceptibility to stressors. However, this effect depended on the individual's genetic make-up: the exact form of a gene on chromosome 17 influenced whether the children developed resilience. In a companion study, Caspi and colleagues (2002) found that childhood mistreatment interacted with a polymorphism of the gene that encodes the neurotransmitter-metabolizing enzyme monoamine oxidase A to influence antisocial behaviour. Both the gene and childhood mistreatment were risk factors for conduct disorder and convictions for violent behaviour, but the two together generated an even higher (i.e., greater than additive) risk.

What such examples show is that nature and nurture are the ends of a continuum and are representative of probably no significant types of behaviour. Instead, behaviours are determined by a constant gene–environment interaction. As noted in this chapter, the genes they describe as having a role in maternal behaviour do not operate independently of environment but confer a degree of susceptibility to a range of environmental influences. This raises the important—and in realms such as intelligence controversial—question of how specific the gene influences are. Is the gene on the X-chromosome claimed by Hamer, Hu, Magnuson, Hu, and Pattatucci (1993) to be related to intelligence[1] truly a gene for intelligence, or is it related to something far more general, such as speed of neural transmission? What is the appropriate characterization of the function of a gene such as *Dbh*? As the authors of this chapter observe, the reward systems of the brain seem to be related to aspects of maternal behaviour inasmuch as lesions of these pathways can lead to impairments in grooming and pup retrieval. But these reward pathways are involved in an enormous range of behaviours, and so the same will be true of the genes that contribute to their functioning. A significant challenge, then, is to be more precise about what each gene is doing at a functional level and how that function contributes to maternal behaviour. At present we are far from being able to do this. I comment below on the related issue of the cognitive processes mediating maternal behaviour.

There can be little doubt that non-genetic determinants of behaviour are very powerful. In addition to demonstrations of the intergenerational transmission of environmentally induced individual differences in maternal behaviour, Francis and her colleagues (Francis et al., 2003; see also Denenberg, Hoplight, & Mobraaten, 1998) have shown that such basic cognitive capacities as learning and memory can be powerfully modulated by environmental interventions. Studies involving mouse prenatal embryo transfer show that performance in the classic Morris water maze and in tests of discrimination learning is very different in genetically identical mice depending on their pre- and post-natal environment. These are not small differences: in the Francis et al. (2003) study, the time required to swim to a hidden platform in a water maze after 8 learning trials differed by a factor of 2:1 in mice developing in the "bad" versus "good" environments. Of course, we know that genetic influences on learning and memory (and many other cognitive processes and behaviours) can also be potent—we can genetically engineer clever mice, for instance (Tang et al., 1999)—but what is less clear is (a) the relative importance of normal variations in genetic makeup and environment on cognitive development; and (b) the specificity of genetic influences. Even Tang and colleagues' (1999) intelligent knock-in mice, with overexpression of the NMDA-receptor gene, show non-specific effects such as heightened sensitivity to pain (Wei et al., 2001).

In humans, the influence of genes on behaviour may have been overestimated in twin studies as these typically do not control for chorionicity. It must be borne in mind that the monozygotic (MZ)–dizygotic (DZ) difference found on virtually all behavioural measures is evidence for a genetic contribution only if it can be convincingly argued that the environment is as similar for a pair of DZ twins as it is for a pair of MZ twins. Certainly, this will commonly be the case with respect to important factors such as the attachment-related behaviours and the amount of intellectual stimulation the parents provide: regardless of whether twins are MZ or DZ, their interactions with their parents will be highly similar.

Thus it is unlikely that differences in the post-natal environment of MZ and DZ twins can explain the fact that MZ twins tend to be more similar. But what about the pre-natal environment? One important question is whether or not the twins shared a chorion in the womb. The chorion is part of the placenta and constitutes an important component of the pre-natal environment. A shared chorion implies a shared blood supply and a higher probability of infections passing between the twins. Dizygotic twins are always dichorionic: each twin has his or her own chorion. However, about 60% of MZ twins are monochorionic, sharing a single chorion. This means that on average the pre-natal environment is more similar for MZ than for DZ twins. Is it possible that the greater similarity of MZ compared to DZ twins in measures of behaviour is due to this? The critical test comes from comparisons of dichorionic MZ and DZ twins. Such twins have roughly comparable pre-natal environments, so if the MZ twins still show higher concordance than the DZ twins, that would bolster the case for a genetic contribution. On the other hand, if such twins are equally similar, that would suggest that the standard MZ–DZ difference is largely due to the fact that some of the MZ twins share a chorion, which makes them especially similar.

Unfortunately, chorionicity is rarely measured in twin studies, and researchers tend to lump together mono- and dichorionic MZ twins. A very small number of studies (e.g., Jacobs et al., 2001; Wichers et al.,

2002) have measured concordance rates as a function of both zygosity and chorionicity and have observed a greater rate in dichorionic MZ than DZ twins (consistent with a genetic contribution), but it is far too early to say whether this pattern holds across all forms of behaviour.

Nevertheless, work such as that described in this chapter, with its demonstration both of (a) the many levels of analysis (genes, physiology, neurochemistry, cognition) at which behavioural questions can be addressed and of (b) gene–environment interactions, points to the sort of position on nature/nurture persuasively elaborated by Elman and co-authors in their book *Rethinking Innateness* (1996). The role of genes in behaviour is the result of a complex set of interactions at many levels. Genes do not directly code for behaviours or particular forms of representation. In no sense is a given gene or even set of genes a necessary and sufficient condition for having high intelligence or a particular type of maternal nurturing. Rather, genes, in response to environmental events, constrain the architecture of the brain (e.g., the types of cells that develop), their connectivity, and the timing of developmental events in the brain and hence stages of mental development. No "modules" for specific genetically pre-programmed behaviours exist. This view on nature/nurture allows for the influence of genetic makeup on the phenotype while also accommodating evidence on the plasticity of the brain and the cases described above of gene–environment interactions.

Studies have shown extraordinary plasticity in the developing brain and that cortex is close to being equipotential in the sense that any area of cortex can, with appropriate input, develop adequate computational sensitivity to that input. Groundbreaking studies by Sur and his colleagues (see Sur & Leamey, 2001) involve rewiring of auditory and visual pathways in ferrets. Sur induced retinal projections to connect to auditory cortex and found that this area became functionally like visual cortex—that is to say, it developed a spatial map of the visual world. This extraordinary work suggests very strongly that even large-scale brain structures are not genetically determined to evolve a given function. Rather, genetically coded architectural and developmental constraints interact with input to fix function.

Cognitive modelling

In some aspects of behaviour such as language acquisition and reading, we can not only say a great deal about genes, neurochemistry, social/environmental influences (e.g., the effects of deprivation), and so on, but also about the functional and computational properties of the neural networks that directly control behaviour. This can only be achieved by bringing an additional community of researchers into the programme: namely, computational modellers. This type of modelling takes as its goal the mechanistic explanation of how it is that a particular piece of brain hardware, wired up as it is and receiving the inputs that it does, can generate the relevant output. For instance, in a real language problem, computational modellers (e.g., Seidenberg & McClelland, 1989) have attempted to understand how a piece of neural machinery can take as its input from the visual system a description of marks on a page (that is to say, the letters that make up a word, such as b—a—b—y) and turn these into a different form (the spoken word "baby"). At first glance this capacity seems very mysterious: how could a network of computing elements (neurons) that simply transmit activation among themselves achieve such a complex task as reading written words? The answer, of course, has been one of the great achievements of modern science, the field of neural computation. The emergence of intelligent structured behaviour from simple computing elements, now well understood thanks to the work of Hopfield, McClelland, Rumelhart, Hebb, Hinton, and many others (Hebb, 1949; Hopfield & Tank, 1985; McClelland & Rumelhart, 1986; Rumelhart & McClelland, 1986), provides the key missing piece in the jigsaw relating molecular events to behaviour (see Figure 3.1). Without this piece, we can never claim to have a full understanding of the causes of behaviour, no matter how detailed our knowledge of genes or neurotransmitters.

In the case of maternal behaviour, the challenge of providing a description of the underlying computational or cognitive characterization of the relevant brain systems such as the paraventricular nucleus (PVN) of the hypothalamus is formidable. The first problem is that we don't as yet really know, even in global terms, what it is that systems such as this are doing. We may know that they are involved in the regulation of certain behaviours, but, as mentioned above with respect to gene function, it is very difficult to go beyond this. We know, for example, that the oxytocin pathways are involved in maternal behaviour. Does this mean that oxytocin turns up the attentional "gain" on relevant stimuli such as the sight or smell of offspring? A function such as this could readily be instantiated computationally. But we also know that oxytocin relates to mood and anxiety, so its function must be

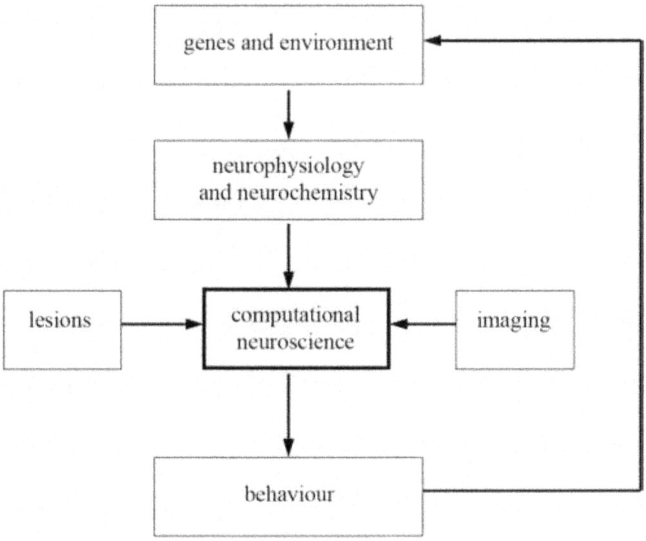

Figure 3.1. At the centre of the complex pattern of causal processes mediating between genes/environment and behaviour lies computational neuroscience. This is the study of brain structures with distinct input and output pathways that instantiate some computational process. Although their function can be elucidated by imaging and lesion techniques, only formal modelling can yield a full characterization of their contributions to behaviour.

broader than this. A major challenge to researchers studying maternal behaviour will be to try to increase the specificity of the functions they attribute to different brain systems so as to allow those functions to be computationally implemented.

NOTE

1. The validity of this claim has been disputed (Rice, Anderson, Risch, & Ebers, 1999).

CHAPTER FOUR

Exploring the neurobiology of attachment

Lane Strathearn

The mother–infant relationship has been characterized as one of the most important relationships affecting the health and development of the human species (Schore, 2001). When that relationship involves abuse or neglect, it is associated with a diverse range of adverse neurodevelopmental outcomes in the offspring (Cahill, Kaminer, & Johnson, 1999), including long-term cognitive and academic delays (Singer & Ryff, 1999; Strathearn, Gray, O'Callaghan, & Wood, 2001), psychiatric illness (Johnson, Cohen, Brown, Smailes, & Bernstein, 1999; Widom, 1999), social impairment, and delinquency (Dubowitz, 1999).

Yet when this relationship is characterized by secure attachment between infants and their primary caregivers, and in the absence of other mitigating factors, these infants go on to manifest higher levels of self-esteem and self-reliance and show more effective self-regulation of impulses and emotions from preschool through to adolescence. They are better able to form close relationships, and this evolves into an enhanced capacity for intimacy and self-disclosure in adulthood (Sroufe, 1983; Sroufe, Carlson, & Shulman, 1993). In contrast, insecure disorganized patterns of attachment, most often seen in cases of maltreatment or emotional unavailability, are associated with a higher risk for anxiety disorders, aggression, conduct disorder, and other forms of psychopathology (Carlson, 1998; Sroufe, 1997; Warren, Huston, Egeland, & Sroufe, 1997).

So, what is it about this early relationship that can have such a profound influence on subsequent behaviour and development?

The purposes of this chapter are:

1. to summarize the evidence from animal research linking maternal care and infant development, as well as how infant cues may enhance maternal behaviour;
2. to explore possible neuroendocrine correlates underlying the development of attachment behaviour;
3. to discuss the role of functional neuroimaging in testing these hypotheses in human populations.

Maternal care and infant development

The central role of maternal behaviour in development has been most clearly demonstrated in rodent studies, which provide a neuroendocrine model of maternal behaviour. In order to survive, newborn rodents are totally dependent on the initiation of a specific set of maternal behaviours, such as nest repair, pup retrieval, licking, grooming, and "arched-back nursing" (Leckman & Herman, 2002). These behaviours are a response to a variety of sensory stimuli emitted from the rodent pup, including vocalization, pup odours, and somatosensory cues from nippling. Overall, these maternal responses represent a pattern of responsive, contingent behaviours attuned to the needs of the offspring (Figure 4.1 [A]).

From these studies, maternal behaviour has been shown to influence infant neural development in three specific areas: stress reactivity, cognition, and maternal behaviour in female offspring.

• *Stress reactivity*

One critical observation has been that differences in maternal behaviour—both naturally observed and experimentally induced—correlate with altered stress reactivity and behaviour in the offspring (Champagne & Meaney, 2001; Francis, Caldji, Champagne, Plotsky, & Meaney, 1999; Francis & Meaney, 1999). For example, in adulthood, rodent pups that had received higher levels of licking, grooming, and arched-back nursing in infancy showed reduced levels of stress hormones corticotropin (or ACTH) and corticosterone in response to restraint stress.

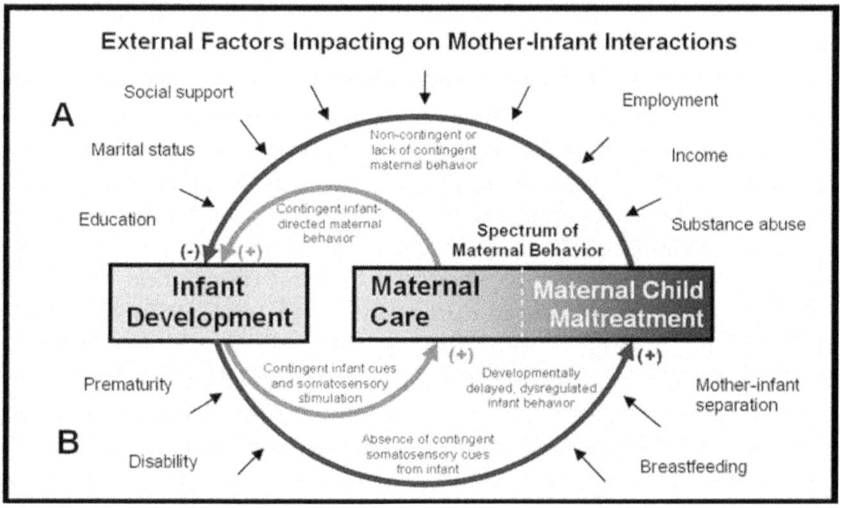

Figure 4.1: Model of interdependent relationships between maternal behaviour and infant development

There were also decreased levels of corticotropin-releasing factor (CRF) messenger RNA (mRNA) in the brain's hypothalamus and central nucleus of the amygdala, indicating reduced production of this stress-hormone-releasing factor. In addition, they showed increased levels of the protective glucocorticoid receptor mRNA in the hippocampus, which facilitates feedback inhibition of CRF. The magnitude of these differences was significantly correlated with the frequency of maternal licking and grooming ($r = -0.61$) and arched-back nursing ($r = -0.64$) during the first 10 days of life (Liu et al., 1997). A more recent study has identified epigenetic mechanisms by which these long-lasting changes may occur, with maternal care altering DNA methylation and histone acetylation patterns, which result in increased glucocorticoid receptor gene expression (Weaver et al., 2004). Thus, differences in early patterns of maternal care appear to alter the DNA structure and subsequent gene expression, which affects the brain's ability to modify the physiological stress response.

Animals who received higher levels of maternal care also exhibit behavioural differences in adulthood, including decreased startle response and increased open field exploration, consistent with reduced levels of anxiety and fearfulness (Caldji et al., 1998). Cross-fostering studies, including a study using embryo transfer technique (Francis, Szegda, Campbell, Martin, & Insel, 2003), have convincingly demonstrated that maternal behaviour is a critical mode of transmission, rather than genetic inheritance alone (Francis, Diorio, Liu, & Meaney, 1999; Liu, Diorio, Day, Francis, & Meaney, 2000).

In parallel to these findings, prolonged periods of maternal separation, resulting in reduced levels of responsive caregiving, significantly increase the magnitude of neuroendocrine and behavioural responses to stress (Francis, Caldji, et al., 1999). Comparable findings have been reported in rhesus monkeys exposed to varying degrees of maternal deprivation (Suomi, 1997). The behavioural profiles of these monkeys were remarkably similar to Bowlby's original description of secure versus anxious attachment in human infants (Suomi, 1995). In human populations, children exposed to abuse also manifest higher levels of cortisol and catecholamine stress hormones (De Bellis et al., 1999), and infant attachment security correlates with cortisol reactivity to stress (Gunnar, Brodersen, Nachmias, Buss, & Rigatuso, 1996).

- *Cognition*

In rat models, these highly contingent maternal behaviours are also strongly linked with infant cognitive development (Liu et al., 2000; Weaver, Grant, & Meaney, 2002). Mechanisms may include increases in the formation of new synaptic connections within the hippocampus (Liu et al., 2000), and reduced cell loss through apoptosis (Weaver, Grant, & Meaney, 2002). Prolonged maternal separation, in contrast, has a negative effect in both rodent and primate studies (Dettling, Feldon, & Pryce, 2002; Huot, Plotsky, Lenox, & McNamara, 2002).

My previous longitudinal human research examined cognitive outcomes in extremely premature infants who were exposed to abuse or neglect. These data revealed that neglected infants experienced a progressive decline in cognitive functioning over the first 4 years of life, which was also associated with significantly reduced head circumference *z*-scores at 2 and 4 years (Singer & Ryff, 1999). These results have since been replicated in a cohort of over 7,000 mother–infant dyads, followed over 14 years (Strathearn et al., 2002).

- *Maternal behaviour in the offspring*

Differences in maternal behaviour have also been shown to influence patterns of maternal behaviour in the female offspring, mediated via differences in central oxytocin and oestrogen receptor expression (Champagne, Weaver, Diorio, Sharma, & Meaney, 2003; Francis, Champagne, & Meaney, 2000; Lovic, Gonzalez, & Fleming, 2001; Pedersen

& Boccia, 2002). An increased level of licking and grooming in rats is associated with enhanced oxytocin receptor expression in brain areas functionally related to maternal behaviour (Champagne, Diorio, Sharma, & Meaney, 2001), including the bed nucleus of the stria terminalis and the central nucleus of the amygdala in females (Francis, Young, Meaney, & Insel, 2002). Naturally occurring variations in maternal behaviour are associated with similar differences in oxytocin receptor levels in the female offspring (Francis, Champagne, & Meaney, 2000). With oxytocin known to be important in the initiation of maternal behaviour in several mammalian species, these studies strongly suggest a link between rearing experience, oxytocin receptor expression, and subsequent maternal care in adulthood (Pedersen & Boccia, 2002).

Infant cues and maternal behaviour

While maternal behaviours may act to promote infant development, infant cues (such as suckling, auditory, and visual stimuli) may also stimulate maternal care, even modifying pre-existing behaviour patterns (Rosenblatt, 1994; Stern, 1997b). Nursing and/or somatosensory stimulation of rat dams are thought to promote maternal care via increased expression of oxytocin receptors in specific brain areas (Francis, Champagne, & Meaney, 2000), whereas long periods of mother–infant separation inhibit maternal behaviour (Boccia & Pedersen, 2001). Similarly, in human mothers breastfeeding stimulates oxytocin release, which is associated with reduced levels of maternal anxiety, an attenuated physiological stress response (Chiodera & Coiro, 1987; Legros, Chiodera, & Geenen, 1988), and more attuned patterns of maternal behaviour (Champagne & Meaney, 2001; Uvnas-Moberg, 1998; Uvnas-Moberg & Eriksson, 1996). In contrast, prolonged mother–infant separation has been associated with reduced maternal sensitivity and more negative patterns of mothering throughout the first 3 years of life (NICHD Early Child Care Research Network, 1999) (Figure 4.1 [B]).

Thus, it is proposed that variation in human maternal behaviour, ranging from contingent infant care to abuse or neglect, may contribute to differences in infant development. In a reciprocal fashion, infant cues and somatosensory stimulation received by the mother may actually enhance maternal care (see Figure 4.1). Where stimuli are reduced (due to mother–infant separation, maternal depression, or substance abuse, for example) or dysregulated (e.g., in cases of extreme prematurity, illness, or birth defects), there may be an increased risk of disturbed attachment or maltreatment (Singer & Ryff, 1999; Weinfield, Sroufe, & Egeland, 2000). Differences in temperament as well as socio-economic and environmental factors may also impact on the integrity of this mother–infant relationship.

Attachment theory

After first studying associations between maternal deprivation and juvenile delinquency, John Bowlby formulated his attachment theory, postulating a universal human need to form close affectional bonds, primarily between mother and infant (Bowlby, 1969; Fonagy, 2001). He strongly argued, from an evolutionary perspective, that attachment was an innate biological system promoting proximity-seeking between an infant and a specific attachment figure, in order to increase the likelihood of survival to a reproductive age. As a result of this powerful biological instinct, he hypothesized that all human infants become attached to their caregiver—even if the care is harsh or neglectful—but that these children manifest different patterns of attachment "security". Infants of caregivers who are available, responsive, and sensitive to their emotional and physical needs tend to manifest patterns of "secure attachment". However, if the care provided is chaotic, unpredictable, rejecting, or neglectful, or where the caregiver consistently provides non-contingent responses to the child, an anxious, insecure, or disorganized pattern of attachment evolves.

While acknowledging that these "internal working models" develop in response to ongoing experience, Bowlby considered the foundation of attachment to be established in early childhood. The initial pattern of attachment security was seen as a developmental pathway of major significance throughout the child's life course, with longitudinal research verifying many of these initial hypotheses (van IJzendoorn, 1995).

Over the past decade, a diverse spectrum of research has begun to explore the neural basis of attachment—at molecular, cellular, and behavioural levels (Insel & Young, 2001). This research, using research techniques as diverse as molecular genetic probes and fMRI, has uncovered many parallels between Bowlby's original thesis and the biological systems that may underlie attachment and stress reactivity. Understanding the neurobiology of attachment may help us to better formulate and address the pervasive problem of child abuse and neglect.

Exploring the neurobiology of adult attachment patterns

Since Bowlby first published his seminal work on attachment theory, numerous research methods have been developed to systematically classify attachment styles, as observed in infancy through to adulthood. The two most accepted and empirically tested instruments are the Strange Situation Procedure in infancy (Ainsworth & Bell, 1970) and the Adult Attachment Interview (AAI) (George, Kaplan, & Main, 1996). The AAI is a semi-structured interview designed to identify differences in "state of mind with regard to overall attachment history" by examining the subject's ability to describe attachment-related memories while simultaneously maintaining a coherent, cooperative discourse (Main, 1997). From an analysis of the transcribed discourse, three basic attachment patterns—summarized as "secure", "dismissing", and "preoccupied"—emerge. Numerous longitudinal studies have demonstrated the unique capacity of a caregiver's AAI to predict infant attachment patterns, although the transmission mechanisms are still unclear (van IJzendoorn, 1995). Understanding the neurobiological differences between these adult attachment patterns may help us better understand the mechanisms behind its intergenerational transmission.

Crittenden has suggested that these basic attachment patterns may, in fact, represent differences in how the brain processes sensory information (Crittenden, 2002). She proposed that sensory stimulation is transformed into one of two basic forms of information: temporally ordered "cognitive" information and intensity-based arousal or "affective" information. The first is believed to be the predominant mechanism in "dismissing" attachment organization, whereas the second is most predominant in "preoccupied" attachment. "Secure" organization is thought to be a balanced integration of both sources of information. For example, "dismissing" adults tend to dismiss their own feelings, intentions, and perspectives and rely more upon rules and learned temporal relations in predicting future reward. These individuals behave as if following the rule: "Do the right thing—from the perspective of other people, without regard to your own feelings or desires" (Crittenden, 2004). "Preoccupied" adults, in contrast, organize their behaviour around affective information, such as fear, anger, or desire for comfort. They tend to be preoccupied by their own feelings and perspectives while omitting or distorting cognitive or temporally ordered information. They function as if under the dictum: "Stay true to your feelings, and do not delay, negotiate or compromise" (Crittenden,

2004). Adults with "secure" or balanced patterns of attachment are able to integrate temporally ordered information regarding causal effect as well as more affect-based information, such as emotional states and imaged memory, in order to form close relationships, make accurate decisions, and predict future reward.

The organization of attachment may also involve the differential development of specific memory systems within the brain, such as procedural and semantic memory (processing temporally ordered or cognitive information), imaged memory (processing more affect based information), and episodic and working memory systems (which integrate cognitive and affective information), each of which may be represented in particular brain regions (Crittenden, 2004).

Two neuroendocrine systems that may be related to these forms of information processing are the dopaminergic and oxytocinergic systems, the development of which appears to be influenced by early life experience, such as variations in maternal behaviour (Champagne et al., 2004; Francis, Young, et al., 2002; Meaney, Brake, & Gratton, 2002; Pruessner, Champagne, Meaney, & Dagher, 2004). The dopaminergic system is involved in reinforcement stimulus–reward learning and in decision making based on future predicted reward (McClure, Daw, & Montague, 2003). The oxytocinergic system is important in the formation of social and spatial memories, affiliative behaviour, and emotion regulation (Ferguson, Young, & Insel, 2002).

Recent data have indicated an interactive effect between the mesocorticolimbic dopamine system, the oxytocinergic system, and the physiological stress system (Insel, 2003; Meaney, Brake, & Gratton, 2002). Oxytocin receptor blockade results in an exaggerated ACTH and corticosterone stress hormone response in rats (Neumann, Torner, & Wigger, 2000), and similar results are seen in oxytocin-deficient knock-out mice (Amico, Mantella, & Vollmer, 2002). The mesocortical dopamine system is likewise thought to have a stress inhibitory effect via the medial prefrontal cortex (Charmandari, Kino, Souvatzoglou, & Chrousos, 2003). Thus, one primary role of these neuroendocrine systems may be to modulate human stress responses and thus facilitate optimal social bonding and attachment through two different but complimentary mechanisms.

Oxytocinergic system

The neuropeptide hormone, oxytocin, is synthesized in the paraventricular nucleus of the hypothalamus and has projections to the posterior pituitary gland, where it is released into the blood stream. This accounts for its well-described peripheral actions, including uterine contraction at childbirth and milk ejection during lactation. However, over more recent years central actions relating to maternal behaviour have also been demonstrated. In several mammalian species, oxytocin has been shown to facilitate physical proximity and nurturant care between the mother and infant (Insel & Young, 2001). For example, in virgin rats, which normally exhibit aversive behaviour towards rat pups, a brain injection of oxytocin stimulates a broad range of maternal behaviours, whereas an oxytocin antagonist blocks these effects. In the amygdala, oxytocin is critical for the formation of social memories and also has an anxiolytic effect, which helps to promote social bonding (Ferguson, Aldag, Insel, & Young, 2001). It is an important factor in the development of long-term spatial memories in the hippocampus (Tomizawa et al., 2003). Oxytocin receptors are enriched in brain areas that are significant in the manifestation of social and maternal behaviour, such as the bed nucleus of the stria terminalis, hypothalamic paraventricular nucleus, central nucleus of the amygdala, ventral tegmental area, and lateral septum (Francis, Champagne, & Meaney, 2000) (see Plate 4A). It is hypothesized that oxytocin production in the human maternal brain may be similarly associated with attachment patterns in adulthood, being relatively deficient in "dismissing" attachment patterns.

Dopaminergic system

Dopaminergic neurons respond to temporally ordered prediction errors signals, facilitating stimulus–reward learning in the brain (Montague, Hyman, & Cohen, 2004). Positive prediction errors (i.e., unanticipated rewarding events) result in an increase in the firing rate of dopaminergic neurons, whereas negative prediction errors (i.e., failure to receive an anticipated reward) result in a marked decrease in the firing rate (Schultz, 1998). These signals generally originate in the ventral tegmental area of the midbrain and project to a variety of regions throughout the brain, including the nucleus accumbens, dorsal striatum, prefrontal cortex, and the anterior cingulate cortex (Montague, Hyman, & Cohen, 2004).

Repeated episodes of early maternal separation in rats result in altered dopamine functioning in infancy and adulthood (Meaney, Brake, & Gratton, 2002), whereas elevated levels of pup licking/grooming is associated with increased dopamine receptor expression and enhanced dopamine production in the mothers (Champagne et al., 2004). Altered activity of the dopaminergic system has been associated with a wide range of human diseases and psychopathology, including drug addiction, attention-deficit hyperactivity disorder, obesity, compulsive gambling, and several personality traits (Comings & Blum, 2000; Montague, Hyman, & Cohen, 2004), all of which may also be associated with adverse early life events. A recent PET study showed that dopamine production in the human brain was associated with reduced self-reported maternal care in childhood (Pruessner et al., 2004). It is hypothesized that abnormal development of the dopaminergic system may also be associated with differing patterns of adult attachment, with a relative deficit seen in "preoccupied" patterns and an excess in "dismissing" types.

Recent data from female prairie vole experiments have demonstrated that, in the nucleus accumbens, both dopamine and oxytocin are critical for the formation of social attachment (Liu & Wang, 2003). It is hypothesized that a balanced and integrated response from both the oxytocinergic and the dopaminergic brain systems is required for the formation of optimal attachment relationships in humans. While this hypothesis is difficult to test directly in human subjects, functional neuroimaging techniques are now permitting us to "eavesdrop" on the brain and observe patterns of brain activation in response to specific social and maternal cues. Activation of brain regions rich in oxytocin and/or dopamine receptors may suggest involvement of these neurotransmitter systems in responding to particular attachment cues (Bartels & Zeki, 2004).

Attachment and the brain: functional MRI research

Functional MRI (fMRI) is a brain imaging technique that involves the presentation of a series of sensory stimuli to the subject being scanned, and then determining which brain regions are preferentially activated in response to that stimulus type. Regions of brain activation are accompanied by changes in blood flow, with differences in oxygenated versus deoxygenated haemoglobin in a particular region altering the magnetic field signal detected by the scanner. These signals are transformed statistically into activation maps within the brain, specifying regions of probable brain activity.

In animal models of maternal behaviour, mother–infant attachment is initially stimulated by specific sensory cues exchanged between the mother and infant. For example, in rat dams and sheep, olfactory learning is important (Insel & Young, 2001), with oxytocin playing a role in facilitating the transition from avoidance to approach. Pup somatosensory stimulation of rat dams appears to stimulate the production of dopamine, which leads to pup licking and grooming behaviour (Champagne et al., 2004). However, in human mothers, visual and auditory cues appear to play a more central role. Over the past few years, studies using fMRI have begun to explore maternal brain responses to auditory and visual infant cues, with distinctive patterns of brain activation identified.

In examining brain responses of mothers to their own children's facial expressions (compared to other familiar children's faces), Bartels and Zeki (2004) identified regions of activation mapping closely onto areas rich in oxytocin receptors (Loup, Tribollet, Dubois-Dauphin, & Dreifuss, 1991). Some regions of activation, such as the thalamus, substantia nigra, and retrorubal fields, paralleled those activated when adults saw pictures of their romantic partner. However, the periaqueductal grey (PAG), which has been strongly associated with maternal behaviour in animal studies, was uniquely activated by mothers responding to their own children. Other important regions of activation included the lateral orbitofrontal cortex, which is involved in the processing of pleasant visual, tactile, and olfactory stimuli; the middle insula, a subdivision involved in visceral sensations and the "gut feelings" of emotions; and the ventral anterior cingulate, which is also associated with processing social or emotive stimuli. Overall, the study showed that when mothers passively viewed images of their own children, various brain regions rich in oxytocin receptors and known to process positive affective stimuli were activated. More cognitive regions dealing with theory of mind and moral judgement appeared to be inhibited or deactivated in this study.

However, in a similar study of mothers viewing pictures of their children's faces, which also included a cognitive task (pressing a button to indicate face identity) (Leibenluft, Gobbini, Harrison, & Haxby, 2004), the deactivated regions from the previous study (Bartels & Zeki, 2004) now showed significant activity. These regions included the anterior paracingulate, posterior cingulate, and superior temporal sulcus.

Similar brain areas were also activated when mothers heard infant cries compared to a control noise (Lorberbaum et al., 2002), including the right medial prefrontal and orbitofrontal cortices, anterior cingulate, and periaqueductal grey. Other activated areas associated with maternal behaviour in animal models included the ventral tegmental area, hypothalamus, and bed nucleus of the stria terminalis. Some regions of dopaminergic innervation were also strongly activated, including the dorsal striatum and the nucleus accumbens, suggesting that infant cries may also activate the dopaminergic system.

Using functional MRI study to study differences in attachment

Our own work in this area originated with a pilot study of healthy mother–infant dyads, using fMRI to examine maternal brain regions activated in response to infant facial cues of varying affect (smiling, neutral, and crying) and to explore the possible roles of oxytocin in facilitating this interaction (Strathearn & McClure, 2002). A total of 8 healthy right-handed mothers, without a history of psychiatric impairment or child maltreatment, were enrolled, along with their infants, aged between 3 and 8 months. Serum oxytocin levels were obtained sequentially from the mothers during a standardized period of mother–infant interaction, during which the infants' facial expressions were videotaped. Functional MRI was then used to measure maternal brain activity in response to the facial images of their own infant, compared with familiar and unknown infant facial images (Plate 4B).

In comparing responses to the mothers' own infants versus familiar but unknown infant faces, a unique pattern of neural activation was evident, with areas of activation, including brain reward areas with dopaminergic projections (ventral striatum, thalamus, and nucleus accumbens), areas containing oxytocin projections (amygdala, bed nucleus of the stria terminalis and hippocampus), the fusiform face area (involved in face processing), and areas involved in episodic memory processing (bilateral hippocampi) (all $p < .005$, uncorrected) (Plate 4C). A positive but non-significant trend was seen in serum oxytocin concentration during mother–infant interaction (Figure 4.2), suggesting a possible correlation between brain activation and peripheral hormone production.

One aspect that has not been addressed in any prior research is how these patterns of brain activation may differ between attachment groups. Do mothers with insecure patterns of attachment respond in a different way to their infant cues? Are neglecting mothers unresponsive to these cues, or do they fail to receive reward signals in the brain? Our current longitudinal research aims to explore some of these questions by first assessing maternal attachment patterns during pregnancy using the Adult Attachment Interview. We are then exploring how

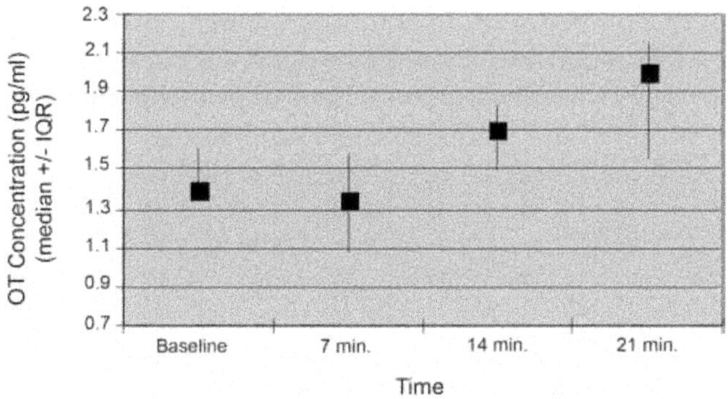

Figure 4.2: Changes in peripheral oxytocin (OT) concentration with mother–infant interaction.

these differing patterns are related to a variety of neuroendocrine parameters, including fMRI responses to infant facial cues and endocrine responses to an infant-related stressor (measuring peripheral oxytocin, cortisol, and catecholamines). The study is also examining longitudinally how these attachment patterns are associated with infant behaviour, using a modified still-face procedure at 6 months post-delivery (Koós & Gergely, 2001) (Plate 4D), and the Strange Situation procedure to determine 12-month-old infants' attachment patterns (Ainsworth & Bell, 1970). It is hypothesized that different attachment styles will be distinguishable by patterns of brain activation, as well as endocrine response, to infant-related cues.

Conclusion

Each year in the United States over 900,000 children become victims of abuse or neglect, with the biological mother identified as a perpetrator in two-thirds of these cases (U.S. Department of Health and Human Services, Administration on Children Youth and Families, 2003). Abuse and neglect perpetrated by a child's biological mother represents a fundamental breakdown in this important attachment relationship, resulting in serious long-term consequences for the offspring. Accumulating evidence from basic, clinical, and epidemiological research indicates that the mother–infant relationship may be a critical target in optimizing developmental outcomes and preventing child maltreatment (Meaney, 2001; Olds et al., 1997; Sanchez, Ladd, & Plotsky, 2001).

It is hoped that by better understanding the neurobiological processes underlying this reciprocal attachment relationship, we may be able to better understand—and ultimately help to prevent—child abuse and neglect.

NOTE

I would like to acknowledge the support of the National Institute of Child Health and Human Development (K23 HD043097), the Baylor CHRC: Pediatrics Mentored Research Program (K12 HD41648), and the South Central MIRECC

Commentary

Arietta Slade

The search for physiological correlates of psychological experience is one that has existed—at least in the imagination of scientists and scholars—for well over a century. Freud himself suggested that the topographical model he used to describe the psychic apparatus would one day find its analogue and indeed roots in actual brain structures. He opened one of his earliest papers on psychoanalysis, "Project for a Scientific Psychology" (Freud, 1950 [1895]), with a bold ambition for the new science of psychoanalysis:

> The intention is to furnish a psychology that shall be a natural science: that is, to represent psychical processes as quantitatively determinate states of specifiable material particles, thus making those processes *perspicuous and free from contradiction*. [p. 295; italics added]

While he was later to abandon this notion of specificity, he nevertheless clearly believed throughout his career that there were brain analogues for psychological phenomena.

The day Freud envisioned is indeed dawning. Over the past decade, psychoanalytic scholars have joined with basic scientists to forge an increasingly sophisticated and convincing picture of potential links between particular kinds of brain activity and psychological processes (chapters 3 and 5, this volume; Mayes, Swain, & Leckman, 2005). This is not to say that such links are clear and easily specified; if anything, the work of these scholars illuminates the extraordinary complexity inherent in all brain–behaviour relationships.

In this chapter, Lane Strathearn provides a clear example of the kinds of complex dialogues that are beginning to take place between neuroscientists and social scientists. He begins with a review of animal studies documenting a relationship between behaviour and neural development in offspring and mothers; in particular, he highlights the effect of maternal behaviour on infant neural development, as well as the reciprocal impact of infant behaviour on neural activity in the mother. The quality of maternal care is crucially related to the development of stress reactivity, cognition, and caregiving behaviours in her offspring, while nursing and other careseeking behaviours in infants trigger the release of oxytocin, a neuropeptide associated with "reduced levels of maternal anxiety, an attenuated physiological stress response, and more attuned patterns of maternal behaviour". These findings provide empirical validation for dynamic relationships long appreciated by clinicians: (a) the relationship between a mother's caregiving capacity and a range of crucial developments in her child, as well as (b) the reciprocal impact of an infant upon his caregiver's availability and readiness to nurture.

Strathearn then extends this research to the study of human attachment, hypothesizing that the relationship between maternal care and neural activity is of particular importance in the development of an individual's characteristic way of regulating fear, stress, and proximity seeking—*that is, in the development of internal working models of attachment.* Attachment patterns, he proposes, are behavioural and psychological manifestations of the shaping of the neuroendocrine systems that are involved in affiliation and reward systems. Such shaping is the direct result of early maternal care. In other words, both child and adult attachment classifications reflect differences in underlying brain chemistry, differences that emerge as a function of early caregiving experience.

Until recently, it would have been very difficult to test such hypotheses in humans. However, thanks to developments in the use of fMRI, the means may now exist to explore hypothesized relationships between attachment organization and the functioning of neuroendocrine systems and to examine the neural bases for the intergenerational transmission of attachment. Over the past five years, researchers have used neuroimaging studies to study attachment processes by tracking the activation of particular areas of a mother's brain when she is presented with visual or auditory images of her child (see chapter 3, this volume; see also Mayes, Swain, & Leckman, 2005, for reviews). What they have discovered is that both reward and affiliation centres in the brain "light up" in distinct ways when mothers are hearing or seeing their own babies. These patterns of brain activation are quite different when mothers are exposed to the cries or faces of unfamiliar infants; there are also differences between mothers and fathers in their responses to these same stimuli. Researchers also report that these patterns of activation change over the course of the early mother–child relationship; thus, the *development* of the relationship is reflected at a neural level. Finally, early anecdotal evidence suggests that there may be individual differences in these patterns of neural activation. These findings led Strathearn to propose that individual differences in adult attachment organization will be linked to differences in patterns of brain activation in mothers. Such patterns of brain activation would then presumably be tied to particular patterns of neural system development in babies.

The research Strathearn proposes would be the first to examine the neural bases of attachment processes, and thus promises to greatly illuminate our understanding of some of the biological foundations of parental love and attachment. In the discussion that follows, I begin by considering the experiential correlates of the patterns of brain activation Strathearn describes. What are the *feelings* that accompany particular patterns of brain activation? I then turn to methodology, and particularly the question of how to best measure attachment phenomena in his proposed study. In particular, I suggest that assessing reflective functioning *in addition* to attachment classification will greatly broaden the measurement of attachment processes. This measure may in fact be better suited to assessing the experiential correlates of the neural activity Strathearn is measuring. I then extend the question of individual differences to consider some of the ways that neuroimaging techniques may be used to assess change in parenting interventions. Finally, I close with a cautionary note about the interpretation and generalizability of neuroimaging studies.

An ineffable combination

When I first read this chapter, I immediately began wondering what the experiential correlates of the patterns of neural activation Strathearn described might be. What were mothers *feeling* when they saw the pictures of their babies or heard their babies' cries? Strathearn tells us that the reward, affiliation, and protection/stress centres of their brains "light up" in unison when normal mothers in the magnet see or hear their very young babies. I wondered: is this parental love? The complex interaction of pleasure, affiliation, and protection made enormous sense to me, for there is a certain something that many parents feel for their children, an *ineffable combination* of great pleasure, longing for closeness, desire for nurture, and an instinct to protect that is so difficult to put into words, but that we know when we see or hear it, and know when we feel it in ourselves or in observing others. These are the *particular pleasures* of parenthood—experiences of love that are like none other and that occur *in concert*: not one feeling alone, but many intense feelings in relation to each other. While something like romantic love, they are nevertheless different, with erotic feelings replaced (or transformed) by the urge to protect.

Psychoanalysts have long recognized that these complex feelings of pleasure, affiliation, and protectiveness (which, for lack of a better term, we will call maternal love) provide a crucial balance to the other, inevitable, and darker side of mothering. Variously defined by terms as diverse as "cathexis", "primary maternal preoccupation", and "attachment", these feelings help the mother contain and regulate the many other intense emotions of motherhood, which can be terrifying and overwhelming when unmodulated by love. Such experiences of pleasure also ensure that she is rewarded (at a physiological as well as psychological level) for providing a secure base for her child—a base that is crucial to his survival, and to the development of his own capacities for love and closeness.

Developmental researchers and clinicians have had an enormously difficult time quantifying the positive parental qualities that make for smooth child adaptation (Cassidy et al., 2005), for they are nearly impossible to operationalize behaviourally. Nevertheless, we know that there is a certain "gleam in the eye" (Mary Dozier, personal communication, April 2003) that we recognize in "good-enough mothers" and that we miss in mothers who have disrupted relationships with their children. When we experience this certain something in mothers and babies, it makes us, as observers, feel good, too; when it is missing, we feel distressed and uneasy, at the least. Are the complex patterns of neural activation Strathearn describes the neurological analogues of such complex feelings of passionate love, great pleasure, intense connectedness, and the desire to know and protect?

A mother we interviewed for our research over 20 years ago came close to describing this ineffable combination when she was asked to pick five adjectives to describe her relationship with her 2-year-old daughter:

> "Close, passionate, dependent, independent, terrific. Close because I sense with her that I'm the closest person to her in the world, but I probably never knew before so much what was in another person's

mind and understood so much another person as I do with Annie. I can figure out what it is that she wants, and I can usually satisfy what she wants, which is a wonderful feeling, so, it's very close.... Um, it's passionate because I just never loved anybody the way I feel about, the way I love Annie. I mean just sitting here thinking about her, I can feel tears welling up, and I sorta', you know, I lie in bed at night saying to my husband, "Can you believe what she did today?" You know, I just can't believe it, and it's just, just a passionate kind of love, you know. I can't bear to be away from her and I've been married for ten years, so I, you know, maybe I'll feel differently about it when she's 10.... But I can be away from my husband for three days easier than I can be away from Annie."

Another mother put it more succinctly:

"There's an *indescribable* feeling when I pick her up and she gives me a little squeeze, her little arms around my neck ... that is just a *tremendous* feeling."

In disturbed mother–child relationships this balance between pleasure and more destructive emotions is disrupted, such that feelings of parental love are overwhelmed by the mother's malevolent projections or indifference. For instance, I recently observed a mother and her son as they arrived at the Anna Freud Centre for their weekly Parent–Infant Program meeting.

I noticed her son first. About 18 months old, he ran exuberantly ahead of her down the hall and headed straight for an exit door, courting risk as he tried to open it onto the icy steps and street. Patty was rail thin and waiflike, and very young—likely no older than 18. She followed him listlessly, and I at first smiled at her as one so often does passing a mother with a small, winning child. But she was like a shadow, nothing behind her eyes but a kind of vacancy and despair; her face looked blotchy and wan, and I found myself wondering whether these were faded bruises. As her son barrelled towards the door, she shrank away and made no move to protect him. The receptionist, by contrast, immediately sensed the danger and leapt from her desk and led him away from the door and back into the waiting-room. Mother said dully, but harshly, without ever moving towards him or making eye contact, "Harrison, will you get over here right now." There was no sparkle, no impulse to protect, or to draw the child closer; that ineffable combination was missing. This is not to say she did not love her child, but certainly all the feelings that might move her to protect her child, to take delight in him, and to long for his presence were muted or undeveloped.

Attachment, reflective functioning, and the complexities of parental love

Attachment researchers have thought of such individual differences in parents, which are palpable at both the representational and behavioural levels, as linked to underlying differences in attachment organization. These differences are most readily captured by the well-validated attachment classification system developed by Main, Kaplan, and Cassidy (1985). Strathearn intends to use this system as his primary method of grouping mothers, presumably because it distinguishes mothers in ways that predict their own children's attachment classification at one year. In essence, he is suggesting that adult attachment security is a *representational manifestation* of particular patterns of neural activation, notably the coincident activation of pleasure, affiliation, and protection centres of the brain. These patterns, and particularly their co-occurrence with the activation of centres that regulate distress and negative emotions, would presumably be different in insecure mothers. Differences in these patterns of activation in mothers will presumably lead to differences in both parenting behaviour and child outcome.

In line with my previous discussion of that ineffable combination of pleasure, longing, and anxiety that characterizes parental love, however, it is important to note that attachment theorists have noted again and again that one of the things that most readily distinguishes secure, dismissing, preoccupied, and disorganized adults from each other is the capacity to *integrate* and *regulate* complex affect states—in particular, to balance the positive affects of mothering (those described as parental love) with negative affects, such as fear and anger. That is, adult attachment categories not only distinguish mothers on the basis of child outcome, but also describe differences in mothers' ability to fully experience and adaptively express parental love.

The notion of mentalization or reflective functioning (Fonagy, Gergely, et al., 2002) provides another and likely complementary way of thinking about the capacity to fully and flexibly experience a range of parental emotions, and in particular to modulate the fragmenting effects of negative affects with understanding and reflectiveness (Slade, 2005). Fonagy and his colleagues (1995) have suggested that adult attachment classificatory schemes actually measure underlying differences in the capacity to hold complex emotional experiences in mind. That is, "security" implies that one viscerally understands the nature and function of mental states, in particular their dynamic, temporal, and transactional properties; it is, in essence, a sophisticated form of emotional and interpersonal understanding, one crucial to the formation and maintenance of attachment relationships. While different attachment categories are useful in identifying *differences* in the quality and nature of defensive organization (for instance, dismissing adults defend again attachment-related thoughts and feelings in a different way than those classified as preoccupied or disorganized), they may in many ways simply be proxies for underlying differences in mentalizing capacities. Fonagy's research clearly linked adult attachment organization and narrative coherence to underlying mentalizing capacities; in related research, we have likewise linked parental reflective functioning to parental attachment status as well as maternal behaviour (Grienenberger, Kelly, & Slade, 2005; Slade, Grienenberger, Bernbach, Levy, & Locker, 2005).

Would developed capacities for reflective functioning make it possible for a parent to experience parental love? Does the perspective and balance afforded by mentalizing capacities make the neutralization of aggression and the full expression of that "ineffable combination" possible? This is certainly an important question, and one that would nicely complement the question of the neural correlates of attachment categories. Personally, I think that the construct of reflective functioning offers more analytic and conceptual flexibility than does the construct of adult attachment organization (Slade, 2005). At the very least, these two approaches provide complementary views of crucial attachment processes. In any event, I think it would make sense for Strathearn to measure reflective functioning as part of his initial screening of mothers. Would differences in patterns of neural activation be linked to differences in mentalizing ability? Might the capacity to hold diverse and contradictory experiences in mind be manifest at the neural level in the integrated activation of multiple, diverse brain centres, including those associated with both positive and negative attachment experiences?

Implications for intervention

Another set of crucial questions that follow logically from Strathearn's work is whether early intervention might affect patterns of neural activation in referred parents. We know that mother–infant psychotherapy, however defined, often has dramatic effects upon maternal behaviour and representation. In recent years, a number of researchers and clinicians have suggested that one of mechanisms of change in mother–infant psychotherapy is the freeing of the parent's representation of her child from malevolent projections and distortions as a function of the development of parental reflective functioning or mentalization (Bateman & Fonagy, 2004b; Fonagy, Gergely, et al., 2002; Grienenberger et al., 2004; Slade, 2002, in press; Slade, Sadler, de Dios-Kenn, et al., 2005; Slade, Sadler, & Mayes, 2005). The development of these capacities—which, whether or not they are specifically targeted, are typically an outcome of most successful parent–infant psychotherapies—presumably allows for the development of positive parental attachment. Are these changes overt manifestations of underlying brain changes? Would the mother's developing capacities to mentalize and hold the baby in mind be reflected in changes in patterns of brain activation? Is one of the functions of treatment the activation of pleasure and affiliation centres in the brain? To activate a mother's concern for her child's safety? To help a mother neutralize the impact of negative emotions via the activation of feelings of love and connection?

Another of the clear implications of the work described by Strathearn, as well as that described by Leckman and colleagues in chapter 3 (see also Mayes, Swain, & Leckman, 2005), is that interventions be started as early as possible. They suggest that patterns of brain activation in mothers change dramatically during the earliest months of life; thus, the earlier we begin, and the more directly we begin developing mentalizing capacities in mothers, the more impact we can expect to have at the neural level, for both mothers *and* babies.

Closing remarks

Clinicians vary in the degree to which they value the specification of the neural correlates for psychological experience. Some see this work as invariably simplifying complex dynamic processes, and as diminishing the multiple challenges of bringing about change in individuals and in relationships. While I can understand this concern, I see neuroscientists and clinicians willingly embracing complexity on a number of levels. Certainly the documentation of neural bases for observed differences in attachment organization or parental reflective functioning would be an enormous scientific achievement, for it would validate many of the basic assumptions of attachment and psychoanalytic theory, and would pave the way for the expansion of both theory and practice. Neuroimaging research offers a particular kind of "hard" evidence for phenomena that cannot easily be described, and that have in many instances been derided and undervalued by "real" scientists who view clinical phenomena as ephemeral and poorly defined. But, as we can see from Strathearn's research, these phenomena are as real as any others. What neuroscience provides are increasingly rich tools to measure them and describe them, tools that reflect the inherent complexity of attachment processes. A continuing and rich dialogue between clinicians and neuroscientists will only enrich the way both think about and make meaning of human experience.

As exciting as these developments are, I would like to close by raising a cautionary note. I live in a country where our current government makes policy decisions using data that they twist and distort to their own political ends. To a disturbing extent, for instance, US policymakers sometimes use "hard" evidence about the poor and disenfranchised to oppress them even more than they already are. As scientific efforts such as those described by Strathearn move forward, we must make every attempt to separate scientific research that illuminates basic relational processes from any effort to use such methods as screening or diagnostic devices, or to incorporate them into real-life decision-making processes. It has often been suggested, for example, that attachment assessments such as the Strange Situation (Ainsworth, Blehar, Waters, & Wall, 1978) or the Adult Attachment Interview (George, Kaplan, & Main, 1996) should be administered as a means of determining a mother's capacity to care for her child. Attachment researchers have resisted this with all their might. These measures, like neuroimaging techniques, are—at least for the foreseeable future—research devices, tools of a basic science that can never be mistaken for absolute knowledge. For those of you who remember Winnie the Pooh, I don't mean to sound like Eeyore, but I am not yet ready to embrace this with the irrepressible zeal and mania of Tigger. For the time being, like Pooh, I will watch, wonder, and be very curious.

NOTE

Earlier versions of this chapter were presented at the Anna Freud Centre as part of the Developmental Science and Psychoanalysis: Integration and Innovation Conference, London (31 January 2004).

CHAPTER FIVE

The Interpretation of Dreams and the neurosciences

Mark Solms

Shortly after Freud's death, the study of dreaming from the perspective of neuroscience began in earnest. Initially, these studies yielded results that were difficult to reconcile with the psychological conclusions set out in his great book, *The Interpretation of Dreams* (1900a). The first major breakthrough came in 1953, when Aserinsky and Kleitman discovered a physiological state that occurs periodically (in 90-minute cycles) throughout sleep and occupies approximately a quarter of our sleeping hours. This state is characterized, among other things, by heightened brain activation, bursts of rapid eye movement (REM), increased breathing and heart rate, genital engorgement, and paralysis of bodily movement. It consists, in short, in a paradoxical physiological condition in which one is simultaneously highly aroused and yet fast asleep. Not surprisingly, Aserinsky and Kleitman suspected that this REM state (as it came to be known) was the external manifestation of the subjective dream state. That suspicion was soon confirmed experimentally (Aserinsky & Kleitman, 1955; Dement & Kleitman, 1957a, 1957b). It is now generally accepted that if someone is awakened from REM sleep and asked whether or not they have been dreaming, they will report that they were dreaming in as many as 95% of such awakenings. Non-REM sleep, by contrast, yields equivalent dream reports at a rate of only 5–10% of awakenings.

These early discoveries generated great excitement in the neuroscientific field: for the first time it appeared to have in its grasp an objective, physical manifestation of dreaming, one of the most subjective of all mental states. All that remained to be done, it seemed, was to lay bare the brain mechanisms that produced this physiological state; then we would have discovered nothing less than how the brain produces dreams. Since the REM state can be demonstrated in almost all mammals, this research could also be conducted in nonhuman species (which has important methodological implications, for brain mechanisms can be manipulated in animal experiments in ways that they cannot in human research).

A sequence of studies followed, in quick succession, in which different parts of the brain were systematically removed (in cats) in order to isolate the precise structures that produced REM sleep. On this basis, Jouvet was able to report in 1962 that REM (and therefore dreaming) was produced by a small region of cells in a part of the brainstem known as the "pons". This part of the nervous system is situated at a level only slightly above the spinal cord, near the nape of the neck. The higher levels of the brain, such as the cerebral hemispheres themselves, which fill out the great hollow of the human skull, did not appear to play any causal role whatever in the generation of dreaming. REM sleep occurs with monotonous regularity, throughout sleep, so long as the pons is intact, even if the great cerebral hemispheres are removed completely.

Neuroscientific research into the mechanism of REM sleep continued along these lines, using a wide variety of methods, and by 1975 a detailed picture of the anatomy and physiology of "dreaming sleep" had emerged. This picture, which was encapsulated in the *reciprocal interaction* and *activation-synthesis* models of McCarley and Hobson (1975, 1977), has dominated the field ever since: or, at least, as we shall see, until very recently. These authoritative models proposed that REM sleep and dreaming were literally "switched on" by a small group of cells situated deep within the pons, which excrete a chemical called "acetylcholine". This chemical activates the higher parts of the brain, which are thereby prompted to generate (intrinsically meaningless) conscious images. These meaningless images are nothing more than the higher brain making "the best of a bad job . . . from the noisy signals sent up from the brainstem" (Hobson & McCarley, 1977, p. 1347). After a few minutes of REM activity, the cholinergic activation arising from the brainstem is counteracted by another group of cells, also situated in the pons, which excrete two other chemicals: noradrenaline and serotonin. These chemicals "switch off" the cholinergic activation (and thereby, according to the theory, the conscious experience of dreaming).

Thus all the complex mental processes that Freud elucidated in his dream book were swept aside and replaced by a simple oscillatory mechanism by means of which consciousness is automatically switched on and off at approximately 90-minute intervals throughout sleep by reciprocally interacting chemicals that are excreted in an elementary part of the brain that has nothing to do with complex mental functions. Thus, even the most basic claims of Freud's theory no longer seemed tenable:

> The primary motivating force of dreaming is not psychological but physiological since the time of occurrence and duration of dreaming sleep are quite constant suggesting a pre-programmed, neurally determined genesis. In fact, the neural mechanisms involved can now be precisely specified. If we assume that the physiological substrate of consciousness is in the forebrain, these facts [i.e., that REM is automatically generated by brainstem mechanisms] completely eliminate any possible contribution of ideas (or their neural substrate) to the primary driving force of the dream process. [Hobson & McCarley, 1977, pp. 1346, 1338]

On this basis, it seemed justifiable to conclude that the causal mechanisms underlying dreaming were "motivationally neutral" (McCarley & Hobson, 1977, p. 1219) and that dream imagery was nothing more than "the best possible fit of intrinsically inchoate data produced by the auto-activated brain-mind" (Hobson, 1988, p. 204). The credibility of Freud's theory was, in short, severely strained by the first wave of data about dreaming that was obtained from "anatomical preparations" (Freud, 1900a, p. 536): and the neuroscientific world (indeed the scientific world as a whole) reverted to the pre-psychoanalytic view that "dreams are froth" (Freud, 1900a, p. 133).

However, alongside the observations just reviewed, which provided an increasingly precise and detailed picture of the neurology of REM sleep, a second body of evidence gradually began to accumulate, which led some neuroscientists to recognize that *perhaps REM sleep was not the physiological equivalent of dreaming after all* (Solms, 2000).

The notion that dreaming is merely "an epiphenomenon of REM sleep" (Hobson, Stickgold, & Pace-Schott, 1998, p. R12) rested almost exclusively on the observation that arousal from the REM state yielded dream reports on 70–95% of awakenings, whereas non-REM awakenings yielded equivalent reports in only 5–10% of attempts. Considering the vagaries of subjective memory (and especially memory for dreams), this is as close to a perfect correlation as one could reasonably expect. However, the sharp division between REM ("dreaming") sleep and non-REM ("non-dreaming") sleep began to fray when it was discovered that reports of complex mentation could, in fact, be elicited in as many as 50% of awakenings from non-REM sleep. This became apparent when Foulkes awakened subjects from non-REM sleep and asked them, "What was passing through your mind?" rather than, "Have you been dreaming?" (Foulkes, 1962). The resultant non-REM dream reports were more "thought-like" (less hallucinatory) than the REM dream reports, but this distinction held only for the statistical average. The fact remained that at least 5–10% of non-REM dream reports were "indistinguishable by any criterion from those obtained from post-REM awakenings" (Hobson, 1988, p. 143). These findings "do not support a dichotomic distinction between REM and NREM mentation, rather they suggest the hypothesis of the existence of continuous dream processing characterized by a variability within and between sleep stages" (Cavallero et al., 1992, p. 563).

The non-REM dream reports could not be explained away as misremembered REM dreams, for it soon became apparent that dream reports could regularly be obtained even before the dreamer had entered the first REM phase. In fact, we now know that dream reports are obtainable from as many as 50–70% of awakenings during the sleep-onset phase—that is, in the first few minutes after falling asleep (Foulkes & Vogel, 1965; Foulkes, Spear, & Symonds, 1966; Vogel, Barrowclough, & Giesler, 1972). This is a far higher rate than at any other point during the non-REM cycle, and almost as high as the REM rate. Similarly, it was recently discovered that non-REM dreams appear with increasing length and frequency towards the end of sleep, during the rising morning phase of the diurnal rhythm (Kondo, Antrobus, & Fein, 1989). In other words, non-REM dreams do not appear randomly during the sleep cycle: dreaming is generated during non-REM sleep by specific non-REM mechanisms.

The only reliable difference between REM dream reports, sleep-onset reports, and certain other classes of non-REM dream report is that the REM reports are longer. In all other respects, the non-REM and REM dreams appear to be identical. This demonstrates that fully fledged dreams can occur independently of the unique physiological state of REM sleep. Therefore, whatever the explanation may be for the strong correlation that exists between dreaming and REM sleep, it is no longer accepted that dreaming is caused exclusively by the REM state.

The presumed isomorphism between REM sleep and dreaming was further undermined by the emergence, very recently, of new and unexpected evidence regarding the brain mechanisms of dreaming. As already noted, the hypothesis that dreaming is merely an epiphenomenon of REM sleep rested on the high correlation between REM awakening and dream reports. But this does not necessarily imply that REM and dreaming share a unitary brain mechanism. In the light of the discovery that dreams regularly occur independently of REM sleep, it is certainly possible that the REM state and dreaming are controlled by independent brain mechanisms. The two mechanisms could well be situated in different parts of the brain, with the REM mechanism frequently triggering the dream mechanism. A two-stage causation of REM dreaming implies that the dream mechanism could also be stimulated into action by triggers other than the REM mechanism, which would explain why dreaming so frequently occurs outside REM sleep.

This hypothesis, that two separate mechanisms—one for REM and one for dreaming—exist in the brain, can easily be tested by a standard neurological research method known as clinico-anatomical correlation. This is the classical method for testing such hypotheses: the parts of the brain that obliterate REM sleep are removed, and the investigator observes whether or not dreaming still occurs; then the parts of the brain that obliterate dreaming are removed, and the investigator observes whether or not REM still occurs. If the two effects dissociate, then they are caused by different brain mechanisms. If they are affected simultaneously by damage to a single brain structure, then they are served by a unitary mechanism.

It is known that destruction of parts of the pons (and nowhere else) leads to a cessation of REM sleep in lower mammals (Jones, 1979), but such experiments cannot, of course, be performed on humans—the only species that is in a position to tell us whether or not destruction of those parts of the brain leads simultaneously to a cessation of dreaming. Fortunately (for science), the relevant brain structures are occasionally destroyed in human cases by naturally occurring damage, due to spontaneous illness or traumatic injury to the brain. In the neurological literature, 26 such cases have been reported with damage to the pons, which resulted in a total or near-total loss of REM sleep.[1] Surprisingly, the elimination of REM in these cases was accompanied by reported loss of dreaming in only one of the 26 patients (Feldman, 1971). In the other 25 cases, the investigators either could not establish this correlation or they did not consider it. By contrast, in all the other cases ever published in the neuroscientific literature in which damage to the brain did result in a reported loss of dreaming (a total of 110 patients), a completely different part of the brain was damaged, and the pons was spared completely.[2] Moreover, it has been proven that REM sleep is completely preserved in these cases, despite their loss of dreaming.[3] This dissociation between cessation of REM and cessation of dreaming seriously undermines the doctrine that the REM state is the physiological equivalent of the dream state.

The parts of the brain that are crucial for dreaming and those that are crucial for REM sleep are widely separated, both anatomically and functionally. The parts of the brain that are crucial for REM are in the pons, which is located in the brainstem, near the nape of the neck. The parts of the brain that are crucial for dreaming, by contrast, are situated exclusively in the higher parts of the brain, in two specific locations within the cerebral hemispheres themselves.

The first of these locations is in the deep white matter of the frontal lobes of the brain, just above the eyes (Solms, 1997). This part of the frontal lobes contains a large fibre-pathway, which transmits a chemical called "dopamine" from the middle of the brain to the higher parts of the brain. Damage to this pathway renders dreaming impossible, but it leaves the REM cycle completely unaffected (Jus et al., 1973). This suggests that dreaming is generated by a mechanism different from the one that generates REM sleep—a conclusion that is strongly supported by the observation that chemical stimulation of this dopamine pathway (with drugs like L-DOPA) leads to a massive increase in the frequency and vividness of dreams without it having any effect on the frequency and intensity of REM sleep (Hartmann, Russ, Oldfield, Falke, & Skoff, 1980; Klawans, Moskowitz, Lupton, & Scharf, 1978; Nausieda et al., 1982; Scharf, Moskovitz, Lupton, & Klawans, 1978). Likewise, excessively frequent and vivid dreaming caused by dopamine stimulants can be stopped by drugs (like anti-psychotics), which block the transmission of dopamine in this pathway (Sacks, 1985, 1990, 1991). In short, dreaming can be switched "on" and "off" by a neurochemical pathway that has nothing to do with the REM oscillator in the pons. What, then, is the function of this higher brain pathway, which is so crucial for the generation of dreams? Its main function is to "instigate goal-seeking behaviours and an organism's appetitive interactions with the world" (Panksepp, 1985, p. 273)—that is, to motivate the subject to seek out and engage with external objects that can satisfy its inner biological needs. These are precisely the functions that Freud attributed to the "libidinal drive"—the primary instigator of dreams—in his (1900a) theory. Accordingly, it is of considerable interest to note that damage to this pathway causes cessation of dreaming in conjunction with a massive reduction in motivated behaviour (Solms, 1997). In view of the close association between dreams and certain forms of insanity, it is also interesting to note that surgical damage to this pathway (which was the primary target of the prefrontal leucotomies of the 1950s and 1960s) leads to a reduction in some symptoms of psychotic illness, together with a cessation of dreaming (Frank, 1946, 1950; Partridge, 1950; Schindler, 1953). Whatever it is that prevented leucotomized patients from maintaining their psychiatric symptoms also prevented them from generating dreams. Contemporary theories of schizophrenia (Kapur, 2003; Silbersweig et al., 1995) attribute a central role in the causation of hallucinations and delusions to the dopaminergic pathway that seems to generate dreams.

In short, the current neuroscientific evidence gives us every reason to take seriously the radical hypothesis—first set out by Freud more than 100 years ago—to the effect that dreams are motivated phenomena, driven by our wishes. Although it is true that the (cholinergic) mechanism that generates the REM state is "motivationally neutral", this cannot be said of the (dopaminergic) mechanism, which generates the dream state. In fact, the latter mechanism is the appetitive (i.e., libidinal) "command system" of the brain (Panksepp, 1985, 1998); and recent evidence confirms that it is maximally activated during REM sleep (Lena et al., 2004).

As stated, it now appears that REM only causes dreaming via the intermediary of this motivational mechanism. Moreover, REM is just one of the many different triggers that are capable of activating this mechanism. A variety of other triggers, which act independently of REM, have exactly the same effect. Sleep-onset dreams and late morning dreams are two examples of this kind. Dreams induced by L-DOPA (and various stimulant drugs) are further examples. Of special interest in this regard is the fact that recurring, stereotyped nightmares can be induced by seizures that occur during sleep.[4] We know from the work of Penfield[5] exactly where in the brain these seizures begin—namely, in the temporal limbic system. This system, which subserves emotional and memory functions, is situated in the higher forebrain and is richly interconnected with the frontal lobe dopamine pathway discussed above. Moreover, we know that such seizures usually occur during non-REM sleep (Janz, 1974; Kellaway & Frost, 1983). The fact that nightmares can be "switched on" by mechanisms in the higher parts of the brain which have nothing to do with the pons and nothing to do with REM sleep is further evidence that dreaming and REM are generated by separate and independent brain mechanisms.

It is surely no accident that what all of these different mechanisms capable of triggering dreams have in common is the fact that they create a state of arousal during sleep. This lends support to another of the cardinal hypotheses that Freud put forward in 1900—namely, the hypothesis that dreams are a response to something that disturbs sleep.[6] But it appears that the arousal stimuli enumerated above trigger dreaming only if and when they activate the final common motivational pathway within the frontal lobes of the brain, for it is only when this pathway is damaged (rather than the arousal triggers themselves, including REM) that dreaming becomes impossible. This relationship between the various arousal triggers and the dream-onset mechanism itself is reminiscent of Freud's famous analogy: dreaming only occurs if the stimulus which acts as the "entrepreneur" of the dream attracts the support of a "capitalist", an unconscious libidinal urge, which alone has the power to generate dreaming (1900a, p. 561).

Thus, Freud's major inferences from psychological evidence regarding both the causes and the function of dreaming are at least compatible with, and even indirectly supported by, current neuroscientific knowledge. Does the same apply to the mechanism of dreaming?

Our current neuroscientific understanding of the mechanism of dreaming revolves centrally around the concept of regression. The prevailing view is that imagery of all kinds (including dream imagery) is generated by "projecting information backward in the system" (Kosslyn, 1994, p. 75). Accordingly, dreaming is conceptualized as "internally generated images which are fed backwards into the cortex as if they were coming from the outside" (Zeki, 1993, p. 326). This conception of dream imagery is based on wide-ranging neurophysiological and neuropsychological research into numerous aspects of visual processing. However the regressive nature of dream processing has recently been demonstrated directly in clinical neurological cases (Solms, 1997).

In order to illustrate this point, it is necessary to remind the reader that loss of dreaming due to neurological damage is associated with damage in two brain locations. The first of these is the white fibre pathway of the frontal lobes that we have considered already. The second location is a portion of the grey cortex at the back of the brain (just behind and above the ears) called the occipito-temporo-parietal junction. This part of the brain performs the highest levels of processing of perceptual information and it is essential for:

> the conversion of concrete perception into abstract thinking, which always proceeds in the form of internal schemes, and for the memorizing of organized experience or, in other words, not only for the perception of information but also for its storage, [Luria, 1973, p. 74]

The fact that dreaming ceases completely with damage to this part of the brain suggests that these functions (the conversion of concrete perceptions into abstract thoughts and memories), like the motivational functions performed by the frontal lobe pathway discussed previously, are fundamental to the whole process of dreaming. However, if the theory that dream imagery is generated by a process that reverses the normal sequence of events in perceptual processing is correct, then we may expect that in dreams abstract thoughts and memories are converted into concrete perceptions. This is exactly what Freud had in mind when he wrote that, "in regression, the fabric of the dream-thoughts is resolved into its raw material" (1900a, p. 543). This inference is supported empirically by the observation that dreaming as a whole stops completely with damage at the highest level of the perceptual systems (in the region of the occipito-temporo junction), whereas only specific aspects of dream imagery are affected by damage at lower levels of the visual system, closer to the perceptual periphery (in the region of the occipital lobe).[7] This implies that the contribution of the higher levels precedes that of the lower levels. When there is damage at the higher levels, dreaming is blocked completely, whereas damage at the lower levels merely subtracts something from the terminal stage of the dream process. This is the opposite of what happens in waking perception, which is obliterated entirely by damage at the lowest levels of the system. In other words, dreaming reverses the normal sequence of perceptual events.

The available neuroscientific evidence, therefore, is compatible with Freud's conception of where and how the dream process is initiated (for example, by an arousing stimulus that activates the emotional and motivational systems), and of where and how it terminates (such as by abstract thinking in the memory and motivational systems, which is projected backwards in the form of concrete images onto the perceptual systems).

In fact, it is now possible to actually *see* where this neural activity is distributed in the dreaming brain. Modern neuroradiological methods produce pictures of the pattern of metabolic activity in the living brain while it is actually performing a particular function, and in the case of dreaming these images clearly show how the brain's energic "cathexis" (as Freud called it) is concentrated within the anatomical areas discussed above—namely, the (frontal and limbic) parts of the brain concerned with arousal, emotion, memory and motivation, on the one hand, and the parts (at the back of the brain) concerned with abstract thinking and visual perception, on the other.[8]

These radiological pictures also reveal something about what happens in-between the initial and terminal ends of the dream process. The most striking feature of the dreaming brain in this respect is the fact that a region of the brain known as the dorsolateral frontal convexity is almost completely inactive during dreams. This is striking, because this part of the brain, which is inactive during dreams, is one of the most active of all brain areas during waking mental activity. If one compares the pictures of the waking brain with those of the dreaming brain, one literally sees the truth of Fechner's (1889) assertion to the effect that "the scene of action of dreams is different from that of waking ideational life" (cf. Freud, 1900a, p. 536). Whereas in waking ideational life, the "scene of action" is concentrated in the dorsolateral region at the front of the brain—"the upper end of the motor system—the gateway from thought to action" (Solms, 1997, p. 223)—in dreams it is concentrated in the occipito-temporo-parietal region at the back of the brain, on the memory and perceptual systems. In short, in dreams, the "scene" shifts from the motor end of the apparatus to the perceptual end.[9]

This reflects the fact that whereas in waking life the normal course of mental events is directed towards action, in dreams this path is unavailable. The "gateway" to the motor systems (the dorsolateral frontal convexity of the brain) is unavailable in dreams (Braun et al., 1997, 1998; Solms, 1997), as are the motor output channels: the alpha motor neurons of the spinal cord (see Pompeiano, 1979). Thus both the intention to act and the ability to act are absent during sleep, and it seems reasonable to infer (as did Freud) that this absence is the immediate cause of the dream process assuming a regressive path, away from the motor systems of the brain, towards the perceptual systems (Solms, 1997).

Finally, due to relative inactivation during sleep of crucial parts of the reflective systems in the frontal parts of the limbic brain, the imagined dream scene is uncritically accepted, and the dreamer mistakes the internally generated scene for a real perception. Damage to these reflective systems (which evidently are not entirely inactive during sleep) results in a curious state of almost constant dreaming during sleep and an inability to distinguish between thoughts and real events during waking life.[10] This provides further evidence of a continuous thought process during sleep, which is converted into dreaming under various physiological conditions, of which REM sleep is just one among many.

The picture of the dreaming brain that emerges from recent neuroscientific research may therefore be summarized as follows: the process of dreaming is initiated by an arousal stimulus. If this stimulus is sufficiently intense or persistent to activate the motivational mechanisms of the brain (or if it attracts the interest of these mechanisms for some other reason), the dream process proper begins. The functioning of the motivational systems of the brain is normally channelled towards goal-directed action, but access to the motor systems is blocked during sleep. The purposive action that would be the normal outcome of motivated interest is thereby rendered impossible during sleep. As a result (and quite possibly in order to protect sleep), the process of activation assumes a regressive course. This appears to involve a two-stage process. First, the higher parts of the perceptual systems (which serve memory and abstract thinking) are activated; then the lower parts (which serve concrete imagery) are activated. As a result of this regressive process, the dreamer does not actually engage in motivated activity during sleep but, rather, *imagines* himself to be doing so. Due to inactivation during sleep of the reflective systems in the frontal part of the limbic brain, the imagined scene is uncritically accepted, and the dreamer mistakes it for a real perception.

There is a great deal about the dreaming brain that we still do not understand. It is also evident that we have not yet discovered the neurological correlates of some crucial components of the "dream-work" as Freud understood it. The function of "censorship" is the most glaring example of this kind. However, we are beginning to understand something about the neurological correlates of that function, and we know at least that the structures that are most likely to be implicated

(Solms, 1998) are indeed active during dreaming sleep (Braun et al., 1997, 1998).

Hopefully it is apparent to the reader from this brief overview that the picture of the dreaming brain that has begun to emerge from the most recent neuroscientific researches is broadly compatible with the psychological theory that Freud advanced. In fact, aspects of Freud's account of the dreaming mind are so consistent with the currently available neuroscientific data that I personally think we would be well advised to use Freud's model as a guide for the next phase of our neuroscientific investigations. Unlike the research effort of the past few decades, the next stage in our search for the brain mechanisms of dreaming must—if it is to succeed—take as its starting point the new perspective we have gained on the role of REM sleep. REM sleep, which has hitherto diverted our attention away from the neuropsychological mechanisms of dreaming, should simply be added to the various "somatic sources" of dreams that Freud discussed in chapters 1 and 5 of his famous book (1900a). The major focus of our future research efforts should then be directed towards elucidating the brain correlates of the mechanisms that Freud discussed in his 6th and 7th chapters: the mechanisms of the dream-work proper:

> We shall feel no surprise at the over-estimation of the part played in forming dreams by stimuli which do not arise from mental life. Not only are they easy to discover and even open to experimental confirmation; but the somatic view of the origin of dreams is completely in line with the prevailing trend of thought in psychiatry to-day. It is true that the dominance of the brain over the organism is asserted with apparent confidence. Nevertheless, anything that might indicate that mental life is in any way independent of demonstrable organic changes or that its manifestations are in any way spontaneous alarms the modern psychiatrist, as though a recognition of such things would inevitably bring back the days of the Philosophy of Nature, and the metaphysical view of the nature of mind. The suspicions of the psychiatrists have put the mind, as it were, under tutelage, and they now insist that none of its impulses shall be allowed to suggest that it has any means of its own. This behaviour of theirs only shows how little trust they really have in the validity of a causal connection between the somatic and the mental. Even when investigation shows the primary exciting cause of a phenomenon is psychical, deeper research will one day trace the path further and discover an organic basis for the mental event. But if at the moment we cannot see beyond the mental, that is no reason for denying its existence. [Freud, 1900a, pp. 41–42]

NOTES

This is a revised and updated version of an essay originally written in German for a centenary reprint of the first edition of Freud's *Traumdeutung* (Frankfurt am Main: Fischer Verlag, 1999).

1. Adey, Bors, & Porter, 1968; Chase, Moretti, & Prensky, 1968; Cummings & Greenberg, 1977; Feldman, 1971; Lavie & Tzichinsky, 1984; Markand & Dyken, 1976; Osorio & Daroff, 1980.

2. Basso, Bisiach & Luzzatti, 1980; Bischof & Bassetti, 2004; Boyle & Nielsen, 1954; Epstein, 1979; Epstein & Simmons, 1983; Ettlinger, Warrington & Zangwill, 1957; Farah, Levine, & Calviano, 1988; Farrell, 1969; Gloning & Sternbach, 1953; Grünstein, 1924; Habib & Sirigu, 1987; Humphrey & Zangwill, 1951; Lyman, Kwan, & Chao, 1983; Michel & Sieroff, 1981; Moss, 1972; Müller, 1892; Neal, 1988; Nielsen, 1955; Peña-Casanova, Roig-Rovira, Bermudez, & Tolosa-Sarro, 1985; Piehler, 1950; Ritchie, 1959; Solms, 1997; Wapner, Judd, & Gardner, 1978; Wilbrand, 1887, 1892.

3. Benson & Greenberg, 1969; Brown, 1972; Cathala et al., 1983; Efron, 1968; Jus et al., 1973; Kerr, Foulkes & Jurkovic, 1978; Michel & Sieroff, 1981; Murri, Massetani, Siciliano, & Arena, 1985.

4. De Sanctis, 1896; Thomayer, 1897; Clarke, 1915; Kardiner, 1932; Naville & Brantmay, 1935; Rodin, Mulder, Faucett, & Bickford, 1955; Ostow, 1954; Epstein & Ervin, 1956; Snyder, 1958; Epstein, 1964; Epstein & Hill, 1966; Epstein, 1967; Boller, Wright, Cavalieri, & Mitsumoto, 1975; Epstein, 1979; Epstein & Freeman, 1981; Solms, 1997.

5. Penfield was able to artificially generate the recurring nightmare scenes by directly stimulating the seizure focus in the temporal lobe (Penfield, 1938; Penfield & Erickson, 1941; Penfield & Rasmussen, 1955).

6. Solms (1995, 1997) provides limited empirical evidence to support the hypothesis that dreams protect sleep: patients who lose the ability to dream due to brain damage report more disturbed sleep than do brain-damaged patients with intact dreaming. More importantly, a recent polysomnographic study of a non-dreaming patient recorded "sleep-maintenance insomnia", just as Freud's sleep-protection would have predicted (Bischof & Bassetti, 2004). Further research into this question is needed.

7. Charcot, 1883; Adler, 1944, 1950; Brain, 1950, 1954; Macrae & Trolle, 1956; Tzavaras, 1967; Kerr, Foulkes, & Jurkovic, 1978; Botez, Gravel, Attig, & Vézina, 1985; Sacks & Wasserman, 1987; Solms, 1997.

8. Braun et al., 1997, 1998; Franck et al., 1987; Franzini, 1992; Heiss, Pawlik, Herholz, Wagner, & Weinhard, 1985; Hong, Gillin, Dow, Wu, & Buchsbaum, 1995; Madsen, 1993; Madsen & Vorstrup, 1991; Madsen, Holm, et al., 1991; Madsen, Schmidt, et al., 1991; Maquet et al., 1990, 1996.

9. It is of utmost interest to note that the major inhibitory systems of the forebrain are concentrated at its motor end, as they were in Freud's (1900a) diagrammatic representation of the mental apparatus.

10. Whitty & Lewin, 1957; Lugaresi et al., 1986; Gallassi, Morreale, Montagna, Gambetti, & Lugaresi, 1992; Morris, Bowers, Chatterjee, & Heilman, 1992; Sacks, 1995; Solms, 1997.

Commentary

Linda C. Mayes

Mark Solms's review of the neurobiology of dreaming is in keeping with his celebrated ability for integration of classical psychoanalytic concepts and models of the mind with contemporary neuropsychological constructs and neuroscientific understanding of the brain. His synthesis is a model for the kind of interdisciplinary bridging in the extended programmes in the joint efforts of the Anna Freud Centre and Child Study Center that are the subject of this volume. Solms has done much to move debates about the relevance of contemporary brain sciences for psychoanalytic models of the mind beyond rhetoric and into data, especially as regards memory, learning, and dreaming.

The dialectic between contemporary neuroscience and either classical or even contemporary models of the mind is an enduring one—far older than psychoanalysis—and, as many analysts point out, a dialectic at the core of psychoanalysis. Psychoanalysts often point to Freud's early grounding in neurology, his interest in the most basic aspects of biology and endowment, and especially the scientific agenda he advanced in his abandoned project as evidence for the compatibility of psychoanalytic theory and practice with the more contemporary sciences of the brain. And, particularly for child analysts, the close relationship between the development of the body and of the representational world places issues of body and mind not only in close theoretical proximity but in lively conversation in every clinical session. In the past decade, the mind–body duality has been increasingly discussed in the guise of the relevance of neuroscience—or the brain and cognitive sciences—for psychoanalysis.

Many analysts have underscored the relevance for psychoanalytic models of the mind of recent advances in the understanding of the neural circuitry of such basic processes as memory, stress regulation and response to trauma, and emotional processing. The journal *Neuropsychoanalysis* and a number of internationally sponsored conferences on the interface of neuroscience and psychoanalysis speak to the growing interest among psychoanalysts for the new brain and cognitive sciences—an interest engendered in no small part by Solms's work. Conversely, some neuroscientists have expressed the hope that the new brain sciences may offer ways to reinvigorate the scholarship on the interface of mind and brain that was so central to the beginnings of psychoanalysis.

So what are the areas that we can point to in contemporary neuroscience that hold relevance for our psychoanalytic models of mind? No doubt in the last ten to twenty years in our understanding of the complexity of brain functioning and of brain development. Contemporary working theories of, for example, learning reveal a much more dynamic model of the brain than heretofore understood—a brain in which structure changes at the cellular level in response to both positive and negative events, new connections and networks are formed throughout life, and apparently new neurons are generated in the healing aftermath of stress and trauma. Neuroimaging techniques allow visualizing neural response in nearly real time, and functional neuroimaging paradigms are becoming ever more psychologically sophisticated so as to permit studying the interface of emotion and cognition, the responses of a parent to the salient cues of a new infant, or of an adult to a romantic partner. Similar advances in genetics have opened up whole new areas of understanding how experiences turn on and off genes regulating aspects of neural function, how there are genetic substrates to such basic processes as parental engagement and attachment and affiliation. Notably while many psychoanalysts are catching on in their conviction of the relevance of neuroscience for psychoanalysis, cognitive and social psychologists have already formed very productive collaborations with the basic neurosciences, particularly around the development of creative neuropsychological paradigms to be used in functional neuroimaging procedures.

Partnerships among the psychological and neural sciences are demonstrating the creative possibilities in collaborations across disciplines that have traditionally worked at different levels of discourse. For example, collaborations between clinicians and neuroscientists working with preclinical models are providing experimental data for how early dyadic experiences shape neural regulatory systems and for the intergenerational transmission of parenting behaviours—the basic biology of how experience impacts on emotional regulation and internalization. These are tenets much discussed by practicing clinicians but partnerships with basic scientists permit detailed study of the possible mechanisms for these clinical phenomena. And especially under Solms's lead, cognitive neuroscientists have also rekindled interest in subjective experience as a legitimate arena for empirical study. In short, these are very exciting times to be thinking about integrating across these fields, and an implicit question raised by Solms today and in much of his work is how psychoanalysts can be better informed about the contemporary neurosciences and also join into productive collaborations.

At the same time, these integrative efforts are fraught with many risks for reductionism. For example, a number of analysts have questioned whether or not new knowledge from basic neurosciences change day-to-day clinical practice with patients—a concern that some may find controversial but that nonetheless bears careful consideration inasmuch as any field, not just psychoanalysis, needs to consider carefully how new knowledge from other fields is incorporated into clinical technique. Several scholars have insisted that although advances in contemporary neuroscience hold the promise of offering significant changes to psychoanalytic metapsychology, the psychoanalytic focus on mental representations and meaning constitutes a very different domain of discourse from the neuroscience focus on cellular processes or on basic cognitive computations. These same scholars caution that attempts to link psychoanalytic concepts to the basic brain sciences exposes psychoanalysis to the levelling, homogenizing effects of reductionism. It is also true that there is a continuing, and sometimes apparently wide, divide between the analytic practitioner and the analytic scholar working as theoretician, empirical investigator, or both. While it may be true that the neurosciences have yet to change clinical practice, it is imperative that as a field we attend to the risks of a continuing divide, real or perceived, between psychoanalytic practitioners and those seeking to advance the interface with the physical brain sciences even if these identities sometimes rest in the same individual. It is also imperative that we wrestle with this question of how integration with contemporary neuroscience and neuropsychology might change clinical practice. For example, how does understanding that dreams may be a product of activation of subcortical salience systems and in turn activation of cortical perceptual systems actually change work with a patient or the metapsychology of dreaming. Solms hints at the latter—that is, some revisions perhaps in the theory of wish fulfilment—but we might ask him to speculate on the former: how best to integrate this new knowledge into clinical practice.

Contemporary methods, such as functional neuroimaging, do offer the promise of visualizing the brain in relative real time in response to various stimulus conditions, including some of interest to psychoanalysts, such as images and sounds from a newborn infant. Not only are advances in contemporary neuroscience of relevance to both psychoanalytic clinicians and theorists, but the neuroimaging techniques may also be sufficiently developed to be appropriate for studying key psychoanalytic concepts such as parental investment. To be sure, there are important distinctions between bottom-up approaches for analysing the molecular components of the brain and top-down approaches relating mental functions to larger networks of neurons, the latter being more compatible with psychoanalytic theory and representing an active area of scholarship among contemporary neuroscientists. Here too, though, there is an appropriate word of caution. All too often, the detailed and colourful images resulting from neuroimaging techniques are taken in without sufficient appreciation of the technical complexity in this rapidly developing science. In an effort to "see" clarity in the images, findings from, for example, fMRI are reduced to which regions of the brain are activated to what stimuli, without a more detailed consideration of the stimuli used and of the basic fact that all neuroimaging studies necessarily compare one set of conditions to another. In other words, the amount of activation is relative to a comparison condition, and some of the greatest creativity in neuroimaging studies is involved in the development of the comparison conditions. Informing the design of such conditions for studies of, for example, structural change in response to psychodynamic treatment is a role in which psychoanalysts may make very important contributions as collaborative members of a research team, a point stressed by a number of psychoanalytic scholars, such as Manfred Beutel, who are working in neuroimaging labs.

Working at the interface of contemporary brain sciences and psychoanalytic models of the mind requires considerable scholarship in both fields, as evidenced by Solms. From the point of view of many psychoanalysts, there is the often expressed fear that the richness of psychoanalytic clinical data is lost in the necessarily more constrained techniques of empirical study, and especially in what is perceived as the "narrow" focus of the neurosciences on cognition and stimulus–response. Underneath this worry is the fear that psychoanalysis as a field cannot hold its own against the machine of "real science"—a concern that mirrors charges from the many critics of psychoanalysis. Thus, in response to this fear, some embrace neuroscience perspectives as the future salvation and vindication of a field that had its origins in neurology, while others shy away, insisting that the discourse of mind and brain cannot be interrelated. Because of these worries, well-placed caution is appropriate. Like psychoanalysis, indeed like most scholarly fields, the neurosciences are vast. Unlike psychoanalysis, the new brain sciences are also rapidly evolving, in both method and application. It is very easy for the informed reader who is nonetheless not a neuroscientist to overinterpret findings or to try to reduce complex methods or data into simple, comprehensible models—to try, for example, to make direct equations between complex psychological constructs and specific brain regions rather than thinking about neural systems. It takes careful study to be informed, as well as active partnering as a student with neuroscience colleagues. It is all too tempting, in our enthusiasm for the promise of the new brain sciences, to neglect developing empirical skills within psychoanalysis and creating a new scholarship that values inquiry, hypothesis testing, and interdisciplinary collaboration. There are many quantitative and qualitative methods well suited to psychoanalytic data, some represented in this volume and others in both the analytic and developmental literature and within our field. It is imperative that we continue to build on this level of scholarship while at the same time working to make transdisciplinary bridges. Ignoring the need to develop an empirical tradition within our own field limits the opportunities to join as partners in scientific collaborations with related disciplines and, even more tragically, ultimately limits the intellectual evolution of psychoanalysis. Solms's work represents a paradigmatic example of how to do this kind of bridging work well, both as a psychoanalytic scholar and a neuropsychologist, and is a positive contribution towards the future shape of psychoanalytic science.

CHAPTER SIX

In the best interests of the late-placed child: a report from the Attachment Representations and Adoption Outcome study

Miriam Steele, Kay Henderson, Jill Hodges, Jeanne Kaniuk, Saul Hillman, & Howard Steele

> Change of the caretaking person for infants and toddlers further affects the course of their emotional development. Their attachments, at these ages, are as thoroughly upset by separations as they are effectively promoted by the constant, uninterrupted presence and attention of a familiar adult. When infants and young children find themselves abandoned by the parent, they not only suffer separation distress and anxiety but also setbacks in the quality of their next attachments, which will be less trustful. Where continuity of such relationships is interrupted more than once, as happens due to multiple placements in the early years, the children's emotional attachments become increasingly shallow and indiscriminate.
>
> Goldstein, Freud, & Solnit (1973, p. 33)

This chapter fits aptly into the celebration of the renewal of collaborative efforts between the Yale Child Study Center and the Anna Freud Centre, as it resonates with the work of the two hallmark figures from each institution: Al Solnit, former Director of the Yale Child Study Center and Anna Freud, founder and former director of the Anna Freud Centre. Together with their Yale colleague, Joseph Goldstein, Solnit and Anna Freud produced the vital trilogy beginning with *Beyond the Best Interests of the Child* (1973). Judges, lawyers, social workers, and child mental health experts continue to rely heavily on this Yale/Anna Freud Centre resource, unlike any other in scope and depth, as they consider the necessary interplay between the psychological and legal issues at stake in making decisions about children who come to the state's attention for decisions about their care.

This chapter summarizes some of the findings from a London-based longitudinal study of attachment representations and adoption outcome. This unique study brings three institutions together—the Anna Freud Centre, the Coram Family Adoption Service, and the Great Ormond Street Hospital for Sick Children—each providing unique areas of expertise. The study has been looking at sources of influence, change, and adaptation in a group of newly formed families—adoptive parents and the maltreated children placed with them—over a three-year time period. The children who participated in this study, and the questions addressed by the research, are very similar to those considered in the Solnit, Freud, and Goldstein trilogy.

The essence of much inquiry, both in academic and in clinical milieus, concerning child psychopathology focuses on the developmental trajectories of adaptation and maladaptation, and the experiences through which the deleterious impact of abuse may respond to amelioration. The intervention of adoption is often cited as being the most dramatic of any that can alter a maltreated child's life course. The "Attachment Representations and Adoption Outcome Study" provides a compelling and unique data set to which questions of outcome and change in attachment representations and overall adaptation in a maltreated group of children under study are possible. The study has focused as much on the change in the child's attachment representations over a two-year period as on the parents' who adopt them. Attachment theory and research is the theoretical and methodological underpinning of the study with ties to broader issues in psychoanalysis and developmental psychology.

Developmental psychology and psychoanalysis have many points of convergence, and none perhaps so evident or urgent as the intergenerational transmission of attachment patterns. This is, of course, a topic that commanded the interest of both Sigmund and Anna Freud, as they pondered the influence of early relationship experiences on later development (e.g., Freud, 1940a [1938]) across generations, and the central role of defence mechanisms in personality (ego) formation and functioning (A. Freud, 1936). Their incisive theorizing was based on clinical and observational evidence. In contrast, more contemporary developmental research, inspired by psychoanalytic object relations theories, has provided empirical evidence of intergenerational patterns of attachment (Fonagy, Steele & Steele, 1991; Steele, Steele & Fonagy, 1996; Van IJzendoorn, 1995).

This work proceeded because of the pioneering and painstaking observations of Mary Ainsworth, who identified patterns of attachment in the defensive behaviour (or relative lack thereof) of 1-year old infants (Ainsworth, Blehar, Waters & Wall, 1978). Links to the attachment patterns of their parents were first reported by Main, Kaplan, and Cassidy (1985) via their detailed study of transcriptions made of interviews with parents about their attachment history. Most importantly, and remarkably, some parents spoke about their family histories, and the meaning of these relationship experiences, in ways that suggested incoherence founded on rigid and restricted defence mechanisms, while others spoke in ways that conveyed mature defence mechanisms and insight. This latter group (whose interviews were called "autonomous/secure") showed spontaneity, humour, and a capacity to reflect on experience and derive meaning that conveyed a valuing of attachment. By contrast, two other groups of adult speakers were identified, whose interviews were called either "dismissing/insecure" or "preoccupied/insecure". The dismissing group showed a consistent reliance on primitive defences, such as denial, avoidance, and isolation of affect, and were generally inclined towards minimizing awareness of negative affect. The preoccupied group showed a reliance on a different group of primitive defences, including fighting (enduring anger) (A. Freud, 1936); they were generally inclined towards maximizing awareness of past hurts, and recriminations abounded. A separate and troubling set of speech responses was evident among some speakers who had experienced significant past loss or trauma and could not speak about these experiences in an ordered way, being at the same time aware of the pain and trauma yet also unable to assign it to the past. These may be people whose characteristic mode of responding to relationship concerns was otherwise autonomous, dismissing, or preoccupied, but who may be particularly vulnerable to a pattern of chronic grief deemed "unresolved with respect to past loss or trauma".

This unresolved group has been found to be highly common in clinical groups (typically more than 60%; see, e.g., Wallis & Steele, 2001), and substantially less frequent (circa 20%) in low-risk community samples (Van IJzendoorn, 1995). These findings are thus of great clinical concern, not only because of the profound distress in the adult with unresolved loss or trauma, but also because of the disorganizing and disorienting effect unresolved parents appear to have on their children (Solomon & George, 1999). In infancy, children of mothers with unresolved loss are prone to show extreme fearful responses, including freezing, hiding, and other primitive self-protective gestures (Main & Hesse, 1990; Main & Solomon, 1990). Once symbolic processes become established and basic language skills are present, children of mothers unresolved with regard to loss or trauma show extreme aggression in their play, as well as controlling or role-reversed behaviour in their interactions with their mothers—this takes the form of placing the parent in a childlike position and then administering either punitive or caregiving actions towards the infantilized parent. In Anna Freudian terms, this is "turning passive into active".

Widely used and previously validated methods for observing these intergenerational patterns include the Adult Attachment Interview (for parents) and various versions of the Attachment Story-Completion Task first reported by Bretherton, Ridgeway, and Cassidy in 1990. Of course, this later story-completion task is a tried and true friend of the child analyst at the Anna Freud Centre or Yale Child Study Center, whose toolbox has long contained human and animal doll figures, used by the analyst interested in how these figures help the child reveal their inner thoughts and feelings, wishes, hopes, and fears. This essential child-analytic aim has been provided an empirical anchor in little more than a decade-old wave of research papers, chapters, and most recently a book about the attachment story-completion method (Emde, Wolf, & Oppenheim, 2003). This literature, to which we have contributed, has yielded fresh and compelling evidence of intergenerational patterns of attachment in low-risk (e.g., Steele, Steele, et al., 2003) and high-risk samples (e.g., Hodges, Steele, Hillman, Henderson, & Kaniuk, 2003; Steele, Hodges, Kaniuk, Hillman, & Henderson, 2003).

The novel feature of our new evidence is the fact that Adult Attachment Interviews have been collected from parents who have no biological connection to their recently adopted children, whose attachment story completions have been shown to relate systematically to the speech patterns of their new parents (see Steele, Hodges, et al., 2003). This work showed that intense aggression in children's story completions obtained three months into placement was related to insecure/

dismissing and insecure/preoccupied Adult Attachment Interviews (AAIs) collected prior to placement. We also showed that emotional themes in children's doll play linked to unresolved mourning in a parent, such as the parent appearing childlike, were also observed for this recently adopted, late-placed sample. Notably, prior to adoption by the parents under study, the children in our study had the kinds of experiences Goldstein, Freud, and Solnit (1973) believed indicated grievous failures or provision, including severe and sustained abuse and neglect. Therefore, our interest in collecting AAIs from the prospective parents was simply to observe individual differences in the parents' attachment patterns, so that we could subsequently observe the children as they accommodated to the adoptive placement, with a view to identifying which parent factors may accelerate the desired outcome of successful adaptation by the child. Our administration of the story-completion task three months into placement was aimed to provide us with a baseline assessment of the children's attachment profile, for subsequent comparison with later assessments one year and two years into placement.

At the same time, we were aware that if we observed associations between AAIs of the adoptive parents and emotional themes in the children's story completions, we would have novel evidence pointing to the social (as opposed to biological) transmission of attachment across generations—something that has been hotly disputed in the developmental literature (see van IJzendoorn, 1995, and the debate engendered by Fox's reply in the same issue of the *Psychological Bulletin*). Thus, we were surprised, but pleased from a psychoanalytic perspective, to have observed that the AAIs from the adoptive parents we were studying had an immediate emotional effect (within three months of placement) upon their newly adopted children's story completions. The central question in this chapter is: how should we understand this "immediate emotional effect"?

We consider below the extent to which the previously reported (Steele, Steele, et al., 2003) intergenerational match between maternal AAIs and their adopted children's story completions was subject to an intervening influence—namely, the adoptive mothers' developing representations of their newly placed children and themselves as parents. We explore this possibility below by first comparing the attachment representations of these adoptive mothers' past family histories (as measured by the AAI) with their representations of attachment in their present (3-month-old) adoptive family context (as measured by the Parent Development Interview or PDI). We then consider whether the PDI could be said to mediate or moderate the influence of the AAI on the child's inner world, as indexed by the story-completion task.

Method

Sample

The sample in this study consist of 43 mothers who had a total of 61 children placed with them. The children ranged in age from 4 to 8 years, with a mean of 6 years. Of the sample of children, 43% were boys, and 85% were white. The children had all suffered serious adversity, including neglect, physical abuse, and sexual abuse. The number of carers they had experienced ranged from 2 to 18 different placements. Five children were placed with single adopters, and the rest were placed within the context of a married couple. The mean age of the mothers was 40 years.

The Adult Attachment Interview

The Adult Attachment Interview is structured entirely around the topic of attachment, principally the individuals' relationship to their mother and father (and/or to alternative caregivers) during childhood. Interviewees are asked both to describe their relationship with their parents during childhood, and to provide specific memories to support global evaluations. The interviewer asks directly about childhood experiences of rejection, being upset, ill, and hurt, as well as loss, abuse, and separations. In addition, subjects are asked to offer explanations for their parents' behaviour, and to describe the current relationship with their parents and the influence they consider their childhood experiences to have had upon their adult personality.

Adult patterns of attachment, identifiable in spoken (recorded and transcribed) responses to the Adult Attachment Interview, refer to different strategies adults rely on when faced with the task of making sense of their childhood relations with parents or caregivers. The signal features of the autonomous strategy are coherence and a strong valuing of attachment. The following is an excerpt from an interview collected from one of the mothers in the sample under study. The pre-placement AAI was ultimately classified autonomous/secure, with evidence for this judgement contained in the fresh, coherent, and genuine speech below:

> "I can remember" [that he was "caring" yet "at times distant"] "because he worked very long hours so mostly I imagine he wasn't round but the example is once when I was ill and it was in the middle of the night and it must have been winter. We didn't have any central heating, so it was a really cold house and I just remember him doing this thing of like he'd get the iron and ironed my sheets so the bed would be warm when I laid down in it so in that sense he was kind of like he seemed to know what you wanted and did little things like that it and it felt like you didn't have to tell to do things, so it's the sense in which I felt like he understood me."

The dismissing and preoccupied patterns each represent different forms of incoherence arising out of negative attachment experiences that appear to not have been integrated evenly into the adult's sense of self. The dismissing strategy leads to global evaluations of a good or normal childhood that cannot be supported by relevant memories. The preoccupied strategy leads to global evaluations of a difficult childhood that are accompanied by an overabundance of memories and affects from childhood and adulthood that lead the speaker to express current feelings of anger, or a sense of resignation to difficulties that cannot be overcome. Finally, the unresolved pattern—which may be present in an otherwise dismissing, preoccupied, or autonomous interview—is evident when an adult shows signs of ongoing grief and disorientation concerning some past loss or trauma. Narratives that are assigned a classification of unresolved with respect to loss and/or trauma include an excessive attention to detail when discussing loss, delayed bereavement reactions, slips in the monitoring of speech, and incoherent contradictions—that is, speaking of the dead person as if still alive.

Beyond the 65% of interviews from non-clinical samples that merit the description of organized, integrated, and autonomous/secure, two insecure patterns are noted. Both of these insecure patterns reveal difficulties with integrating past negative attachment experiences into a current and balanced state of mind concerning attachment. Some of these interviews err on the side of minimizing past difficulties with one or both parents (circa 20% of the non-clinical population), and are thus classified as insecure/dismissing; other interviews err on the side of maximizing and becoming entangled with past attachment difficulties and are thus classified as insecure/preoccupied. In the former "dismissing" case, the speaker seems inexorably focused *consciously* on positive or normal aspects of experience, to the exclusion of what is probably (*unconsciously recognized as*) a much more diverse and negative set of actual experiences. In the latter "preoccupied" case, the speaker seems angrily or passively gripped by past relationship difficulties that intrude upon current thoughts about relationships and are accompanied by confusing and difficult-to-control negative feelings. While this pattern is observed only about 15% of the time in non-clinical samples (van IJzendoorn, 1995), the proportion of interview responses fitting this preoccupied pattern swells to over 50% when clinical psychiatric populations have been assessed (van IJzendoorn & Bakermans-Kranenburg, 1996).

It is a remarkably positive sign when a speaker demonstrates that past trauma has been resolved. Indeed, in the non-clinical population, where childhood experiences have involved trauma, it is not uncommon for the speaker to convey a sense of having moved beyond the fear they felt so often as a child. Additionally, such speakers are capable of progressing towards understanding, though not necessarily forgiving, *caregiving* figure(s) who once perpetrated abuse against them. In these circumstances, the interview often reveals a robust sense of self, interpersonal awareness, and valuing of attachment, so that one can say that the adult who was abused is not likely to become an abuser. Such resilience invariably emerges out of the individual discovering one or more secure bases or refuges beyond the abusive relationship, such as may be provided by an extended family member, spouse, or therapist.

In the current study, the 43 mothers (for whom AAI data was available) adopted 61 children. Of the mothers' interviews, 31 (71%) were judged autonomous/secure, 10 (23%) judged insecure/dismissing, and 2 (5%) judged insecure/preoccupied. Of the 43 interviews, 9 (21%) were judged unresolved with respect to past loss or trauma. This distribution of secure, dismissing, preoccupied, and unresolved mothers is very much in line with samples of non-clinical populations (Van IJzendoorn & Bakersman-Kranenburg, 1996). Notably, with respect to those interviews judged unresolved, 2 were otherwise autonomous/secure, 5 otherwise insecure/dismissing, and 2 otherwise insecure/preoccupied. The first author classified all 43 interviews, without knowledge of the Parent Development Interview or Story Stem Battery results (see below). The sixth author independently classified 11 interviews, and there was 100% agreement with the first author on these cases, which included 5 interviews judged unresolved.

For the most part, the sample of mothers mirrors the frequency of distributions of Adult Attachment Interviews found in the non-clinical population. However, there is a significantly higher proportion of secure mothers represented in the adoption sample. While not surprising, this is very pleasing, as it offers implicit evidence of the careful work of the social workers who undertook the assessment of the adopters, as the majority fall into the secure category. There were still some 18% falling into the dismissing classification. However, this classification has as one its hallmark features higher levels of idealization, which may have sounded convincingly positive to the social workers. Also, given the specific nuances in speech that are required to be classified as unresolved with regard to past trauma, these would not necessarily present as problematic in narratives discussing childhood experiences as explored by the social worker.

The Story Stem Assessment Profile

The child assessments asked the children to respond to a set of story stems (Story Stem Assessment Profile; see Hodges & Steele, 2000; Hodges, Steele, Hillman Henderson, & Kaniuk, 2003), where they were given the beginning of a "story" highlighting everyday family scenarios, each containing an inherent dilemma. Next, children were asked "to show me and tell me what happens next". This allows an assessment of the child's expectations and perceptions of family roles, attachments, and relationships, without asking the child direct questions about their own family, adoptive or biological, that might cause them undue conflict or anxiety. It also has the advantage for younger children of allowing both verbal and nonverbal means of communication. This is important as it allows children to display memories and expectations that are not part of verbally based memory, which they may be anxious about putting into words.

The set of rating scales we developed for scoring the children's story completions looks closely at both what the child says and what the child does in response to the emotionally charged story-beginnings. The set of stems includes five originally designed by Jill Hodges in the context of her work assessing abused children as part of the Child Care Consultation Team at Great Ormond Street Hospital. Eight additional stems were selected from the MacArthur Story Stem Battery (MSSB) (Bretherton, Ridgeway, & Cassidy, 1990; Oppenheim, Emde, & Warren, 1997), which was devised for much wider research uses and has been employed primarily with non-clinical populations. The stems are always administered in the same order, using both a standard doll "family" and animal figures that appear in the Story Stem Assessment Profile (SSAP). The assessment is designed for use with children between the ages of 4 and 8 and generally takes about one hour to complete. Interviews were video- and audiotaped and the tapes transcribed, producing a verbal "script" consisting of what the child and interviewer had said and "stage directions" describing what the child had done—that is, the nonverbal narrative. The rating manual (Hodges, Steele, Hillman, & Henderson, 2002) provides detailed criteria and benchmark examples; raters trained on this system for research purposes achieve good levels of reliability. (For details including a protocol for the SSAP, summaries of the eight MSSB stems, and reliability indices, see Hodges et al., 2003a, 2003b.) To exemplify the narrative story stem process, we provide an example of one late-adopted child's story stem response to a story entitled "Bikes", from the SSAP battery (Hodges et al., 2002). The story involves the Playmobil figures of Child 1, Child 2 (same-sex friend), Mum, Dad, depicted as follows:

> *In the next story, Child 1 is at home. There's a knock at the door, and it's Child 1's friend (Child 2).*
>
> *Child 2 says: "let's go and play on our bikes!"*
>
> *Child 1 says: "I'll go and ask my Mum"*
>
> *So, s/he went and asked her/his Mum.*
>
> *Child 1: "Mum, can we go and play outside on our bikes?"*
>
> *Mum says: "Yes, but be careful!"*
>
> *We have to pretend the bikes.*
>
> *They went really fast on their bikes and they went "wheeeeee" (dramatize wild bike riding), but "oh"—what happened (show Child 1 fallen on ground with friend standing)*
>
> *Show me and tell me what happens now?*
>
> *[Note: "C" denotes child, "I" denotes interviewer, and parentheses denote child's actions.]*

C: "He cries and then . . ." (puts friend doll on the other side of the wall and start banging both dolls on the wall) "They're fighting!"

I: "They're fighting? Are they fighting with one another?"

C: (child nods) (child keeps banging dolls on wall, knocks wall over)

I: "And what happen then?"

C: "The two of them are bleeding."

I: "The two of them are bleeding."

C: (child puts children under the wall) "And then Mummy goes" (bangs Mummy on wall) "and then she bleeds . . ."

I: "How did Mummy get hurt?"

C: "She went like . . ." (bangs mother on wall)

I: "Why was she doing that?"

C: "'Cause she wanted to be naughty."

I: "I see . . . so you know when he fell off the bike what happened to him?"

C: "He bleeded."

This story was coded for a range of themes, including parent appearing childlike, and child aggresses—the two themes that are the focus of the results below. A team of graduate students and researchers coded transcriptions of the story stem responses, independently, without knowledge of the interview material collected from the parents. Interrater reliability for "parent appearing childlike" and "child aggresses" was extremely high ($\kappa > .75$ for both codes), and a prevalence of these themes was pronounced across children and stories.

The parent development interview

With the development of the Adult Attachment Interview (Main, Kaplan, & Cassidy, 1985), and the corollary success in moving the assessment of attachment from the coding of behaviour to the level of representation, there have been several interview protocols designed to explore narrative qualities in adults, which convey representations of their children. Each interview aims to assess the qualities of the parent's narrative, along dimensions crucial to the attachment construct. For example, the Caregiving Parent Interview developed by George and Solomon (1989) focuses on secure base representations (which include understanding the child's specific needs and characteristics), (goal-corrected partnership representations which include being able to provide for the child and their needs and preserve their own autonomy), and self-perceived competence. A second group of researchers have developed the Working Model of the Child Interview (Zeanah, Benoit, & Barton, 1986), which is modelled on the Adult Attachment Interview. The interview probes for the parents' reactions during pregnancy, the infant's personality, and characteristic features of the relationship as seen by the parent. The coding assesses, among other things, the richness of perceptions, coherence, care-giving sensitivity. The narratives are then coded, and each interview is ultimately placed in one of three distinct sub-types: balanced, disengaged, distorted. This interview has been used by a range of researchers exploring mothers' representations of their infants in cases of failure to thrive (Benoit et al., 1997) and maternal depression (Wood, Hargreaves, & Marks, 2004), and has shown impressive associations between those mothers providing balanced interviews and positive features in the mother–infant relationship. Another interview stemming from the approach taken in the AAI, and with promising results, is the Parent Development Interview, developed by Arietta Slade with Larry Aber and their colleagues (Aber et al., 1985; Slade, Aber, et al., 1993, 1994). It is this instrument, in modified form (see below), that we relied on to capture the adoptive parents' representations of their newly placed children.

These various interviews may help explain how it is that the parents' state of mind regarding attachment—namely, in terms of their own attachment history—can predict the quality of their child's attachment behaviour towards them. This widely replicated link (e.g., Main, Kaplan, & Cassidy, 1985; Grossman, Pollack, & Golding, 1988; Steele, Steele, & Fonagy, 1996; Ward & Carlson, 1994) between parents' interviews *about their past* and the *present* infant–parent relationship has been termed the "transmission gap", because we lack a detailed understanding of *how* parents are transmitting their autonomy/security, or lack thereof (Van IJzendoorn, 1995). This question is being investigated by several research teams (see Oppenheim, Goldsmith, & Koren-Karie, 2004), and a likely answer lies, at least in part, with investigating the thoughts, feelings, and more global representations parents form and maintain regarding their children.

We were drawn to the interview and coding system first developed by Arietta Slade, Larry Aber, and their team (Aber et al., 1985), as their approach seemed particularly relevant to adoptive parents. Of primary interest was assessing the initial features of the parent's representation of this newly placed child, dimensions of affect, and its regulation. With Kay Henderson leading this endeavour, we slightly modified the protocol to allow for the unique features of our sample and subsequently changed the original coding manual extensively (see Exhibit 1 for a summary of codes in our revised manual; Henderson, Steele, & Hillman, 2001). The Parent Development Interview protocol (Aber et al., 1985), with our slight modifications, poses the following queries to the parent: (a) what the child was like when she/he first arrived; (b) a scenario when they did—and did not—click with the child during the last week; (c) five adjectives that describe the child, with accompanying examples/incidents for each; (d) from what do they derive the most—and least—amount of pleasure in the relationship. The coding is organized around features relating to how parents sees themselves in the role of parent, their representation of the child, and then several codes originally developed by Charlie Zeanah (Zeanah, Benoit, & Barton, 1986), which include assessing the richness of perceptions and the global features of the narrative, such as the central construct of coherence. We modified the coding, establishing a 4-point scale with operational definitions and anchored points with scores of 1 generally indicating paucity of a construct and 4 indicating high degrees. We included a scale for rating reflective functioning and added other variables of special interest to this group. One such code is "level of child focus". Here we can operationalize where the motivation behind pursuing the adoption lies: for example, to facilitate this particular child's development, to satisfy a wish to become a family, to help consolidate a marital relationship, and so on. Another important dimension included specifically for this sample concerns both the level of, and satisfaction with, emotional support. Given the extensive knowledge of the intense challenges these children bring to their new families (Brodzinsky, 1987; Quinton, Rushton, Dance, & Mayes, 1998; Triseliotis & Russell, 1984), we were convinced that this would be a key issue to explore. A related feature was our wish to explore the parents' level of disappointment and despair in the way the new relationship was developing. For example, in the Parent Development Interview, when asked what she likes least about her newly placed 6-year-old son, one mother said the following:

> "The tantrums have been going on and on and that's the hard bit of it, because it's continuous, every day, I haven't had a day's let-up. Oh, on one day, I think, what a really good day I had with him, and I thought, well, you know, sort of a bit of good and a bit

EXHIBIT 1. Summary of codes for modified experience of parenting coding[a] used with the Parent Development Interview protocol[b]

Parent affective experience codes

Code

1. anger:
   a. degree
   b. expression
2. need for support:
   a. level of need
   b. satisfaction with support
3. guilt
4. joy/pleasure
5. competence
6. confidence
7. level of child focus
8. disappointment/despair
9. warmth
10. attachment promotion
11. hostility

Child affective experience codes

1. child aggression/anger
2. child happiness
3. child controlling/manipulating
4. child affectionate
5. child rejecting

Global codes

1. parent reflection on relationship
2. coherence
3. richness of perceptions
4. description of relationship

List adjectives given:

5. parent discipline style

[a] Henderson, Steele, & Hillman, 2001. [b] Aber et al., 1985.

> of bad. I could, you know—if it were like this every day, I could cope, it wouldn't be so bad. And then there are times when I have been so down and depressed about it all, you know, I just don't think I could go on. It's meant to be a bit easier than this. I know that having children isn't easy, but you know, just thinking, why does it always got to be so difficult. . . . And not because, you know, I think I wish we hadn't adopted, I sometimes think 'Gosh, I wish . . .'; God, that's sounds horrible, but my social worker said it was a natural thing to think. I sometimes think, why did it have to be John, with the problems we've had?"

The despair and disappointment revealed in this small interview segment is obvious and represents one of the more intense examples we encountered.

At the other end of the spectrum, we met with a number of adoptive mothers (the majority) who were able to convey their enjoyment and level of child focus in the following way. Consider this adoptive mother's account of a time she "really clicked in the last week" with her 6-year-old son:

> "We were gardening yesterday, and I found this big, fat green bug in the soil and brought it over for him to see it, and he really liked it. And he likes woodlice, which I can't stand, and he said, 'Feel it on your hand, Mummy, it's all tickly.' And so I let him put a woodlice on my hand, which was against my better judgement, and he really liked the fact that it was running all over me."

This short example manages to convey a positive and secure maternal state of mind, wherein the mother convincingly accesses to a pertinent example of the easy way in which she puts her recently adopted son's needs at the forefront of the interaction.

To follow up on our scoring of the Parent Development Interview narratives, we found impressive psychometric validation for our multi-dimensional approach (Henderson, Steele, & Hillman, 2000). The wide range of 31 rating scales, aimed at tapping all relevant aspects of being an adoptive parent, were applied to the PDI transcripts by a team of coders (kept blind to other data about the children and their parents). They achieved high levels of reliability with one another (r range from .54 to 1.00, with a mean of .75 and a median of .74).

We then subjected the 31 rating scale scores stemming from the PDIs collected at the 3-month assessment to a factor analysis aimed at identifying the latent structure of the maternal responses. Three main factors emerged: positive/reflective parenting, negative/angry parenting, and despair or lack of satisfaction with placement. (a) The PDI rating scales that comprised the items of the positive/reflective composite included the following variables: parents' global reflectiveness on the relationship, the overall richness of perceptions of the child, global coherence, parents' level of child focus, parental warmth and parental joy/pleasure, Chronbach's alpha = .89, accounting for 16% of the variance in PDI ratings. (b) The negative/angry composite comprised the following variables: parent (reporting) showing affection (and believing) child (is) not affectionate, child rejecting, negative global description of relationship, and (confidently reporting) ease of mothering child (alpha = .83, accounting for 13% of the variance in PDI ratings). (c) The despair/lack of satisfaction composite was comprised of parental need for social support, lack of satisfaction with support received, and parental disappointment (alpha = .71, accounting for 12% of the variance in PDI ratings). Together, then, these primary three factors accounted for more than 40% of the variance in PDI ratings and were comprised of coherent, consistent, and reliable sets of rating scales.

Results

Results comprise two sections: (a) correlations between AAI classifications obtained pre-placement from the adoptive mothers and their PDI factor scores three months into placement; (b) identification of story-completion themes emerging from the children with significant correlations to *both* maternal AAIs and PDIs (where these variables were overlapping) with follow-on consideration, in regression analyses, of the possibly mediating role of PDI factors in the link between AAIs and story-completion themes.

Correlations between AAIs and PDIs

Table 6.1 displays the correlations between maternal representations of attachment (AAI classifications) pre-placement and their emerging representations of their adoptive children, and the experience of parenting them (PDI factors) identified at three months.

Table 6.1 reveals a substantial and significant set of correlations between the adoptive mothers' AAIs pre-placement and the factor scores reliably derived from scoring their interview responses to the

Table 6.1. Correlations between pre-placement AAIs and post-placement PDIs

	AAI classifications	
PDI factors	*insecure vs autonomous/secure*	*unresolved vs resolved (re past loss or trauma)*
positive	.31*	–.31*
negative	–.18	.29*
despairing	–.27*	.37**

* 2-sided $p < .05$; **2-sided $p < .01$

Parenthood Development Interview at three months into placement. The most outstanding of these concerns the observed link between unresolved mourning regarding past loss or trauma in the pre-placement AAI and higher scores on the despair/lack of satisfaction with the adoption three months into placement, $r = .37$, p (2-sided) $< .01$. Unresolved status on the AAI was also correlated with higher negative/angry scores, $r = .29$, p (2-sided) $< .05$, and lower positive/reflective scores, $r = .31$, p (2-sided) $< .05$, on the PDI three months into placement.

Table 6.1 also reveals that adoptive mothers presenting with an AAI classified autonomous/secure, as opposed to dismissing/insecure or preoccupied/insecure, were correlated significantly with higher factor scores on the positive/reflective dimension in the PDI, $r = .31$, p (2-sided) $< .05$. Autonomy/security pre-placement was also linked to lower scores on the despair/lack of satisfaction dimension three months into the adoptive placement, $r = -.27$, p (2-sided) $< .05$.

Do adoptive mothers' PDI responses mediate or moderate the link between their pre-placement AAIs and their children's story completions at 3 months?

Here our interest was in identifying features of the adopted children's inner emotional life at three months that linked with both maternal interview measures, such that questions concerning possible mediation of post-adoption representations by the mothers could be put to the data. The candidate list could be narrowed down to a provocative list of 8 emotional themes (indicating intense aggression) in the children's stories that linked with insecurity in the mothers' pre-placement AAIs, and 5 emotional themes (indicating role reversal and fear of abandonment) that linked with unresolved mourning in the mothers' pre-placement AAIs—findings to which we have previously drawn attention (Steele, Hodges, et al., 2003).

Intense aggression from children (in the doll play) was significantly correlated, both with insecurity in the maternal AAIs, $r = .25$ (2-sided) $p < .05$, and with lower scores on the positive/reflective dimension of the PDI, $r = -.26$ (2-sided) $p < .05$, and higher scores on the despair/lack of satisfaction dimension, $r = .29$ (2-sided) $p < .05$. Given that both these PDI factors were significantly correlated with the AAI, we proceeded to consider whether the PDI factors were moderating or mediating the effect of AAI insecurity on this emotional theme of intense aggression from children in the story completions at three months. Tables 6.2 and 6.3 present the regression results testing for mediation and moderation.

For Table 6.2, we entered into the linear regression model "child aggresses" as the dependent variable, and in the first block we entered PDI factor "positive/reflective", with a resulting F-value of 4.1 ($df = 1{,}61$), $p < .05$. At this first step $r^2 = .06$. We then entered AAI "insecurity versus security" in the second block, and while r^2 increased to .09, the F-change = 2.1, $df = 1{,}60$, $p = .16$ pointing to a non-significant increase in variance accounted for. The summary statistics for the models with PDI positive/reflective parenting on its own, and with positive/reflective parenting and AAI security together, are shown in Table 6.2. Notably, the regression summary table indicates that neither PDI (low) positive/reflective parenting nor AAI insecurity remain significant when they are in the model together. This suggests that the partial overlap between AAI security and PDI positive/reflective parenting suppresses the significance of either variable on its own. In other words, each of these variables is moderating or lessening the

Table 6.2. Regression model predicting "child aggresses" in children's story completions at three months from maternal PDI positive and AAI security

Block	*Factor*	*Standardized beta*	*t*	*p*
1	PDI positive	–.25	–2.0	.047
2	PDI positive	–.19	–1.5	.14
	AAI autonomy/security	–.19	–1.4	.16

Table 6.3. Regression model predicting "child aggresses" in children's story completions at three months from maternal PDI despairing and AAI security responses

Block	*Factor*	*Standardized beta*	*t*	*p*
1	PDI despair/lack of satisfaction	.28	2.3	.025
2	PDI despair/lack of satisfaction	.23	1.9	.169
	AAI autonomy/security	–.18	–1.5	.151

effect of the other, suggesting a sufficient number of cases where while the mother's AAI was insecure, she had developed a positive/reflective parenting stance by three months, as well as a similar group of mothers whose AAIs were secure, but who had not developed such a positive stance by three months into the placement.

For Table 6.3. we entered into the linear regression model "child aggresses" as the dependent variable, and in the first block we entered PDI factor "despair/lack of satisfaction", with a resulting F-value of 5.3 ($df = 1{,}61$), $p < .05$. At this first step, $r^2 = .08$. We then entered AAI "insecurity versus security" in the second block, and while r^2 increased to .11, the F-change = 2.1, $df = 1{,}60$, $p = .15$, pointing to a non-significant increase in variance accounted for. The summary statistics for the models with PDI on its own, and with PDI and AAI together, are shown in Table 6.3. Notably, the regression summary table indicates that the AAI insecurity is no longer making a significant contribution to the prediction of "child aggresses" ($p = .15$), whereas PDI "despair/lack of satisfaction" is slightly reduced in significance to the level of a trend ($p = .07$). Overall, the regression results point to a large mediating role for PDI "despair/lack of satisfaction" intervening between AAI insecurity and the emotional theme of "child aggresses" in the story completions. In other words, most of the mothers with high scores on "despair/lack of satisfaction", whose children scored highly on the "child aggresses" theme were also insecure on the pre-placement AAI. Thus, after taking into account the concurrent maternal variable of PDI "despair", the pre-placement maternal AAI does not make an independent contribution to the prediction of "child aggression" emotion themes at three months.

The final set of results pertains to the issue of unresolved mourning concerning past loss and trauma, as evident in the pre-placement

Table 6.4. Regression model predicting role reversing themes of "placing parent in a childlike position" in children's story completions at three months from maternal PDI despairing and AAI unresolved responses

Block	*Factor*	*Standardized beta*	*t*	*p*
1	PDI despair/lack of satisfaction	.38	3.3	.002
2	PDI despair/lack of satisfaction	.28	2.3	.025
	AAI unresolved mourning	.28	2.3	.029

AAIs. Here we explored the extent to which the significant link between unresolved memory and the child emotion theme of role reversal or "placing the parent in a childlike role" was moderated by despair/lack of satisfaction in the PDI at three months. The relevant regression results are shown in Table 6.4.

For the results portrayed in Table 6.4, the presence of role reversal themes, as indicated by the children's depiction of "parents in a childlike position", was entered as the dependent variable. In the first block, parental "despair/lack of satisfaction" in response to the PDI at three months was entered, $F = 10.6$, $df = 1{,}61$, $p = .002$, with 15% of the dependent variable accounted for. In the second block, unresolved mourning in the pre-placement AAI was entered, F change $= 5.0$, $df = 1{,}60$, $p = .029$, with an additional 6% of variance in the dependent variable accounted for. Notably, Table 6.4 highlights how both the pre-placement AAI variable and the PDI variable remain significant in the final model. Thus, of all the AAI variables associated with story-completion themes at three months, the issue of unresolved mourning regarding past loss or trauma stands out as uniquely predictive of a child depicting the parent as childlike and, correspondingly, in need of care or discipline.

Discussion

Three patterns of results deserve consideration here. (a) We have found evidence for a link between adoptive mothers' representations of their attachment history (AAI), and their thoughts and feelings concerning their newly adopted children (PDI). (b) We have found a link between a mother's representations of attachment stemming from her own childhood experiences and her adopted children's story completions assessed within the first three months of placement. (c) Finally, we have results highlighting how the PDI moderated and mediated the influence of the maternal AAI upon one of the children's thematic responses to the story-completion task at three months ("child aggresses") but not another ("child presents parent as childlike"). We discuss these findings in turn below.

The results presented here show, for the first time, that a mothers' thoughts and feelings about adopting a previously maltreated child can be predicted by their pre-placement thoughts and feelings about their own attachment history. This aspect of the findings provided validation of our approach to coding mothers' representations of their children, even in the very early stages of a newly forming attachment relationship. Mothers who provide coherent, organized, reflective narratives in response to the Adult Attachment Interview bring some of these strategies to the discussion of their newly placed adoptive child and are less likely to be overwhelmed with feelings of anger or despair. These findings highlight what may be viewed as a window into the adult's internal working model, and that organizes both attachment representations of their own previous attachment experiences as children, and also in the new role of caregiver to an adopted child. Clues as to what the child brings to this new relationship are expressed in their narratives and play in response to the story-stem assessment.

That the majority of mothers were classified as autonomous/secure, which correlated highly with positive/reflective parenting, is all the more important given the children's adverse histories. All the children in this study have endured maltreatment and have experienced repeated changes of caregivers, often without much forewarning. The task at hand for them is to "attach" to a new and hopefully "forever" parent. These children then bring with them not only the many complicated representations of attachment figures from the failed first relationship with biological parent(s), but also from subsequent experiences with extended family and/or foster carers, which, while possibly benign or even positive, were ultimately deemed non-optimal as a permanent solution. Furthermore, these children lack some of the most basic features normally present in infant–parent relationships—namely, the physical and social predisposition that characterize newly born offspring across the species: small and attractive features, large head-to-body ratios, and big, endearing eyes (Hrdy, 1999). Instead, the adoptive parent has the task of forging ahead with an older child, who may not possess these attachment-facilitating qualities and may display, instead, many challenging behaviours. Still, we found that mothers who provide narratives characterized by coherence and flexible strategies in evaluating their attachment histories are ready to experience their newly placed child in more hopeful, joyful, child-focused and reflective ways.

These mothers are in contrast to those who provide Adult Attachment Interview narratives rated insecure and/or unresolved with respect to trauma. In those interviews classified as insecure/dismissing, descriptions and evaluations of childhood experiences are marked by idealization of caregivers and reluctance or inability to provide compelling evidence for positive features of their purportedly enjoyable childhood. When these mothers are in the new situation of parenting a previously maltreated child, the strategy of pushing the negative aspects of relationships to one side seems to falter. These parents are most apt to describe the new relationship in disappointing and despairing terms. This finding may provide us with strategic empirical support for providing extra help to these parents who, from the very earliest days of becoming adoptive parents, are suggesting they require it.

Further evidence of which group might most benefit from support is provided by the regression findings predicting the "child aggresses" theme at three months into placement. Here we saw that the link between insecurity in the AAI and the "child aggresses" theme was mediated or carried by despair/lack of satisfaction in the PDI. In other words, insecurity in the AAI of an adoptive mother represents a risk factor for her newly placed child, but primarily because some insecure mothers were vulnerable to feelings of despair and lack of satisfaction early in the placement. This result highlights the utility of the Parent Development Interview for identifying adoptive parents who are reflective, coherent, and already (in the first three months) deriving much pleasure from the immense parenting task they have taken on.

In contrast, parents who provide a pre-placement AAI narrative that contains perturbations that give rise to the classification of unresolved with regard to trauma begin this newly forming attachment relationship with a markedly less optimal outlook. This leads on to the main finding that two thematic responses from the children at three months into placement in their story completions linked up with both the pre-placement AAI and the three month PDI provided by the mothers. From a wide range of themes identified in the children's story completions, it is worth asking why two themes alone related to *both* these pre- and post-placement maternal interviews. These themes were "child aggresses" and "child places parent in a childlike role". Anna Freud's account of the ego's mechanisms of defence (A. Freud, 1936) is relevant here, as both these themes can be seen to indicate a turning of "passive into active"—that is, a strategy where the child is depicted as aggressive is most often linked to the portrayal of the child doll figure being active, powerful, and certainly taking charge. By the same token, portraying adults in a childlike role, as weepy, needy, or naughty and thereby deserving punishment, were often characteristic of the code "child places parent in a childlike role". It is understandable for these children to rely on this self-protective and self-enhancing strategy. However, it is remarkable that this defensive position was significantly less in evidence if the adoptive mother lacked despair and was more satisfied with the adoption (in the PDI at three months) *or* was resolved with respect to past loss or trauma (in AAI pre-placement). The final regression analysis predicting "child portrays parent in a childlike role" highlighted an independent contribution made by both these interview-based measures, with no evidence that the post-adoption thoughts and feelings carried the effect of unresolved mourning picked up in the pre-placement interview. This suggests that some of the adopted children were hypersensitive to the sad and angry feelings of their adoptive parents in ways that strengthened their strategy of turning passive into active in the story-completion task; in some cases these children had adoptive mothers who were unresolved with respect to past loss or trauma, and in other cases their adoptive mothers were simply those who felt prey to disappointment and despair early in the placement.

The theme of "placing the parent in a childlike role" is significant not only as it reflects a turning passive into active, but is also suggestive of a strategy relied upon by children with a history of attachment disorganization, namely a controlling stance that is either punitive or caregiving (Solomon & George, 1999). This is not surprising, as it is likely that the original primary attachment for the adopted children in this study would have been classified as disorganized. And the strategy employed by some of the children in the face of distress was maintained in the new attachment relationship, as evidenced in the story completions.

Further research and clinical interventions are needed to promote and encourage reflective/positive security-enhancing characteristics in adoptive parents, given the demonstrated beneficial effects this has on their children's emotional development. It is hoped that the interview measures deployed successfully in this study may come into wider use in the applied fields that were of so much interest to Anna Freud, Albert Solnit, and Joseph Goldstein. This might lead to evidence-based strategies for providing support for those involved in the complicated social and judicial task of deciding how to provide for a child's best interests when birth parents, and perhaps the public care system, have previously failed the child.

Commentary

Arietta Slade

The Anna Freud Centre and the Child Study Center have long been linked by many friendships and rich collaborations, and—perhaps most important—by a set of profoundly shared beliefs about the development of children and their families. Many of these beliefs are beautifully reflected in this complex, integrative chapter by Miriam Steele and her colleagues.

Adoption has been practiced in one form or another since the beginning of time. Across many species, adults regularly adopt parentless, abandoned, or unwanted offspring, so that they, too, can survive (and, in many cases, so that the parents themselves can raise children). For human parents and children, this particular form of parenting raises a number of complex issues. We can see this at the general, epidemiological level: adopted individuals make up a higher proportion of referrals for psychiatric and other forms of mental health treatment than do any other group. We can also see this clinically at the individual and family level: many child clinicians, particularly those of us interested in attachment, are consulted regularly about adoptions that have gone badly—often, these are late adoptions such as those Steele describes. Adoption also makes its way into the psychotherapeutic situation in a number of more subtle ways. In over 25 years of clinical practice, I have found that adoption has been a crucial aspect of the self-experience of every adopted individual with whom I have worked. The same is true of adoptive parents, who routinely struggle with the complexities of their feelings in relation to adopting and with their anxieties about the child's genetic (and cultural) heritage. And the adults I have worked with who long ago gave up their children for adoption continue to be haunted by complex feelings that usually include guilt or shame (and some combination of fear and hope that they will be found by these children).

Despite its commonality and inherent complexity in terms of developmental risk and vulnerability, adoption has—outside the dangerous and radical work of "attachment therapists"—been largely ignored within the clinical and research literatures. The reasons for this may have to do with researchers and practitioners being loath to shed negative light on a practice so crucial to the survival of so many children and to the potential happiness of so many adoptive parents. Regardless of the complex motivations for such ignorance, clinicians and parents are vastly uninformed about how to think about and manage the complexities of adoption, which are—needless to say—quite problematic. The popular press is full of stories of adult adoptees learning—after years of struggle—the sad truth of their own genetic heritage, truths that might have greatly changed the way their difficulties were managed and understood in childhood. Also common, sadly, are stories of adoptions gone "wrong", with children failing to develop sustaining and positive attachments to their adoptive parents.

This failure to fully study adoption must be addressed from the ground up, and in a variety of contexts. Steele's groundbreaking work—the first of its kind—sets the gold standard for such investigations. Located at the intersection of psychoanalytic and attachment theory, her research is broadly aimed at investigating the relationship between the parent's state of mind in relation to attachment—in this particular study, the *mother's* state of mind—and the adopted child's experience of himself and others. The particular research described in this chapter, however, is aimed at examining how the *internal experience of parenting*—that is, the mother's representation of the child and of their relationship—is linked both to her own attachment experiences and to the child's sense of self and others.

The study of parental representations of the child grows out of recent developments in attachment research. In 1985, Main, Kaplan, and Cassidy (1985) began to examine the impact of parental representations of attachment upon child attachment outcomes. The attachment representations they studied were parental working models of *the parents' own parents*; these were found to predict in a number of meaningful ways to child adaptation and socioemotional development (Main, Kaplan, & Cassidy, 1985). Within a relatively short period, researchers also began to focus on parental representations *of the child*; a number of studies have reported that this variable, while related to adult attachment organization, contributes independently to child outcome (Slade et al., 1999; Slade, Grienenberger, Bernbach, Levy, & Locker, 2005; Zeanah, Benoit, Hirshberg, Barton, & Regan, 1994). This, of course, makes enormous intuitive sense: what a parent thinks and feels about the child is going to affect how she behaves and interacts with him, which is, in turn, going to impact on the way he feels about himself.

Steele's research is aimed at studying the impact of parental representations of the child in a very particular kind of population: late-adopted children who had suffered some form of maltreatment prior to their adoption. These children present a set of unique challenges to their adoptive parents, largely because of the presumptive effects of prior trauma and loss upon their capacity to develop new, more secure relationships with their adoptive parents. These are children who have had an experience akin to (if not in fact) the death of a parent, accompanied by the betrayal and violation inherent in abuse. Many have had multiple and sequential caregivers. From the point of view of the adoptive parent, this is a dangerous mix, and indeed one of the assumptions that initially guided Steele's research investigation was that these factors would play a more significant role than the mother's attachment organization in predicting child outcome.

At the same time, of course, adoptive parents bring their own dynamics into the mix. Adults who adopt older, traumatized children are likely to do so for a variety of reasons, altruism being only one of them, and a number of more complex motives—the most apparent of which is often rescue—motivate parents to "save" such traumatized children. Unfortunately, however, the image of the "rescued" child who would of course be "grateful" for his salvation is often sharply contrasted with the angry, disoriented, and insecure abuse survivor who sometimes suffers from a range of psychological and neurological difficulties that are the result of prior maltreatment. This complex terrain forms the background for the research described here.

Steele's research began with the question of whether a parent's own attachment organization, measured before the adoption has taken place, would have an effect on her experience of the adoption and the developing relationship with her child. Steele then asked whether these two variables—her own state of mind in relation to attachment or her internal affective experience of parenting—might, either together or separately, be predictive of the child's experience of himself and relationships, as measured by the nature and quality of the stories told by the child in response to a story-telling task. In analysing her findings, Steele focuses upon two particular features of the story stem data: the child's expression of aggression, and the presence of role reversal and fear of abandonment in the stories.

In previous research with this population, Steele, Hodges, Kaniuk, Hillman, and Henderson (2003) found that the mother's attachment organization—that is, her own internal working model of attachment—was predictive of differences in these two aspects of her child's story-stem data (child aggression and role reversal). Thus, mothers who were either dismissing or unresolved in relation to attachment had children who were more likely to have children who expressed intense aggression or to take on the parental role in their stories at three months post-placement. Interestingly, only a small proportion of the mothers in her sample were insecure (18% dismissing, 10% unresolved, 0% preoccupied); the great proportion of them (70%) were secure. This initial set of findings (Steele, Hodges, et al., 2003) demonstrated in a dramatic way the relationship between the adoptive mother's inner life—explicitly her openness to forming a secure and organized attachment relationship—upon the child's regulation of emotion and, potentially, of relationships. This finding was surprising for the simple reason that—given the particular vulnerability of the population of adopted children studied—one would have expected the child's history, rather than the mother's state of mind in relation to attachment, to account for the apparent variance in children's self-experience.

Steele and her colleagues then set out to discover whether the parent's developing representation of the child might enhance or mediate this relationship—that is, how would the parent's feelings and thoughts about the child affect the child's own internal experience? They analysed the data in two ways, distinguishing mothers along the secure/insecure dimension on the one hand and along the resolved/unresolved dimension on the other. Both dimensions were predictive of differences in the positive/reflective aspects of the representation, as well as mothers' experience of despair in the relationship. The resolved/unresolved distinction was also predictive of negative representations of the child. Thus, as might be expected given prior research (Slade, Belsky, Aber, & Phelps, 1999), maternal representations of attachment were in meaningful ways predictive of parental representations of the child. The next set of analyses then examined how the parental representation variable might affect the documented relationship between AAI and child story stem outcomes. Interestingly, it played a number of different roles. First, when AAIs were analysed along the secure/insecure dimension, the PDI positive/reflective factor played a significant role in "carrying" the mother's state of mind in relation to attachment into the parental representation of the child. What this means is that the parent's representation of the child—rather than her attachment organization—is what most directly accounted for the child's expression of aggression in the story stems. When this same analysis was repeated for the PDI despair variable, however, the outcome changed: with this variable, the parent's insecurity determines the extent to which she will experience despair in the relationship. Finally, AAIs were analysed along the resolved/unresolved dimension; in this analysis, both unresolved status and parental despair in relation to the child predicted child role reversal in the story stems.

What are we to take away from this complex story? First, it matters a great deal what a mother's own state of mind in relation to attachment is *before* she adopts. But what these data also tell us is that a mother's capacity to form a positive and reflective representation of the relationship *also* matters a great deal and may in some instances occur despite a mother's own insecure attachment status. That is, some mothers will rise to the occasion and find pleasure in their adopted child, despite their own prior attachment experience and organization. The two factors that seem to mitigate most directly against such positive outcomes appear, in this sample, to be a parent's lack of resolution of mourning on the AAI and despair in relation to the child post-adoption.

One of the most heartening things about the data reported in this chapter is the observation that by and large the huge majority of adults in her sample seeking to adopt these hard-to-place children are secure in relation to attachment. This bodes well for the children, obviously, but also says something very positive about the psychological organization of the adults seeking to adopt them. Another heartening aspect of the data is the observation that it is sometimes possible for parents with insecure attachment histories to develop positive representations of their children. The relationship between a mother's attachment organization and her representation of the child is not always lawful and may, indeed, have something to do with the child's own capacities. While not measured in this study, it is important to remember that some children are especially able to connect with their caregivers, even after multiple traumas and losses. Such children might be best positioned to connect in a positive way with an adoptive mother, despite her own insecure attachment organization.

But it is the observation that the parent's representation of the child plays a key role in predicting child outcomes that is—to me—the most compelling part of the story. While adoption agencies can learn to watch for danger signs in prospective adoptive parents, they cannot screen out parents who are insecure in their attachment organization. That is a Machiavellian solution, and one that could not possibly be defended except perhaps in the most extreme situations (which adoption agencies probably do intuitively, in any case). After all, children in everyday life survive insecure parents and, in some instances, thrive despite them. But we can teach professionals working with adoptive families to pay close attention to developing parental representations of the child. The experience of pleasure and the emergence of the capacity to hold the child in mind bode well for the child's outcome, whereas experiences of despair and hopelessness in relation to the child do not. When positive representations are lacking or despair has begun to dominate the relationship, intervention is required.

What Steele's research suggests is that these processes can start to go awry as early as at 3 months. They can go awry because of the impact of the mother's own internal working models of attachment, whose lack of resolution of loss or abuse in her own history makes it difficult for her to regulate the negative and difficult affects that are an inevitable part of parenthood. They can go awry because the mother's experience of the child is quickly distorted by anger, disappointment, and despair. The fact that the effects of parental insecurity and despair can be seen so early in the adoption process suggests the importance of continuing to monitor and screen the evolving adoptee/adoptive parent relationship for at least the first six months after adoption, certainly in those cases of late adoption where there has been evidence of prior maltreatment.

When intervention is required, attachment-based or reflective parenting interventions would seem most appropriate (Grienenberger, et al., 2004; Slade, in press; Slade, Sadler, & Mayes, 2005; Slade, Sadler, de Dios-Kenn, et al., 2005), for, as we can see from the data in this chapter, the parent's representations of attachment and of the relationship play a crucial role in determining the success of the child's placement. Unfortunately, agencies eager to place children, especially maltreated and vulnerable children, appear loath to fully apprise parents of the risks of these adoptions or to monitor the new family's progress in an ongoing way. Parents wanting to adopt vulnerable children are often moved by profound rescue fantasies that are both conscious and unconscious; in many instances, as we see from Steele's data, these complexities take place within the framework of essentially secure and positive attachment representations. When they do not, however, the results can be deleterious to both child and parent.

Optimally, we hope that in the years following an adoption, the initial experience of suddenly *becoming* a family will become background rather than foreground for the many participants in the process. From the child's perspective, this will become "his" family, a haven of safety and security; from the mother's (and father's) perspective, this will become "her" child, to be known, protected, and loved. But getting from initial meeting to becoming truly family is a complex process indeed.

I would like to close with two clinical vignettes.

> Many years ago I worked with a young girl who had been sent to boarding school at 12 by her parents. She had been adopted into an upper-middle-class professional family when she was 5, after having been repeatedly abandoned by her biological mother and exposed to a myriad inherently traumatizing events in her native country. The adoptive parents had two biological children who were young teenagers when they adopted Ashley. When she came to the United States, Ashley was given a new name and was no longer addressed in her native tongue (which, given the family's circumstances, would easily have been possible). Indeed, by the time she was 13, she had forgotten her native language completely (to the great consternation of her parents and language teacher). When Ashley came to me, she was entirely shut down: sullen, resistant, and full of barely disguised rage. Lying and stealing were among the primary presenting problems; she was also sexually provocative and inappropriate. There are many things that can be said about Ashley and her family, but what struck me almost immediately upon meeting her parents was how little they understood her *or wanted to understand her*. When she had arrived in their home, she had been expected to assume a new identity, *without any attention or acknowledgement of all that had passed before.* A new name, a new language, a new life, all of which she was expected to be grateful for. There was never any effort made to address the trauma she had endured, or to help her grieve the losses she had suffered. She was 5 years old when she was adopted, obviously a sentient being. What I sensed almost immediately in her parents, particularly her mother, was that *who* Ashley was mattered little to her. She was locked in a struggle to control and dominate her, to obliterate Ashley's experience in whatever way she could. Ashley was fighting for her life, and killing her *self* in the process. It was a heartbreaking situation, and one largely impervious to intervention.

> In contrast, I recently had a young family seek my help in dealing with their 5-year-old adopted daughter. Even before I met Lucy, who had been adopted when she was under a year old, I met her mother, Jane, who *instantly* began to talk about Lucy as a psychological being. She empathized with Lucy's grief over losing her foster family upon being adopted and appreciated that this was an unfathomable loss for a young infant. Jane also understood that the physical setbacks that she herself had suffered following a bicycle accident were also painful and incomprehensible for her daughter, who did not understand why she couldn't be held and carried as much as she'd like. While Lucy's symptoms—also lying and stealing—were very painful for Jane, she so clearly adored Lucy and *understood* the genesis of her confusion and loss. As a mother, she felt anger, frustration, guilt, and anxiety, but she did not feel despair. Treatment, in this instance, was possible, and the opportunities for change and development limitless.

Recently, on a cross-country flight from San Francisco to New York, I happened to be seated behind a group of Korean caregivers and infants; there were three caregivers and three infants. It became clear as the flight progressed that the caregivers were delivering these babies to their new adoptive families. From early in the flight I had noticed how gentle these women were, handling their precious cargo with sensitivity and patience, settling them over and over again as the flight progressed, passing them back and forth as one or the other caregiver tired and needed to stretch her legs. To my amazement, not one of the babies ever fussed more than momentarily; each was easily and readily soothed. And this was the last leg in what had to have been nearly a 24-hour journey. The flight attendants, probably filled with admiration and a sense of the poignancy of the mission, gave the little troupe extra seats, blankets, and pillows. They fussed over the babies and themselves took turns holding and cuddling them.

When I arrived at the airport and walked down the concourse past the security checkpoint, I immediately saw the waiting families: mothers, fathers, grandparents, siblings, other Korean children, already assimilated and at home with their adoptive families. Adoption agency personnel were on hand to manage the transition. As the little band of caregivers and babies approached the waiting families, cheers, gasps, and cries of happiness erupted. Cameras flashed, and soon each baby had a tight cluster of beaming, weeping new mothers and fathers reaching to hold her. The babies, already world travellers, looked stunned and overwhelmed. The caregivers slowly moved away and stood together, their arms full of the detritus of a long trip with a baby—diaper bags, blankets, and stuffed animals—their own clothes dishevelled from the journey, gathering themselves for a few days' rest before the return back halfway around the world.

I couldn't help but wonder: What were they thinking? Did their arms and hearts feel empty? Had these babies been precious to them? Wouldn't they *miss* them? More importantly, had *they* been precious to these babies, beginning a new life in a new and alien world, without a familiar sight, sound, or touch? How could the babies begin to make sense of the loss and of all the newness? Even the small things, the blanket that had covered them for the entire journey and the stuffed animal that had soothed them, were gone, left in the arms of their now departed caregivers. And what of the new adoptive parents? This was the beginning of their dream—what did it feel like? Was it what they had imagined and hoped for? And of course I thought of the future, and of all that lay before each parent, each sibling, and each baby. I was filled with admiration for their courage and with hope for the discoveries that were to follow from this first, extraordinary, meeting.

NOTE

This chapter is based upon a paper delivered at a conference co-sponsored by the Yale Child Study Center and the Anna Freud Centre: Developmental Science and Psychoanalysis: Integration and Innovation. New Haven, CT, 11 December 2003.

CHAPTER SEVEN

Child psychotherapy research: issues and opportunities

Alan E. Kazdin

Psychotherapy for children and adolescents has made enormous advances in the past decade.[1] The advances reflect a heightened interest in evidence and increased accountability for the precise services that are provided to children and families. Much of the child therapy literature has been clinical in the sense of describing treatments and their applications to cases, how treatment is individualized, and what the critical processes may be. Therapies have proliferated in the process. Currently, a conservative count has identified over 550 psychotherapies in use for children (Kazdin, 2000b). The vast majority of these techniques have never been studied. Research has increased accelerated: over 1,500 controlled treatment trials of treatment have been completed (Kazdin, 2000a). With such remarkable attention to child therapy and empirical work obviously well underway, what more could one want? Actually, a great deal.

In this chapter I highlight the current focus of outcome research in child therapy. The purpose is to direct attention to critical areas that are being neglected in child therapy research and what is needed to rectify this. Among the central issues is the need to understand psychotherapy and how it produces change. The chapter ends with a discussion of research opportunities for child psychoanalytic therapy. Lines of psychoanalytic research that might be particularly useful to develop are highlighted both to advance psychoanalysis and child therapy more generally.

Evidence-based treatments

Background

The main focus of contemporary psychotherapy research is on evidence-based treatments (EBTs).[2] These refer to interventions that have empirical research in their behalf. The evidence refers to rigorous tests that the treatments, relative to various control or other treatment conditions, produce therapeutic change.

Several background and contextual factors have played critical roles in current interest in EBTs:

1. There has been a longstanding concern about the effects of psychotherapy. Eysenck's (1952) provocative review of psychotherapy research galvanized opinions about the issue and firmly placed psychotherapy into the empirical arena. The review concluded that approximately two thirds of patients who received psychotherapy improved and that this proportion was the same for individuals who did not receive treatment. The review stirred controversy and prompted greater attention to the evidence on behalf of psychotherapy. Subsequent reviews, including reviews of child therapy (Levitt, 1957, 1963), kept the conclusion very much alive: namely, therapy may not be very effective, if effective at all. The reviews were criticized on several grounds, but the criticisms did not mitigate the impact or concern.

2. The challenges were followed by a great deal of empirical research in the 1960s and 1970s (Bergin & Garfield, 1971; Garfield & Bergin, 1978). Reviewers using different methods of counting studies (e.g., box score, meta-analyses) concluded that therapy was effective and surpassed the effects of no treatment (e.g., Luborsky, Singer, & Luborsky; 1975; Smith & Glass, 1977; Smith, Glass, & Miller, 1980). Currently, there are scores of meta-analyses of psychotherapy. The conclusions are quite similar across treatments for children, adolescents, and adults, namely, various psychotherapies are effective and surpass the effects of no treatment. This seemingly modest conclusion is important historically. Interest in EBTs is a logical step from years of accumulating research on psychotherapy.

3. There has been an enduring hiatus between psychotherapy research and clinical practice (e.g., Hayes, Follette, Dawes, & Grady, 1995; Stricker, 1992). Among the lamentable aspects of this hiatus is

the fact that treatment research has had little impact on clinical practice, and clinical practice has had little impact on treatment research (Kazdin, Bass, Ayers, & Rodgers, 1990). For example, clinical practice does not rely very heavily on EBTs and, indeed, has been accused of showing a "blatant disregard of the empirical literature" (Ammerman, Hersen, & Last, 1999, p. 4) in deciding what treatments to use. This dissatisfaction with clinical practice reflects on the research as well. Perhaps the research cannot be drawn on because it is not seen as being very relevant to clinical practice.

4. Concerns about the spiralling costs of health care provide an important impetus for EBTs. Third-party payers (e.g., businesses, insurance companies, government) have led to managed care and concerns about the costs of diagnosis, assessment, and treatment. The challenges question whether a procedure—diagnostic test, treatment—ought to be provided at all, let alone reimbursed. In relation to psychotherapy, managed care emerged to raise questions such as: Why this treatment? Why this number of sessions? When will treatment end? Why is more treatment needed? What effects will it have? This new accountability underscores the important of having evidence about what is needed for treatment.

Identifying effective treatments

The efforts to identify EBTs traverse many professional organizations and countries (e.g., *Evidence Based Mental Health*, 1998; Christophersen & Mortweet, 2001; Fonagy, Target, Cottrell, Phillips, & Kurtz, 2002; Kazdin & Weisz, 2003; Lonigan & Elbert, 1998; Nathan & Gorman, 2002). They are consistent in seeking rigorous scientific data but differ slightly in the criteria. Typically, the criteria include several characteristics, that is, at least two studies with:

- random assignment of subjects to conditions;
- careful specification of the patient population;
- use of treatment manuals;
- multiple outcome measures (raters, if used, are naïve to conditions);
- statistically significant difference of treatment and comparison group;
- replication of outcome effects, especially by an independent investigator or team.

Many EBTs have been identified—Table 7.1 lists several to illustrate what can be culled from the available reviews. A few points are conspicuous from the table: (a) There *are* EBTs for children. Clearly, a child referred for anxiety, for example, ought to receive one of the EBTs as a treatment of choice. (b) The list of EBTs is not that long; with hundreds of therapies, it is surprising how few are listed. (c) The list is dominated by cognitive-behavioural treatments. This is no coincidence. To be counted as evidence-based, studies must include several methodological features (e.g., random assignment of cases to conditions, use of

Table 7.1. Treatments for children and adolescents that are evidence-based for key problem domains

Problem Domain	*Treatment*
Anxiety, fear, phobias	Cognitive behaviour therapy Modelling Reinforced practice Systematic desensitization
Depression	Cognitive–behaviour therapy Coping with depression course Interpersonal psychotherapy for Adolescents
Oppositional and conduct disorder	Anger Coping Therapy Multisystemic Therapy Parent management training Problem-solving skills training
Attention-Deficit Hyperactivity Disorder	Classroom contingency management Parent management training Psychostimulant medication

Note: The techniques noted here draw from different methods of defining and evaluating evidence-based treatments ((e.g., Lonigan & Elbert, 1998; Nathan & Gorman, 2002; Wasserman, Ko, & Jensen, 2001). The techniques are those that would meet criteria for well established or probably efficacious or those with randomized controlled trials in their behalf. Evaluation of treatments and identification of those that meet criteria for empirical support are ongoing, and hence the above is an illustrative rather than fixed or exhaustive list. Psychostimulant medication is mentioned because this is the standard treatment for attention-deficit hyperactivity disorder (Arnold, 2002).

treatment manuals). These characteristics are much more likely among contemporary than among past studies. Cognitive-behavioural therapies are more popular in contemporary work and are more likely to use the methodology required for establishing treatment.

Overall, there has been palpable progress in identifying EBTs. It is important to bear in mind that EBTs meet the criteria or approximations of the criteria noted in Table 7.1. This does not necessarily mean that the treatments ameliorate the clinical problems to which they are applied, have enduring effects, or are the best treatments—points to which I return later.

Issues in identifying and disseminating treatments

Applicability of research to clinic work

There are several issues that have challenged the evidence for EBTs. The most fundamental and frequently voiced issue is that evidence obtained in well-controlled studies may not apply (generalize) to the conditions of clinical settings. In contemporary writings, this concern has been reflected in the distinction between efficacy and effectiveness research (Hoagwood, Hibbs, Brent, & Jensen, 1995). *Efficacy research* refers to treatment outcomes obtained in controlled psychotherapy studies that are conducted under laboratory and quasi-laboratory conditions (e.g., subjects are recruited, they may show a narrow range of problems, treatment is specified in manual form, and treatment delivery is closely supervised and monitored). *Effectiveness research* refers to treatment outcomes obtained in clinic settings where the usual control procedures are not implemented (e.g., patients seek and present with multiple problems, therapists combine diverse techniques to individualize treatment to the patient).

The concern about whether the findings of therapy research can be generalized to clinical practice has been an ongoing since the 1960s. What is new in contemporary work is an urgency to test treatments in clinical settings now that there are EBTs. Various consensus panels and funding agencies have accorded high priority to tests of EBTs in clinical service settings (e.g., NAMHC, 1999, 2001).

Relative ease of demonstrating efficacy

A limitation in identifying EBTs pertains to what counts as evidence. The criteria for demonstrating treatment efficacy and concluding that treatment is "evidence-based" are not sufficiently stringent. At the level of individual studies, the requirement includes demonstrating that treatment is better than no treatment or treatment as usual. "Better than" means statistically significantly different on some outcome measures. This is not a very difficult obstacle to surmount. Research in adult therapy has shown that almost any active treatment is better—statistically—than no treatment. Expectations, attention, and the common factors associated with coming to therapy alone can produce such a difference. "Fake" treatments in which the patient engages in some activities not considered on *a priori* grounds to have therapeutic value can generate such a difference and surpass the effects of no treatment (Grissom, 1996). Moreover, as the "fake" treatment increasingly resembles the veridical treatment in terms of structure, components, and expectations for change generated in the client, so a difference between them is less likely (Baskin, Tierney, Minami, & Wampold, 2003). If each of us endeavoured to test our favourite treatment versus no treatment, the results might yield statistically significant differences, with reasonable but perhaps not even excessive statistical power.

Statistical significance alone is an odd or limited criterion to establish whether a treatment ought to be anointed as evidence-based. The results of a clinical trial might be evaluated in terms of statistical significance, the magnitude of effect (e.g., effect size), and clinical significance. Statistical significance may have no bearing on the practical impact of treatment on the patient. For example, a statistically significant difference favouring one treatment over another on some measure of anxiety may not reflect genuine differences or improvements on patient anxiety or functioning in everyday life. Similarly, indices of magnitude of effect (e.g., d, r, β) are excellent supplements to statistical significance. Yet, strength of an effect from a statistical standpoint (e.g., in standard deviation units) has no necessary relation to the impact of treatment on patients (Kazdin, 1999). Indeed, effect size can be quite large in cases where impact on the patient is nugatory or where the measure does not reflect symptoms or impairment.

Clinical significance refers to a set of indices designed to evaluate whether the impact of treatment translates to meaningful changes in the patient (Kazdin, 2001; Kendall, 1999). One of several criteria is usually invoked at the end of treatment to decide whether the changes are clinically significant. These include a demonstration that at the end of treatment: (a) the level of symptoms falls within the normative range (i.e., of individuals functioning adequately or well in everyday life); (b) patients no longer meet criteria for a psychiatric diagnosis that was evident at pre-treatment; or (c) the individual has made a large change (e.g., 1–2 standard deviations) on key outcome measures. Fundamental questions remain about what these changes mean and indeed whether the clinical significance of these indices is in name only (Kazdin, 2001).

Measures of clinical significance are not standard criteria for evaluating or establishing EBTs. Consequently, it is quite reasonable to say that a treatment that produces a statistically significant difference in relation to no-treatment control or another treatment may qualify as evidence-based but not really help patients very much or in ways that make a difference. This is a rather stark qualifier to the evidence and the criteria used to establish EBTs.

As researchers and clinicians, we want to be able to say that a given treatment produces change and that the change makes a difference. In some cases, the outcomes of treatment make clear that the treatment is not only evidence-based but also has strong impact on patients. For example, for the treatment of adults with panic attacks, the treatment may eliminate panic for many individuals. The qualitative difference in patient functioning from several to no panic attacks provides a fairly clear verdict on impact. For outcomes of most treatment studies, statistically significant differences may reflect change (e.g., reductions in depression, aggression, or hyperactivity), but we do not have a reliable or valid way at this point of stating whether the differences or changes translate into palpable benefits.

Disparate views among interested parties

Assume for a moment that findings from controlled studies generalize to clinical practice and that statistically significant treatment effects actually make a difference in the lives of patients. This would not by itself lead to adoption of EBTs in clinical work. Different parties or stakeholders in treatment are likely to vary in their views about the value and utility of EBTs. These views may have significant impact on whether EBTs are integrated into clinical practice and if so, the extent, or speed at which they are integrated.

1. *Researchers* are likely to favour greatly EBTs and their integration into clinical work. Indeed, researchers may well view EBTs as the high moral ground and wonder who could be against use of such treatments or delay their integration.

2. *Clinicians* are less likely to favour EBTs. The research identifying EBTs is completed in highly controlled settings where the

participants—patients and therapists—differ from those seen in clinical practice. Patients recruited in research are less likely to reflect the complexity of conditions (e.g., comorbidity) than the patients seen in practice, although this is certainly not always the case (Stirman, DeRubeis, Crits-Christoph, & Brody, 2003). Therapists in research, while less experienced (e.g., often graduate students), are highly trained and supervised to carry out the procedures, have small case loads, and do not depend on providing treatment for their income—a very different situation from what transpires in clinical practice. Also, most clinicians in practice are less likely to know or to be trained in EBTs merely because of the cohort in which they were trained.

3. *Administrators in agencies responsible for reimbursing treatment*—health maintenance organizations, government and insurance agencies—are likely to vary in their views of EBT. If an EBT for a given problem can save costs, the agencies are likely to favour the treatment. For example, an outpatient therapy or medication that averted psychiatric hospitalization would be greatly supported. Yet, an EBT might well increase costs, for example, by showing that a condition not previously covered can be treated effectively or that a longer treatment is effective whereas a shorter one is not.

4. The *public* at large, or at least individuals with some interest in mental health care, could exert considerable influence on the quality and type of care. Adults who have received psychotherapy are generally satisfied with their treatments, independently of the specific treatment they receive (Consumers Union, 1995). Satisfaction with treatment is not highly related to therapeutic change (Ankuta & Abeles, 1993; Lambert, Salzer, & Bickman, 1998; Pekarik & Wolff, 1996). Thus, the public with any experience in psychotherapy is likely to be satisfied and unlikely to scream out for more effective or well-established treatments. They have not been receiving EBTs and have been quite satisfied. Thus, there is not a groundswell of public insistence on treatments that are evidence-based or perhaps even effective.

For purposes of presentation, I have simplified the different roles of stakeholders in treatment. Individuals have different and multiple roles (e.g., a person is a researcher and public citizen) and this increases the variability and complexity. The purpose was merely to convey the point that stakeholder support for EBTs and their extension to clinical practice is mixed at best. There are challenges to conduct the requisite studies that establish treatment as evidence-based. These tasks are relatively straightforward. Much less clear is how to mobilize interest and support for the use of EBTs and their integration into patient care once such treatments have been identified.

Training of therapists

An obstacle to extending EBTs to clinical practice is training. Most clinical training programmes—child psychiatry, psychology, counselling, and social work—do not have the faculty and staff trained in EBTs to serve as models for trainees. Supervisors of therapy often are clinical and volunteer faculty who generously donate their time. Typically, they have not been trained in the latest or indeed any EBT.

Consider as one example of treatment. Parent management training is an intervention that is probably the most studied intervention of all therapies for children (Kazdin, 2005). The usual application of this treatment is for oppositional, aggressive, and antisocial behaviour, but there are other applications as well. There are scores of controlled trials spanning decades. It is very unlikely that trainees in most child psychiatry, psychology, counselling, and social work programmes are exposed to this treatment. At best, the treatment may be mentioned, but there are probably few opportunities for training.

Moving EBTs from the lab to training programmes and to those who eventually will provide services raises many challenges (Shernoff, Kratochwill, & Stoiber, 2003). A key issue is how to place EBTs at the disposal of those involved in training mental health professionals. Perhaps special training curricula could take advantage of the latest technologies (e.g., Web-based training materials). Otherwise one might expect considerable delays between demonstrating that a treatment is suited for clinical work and integrating this treatment into training programmes. Hiring young new faculty—trained in EBTs—is not necessarily a solution if the supervision and training remain in the hands of those who are much further along in their career and trained in less well studied treatments. Integrating EBTs into training remains a critical issue.

Psychotherapy research agenda

Focus on mechanisms and efficacy studies

The interest in EBT has narrowed the focus of therapy research to address primarily two questions: (a) Is a treatment "efficacious" (beneficial in controlled settings)? and (b) Can the treatment be transported to clinical settings? We would like to have a broader set of questions answered about therapy. For a given treatment, we would like to know:

1. What is the impact of treatment relative to no treatment?
2. What components contribute to change?
3. What treatments can be added (combined treatments) to optimize change?
4. What parameters can be varied to influence (improve) outcome?
5. How effective is this treatment relative to other treatments for this problem?
6. What patient, therapist, treatment, and contextual factors influence (moderate) outcome?
7. What processes within or during treatment influence, cause, and are responsible for outcome?
8. To what extent are treatment effects generalizable across problem areas, samples, and settings?
9. What is needed to foster adoption and effective implementation of treatment in clinical settings?

A high priority is the understanding of why treatment works—that is, the mechanisms of change (i.e., Question 7). The study of mechanisms of treatment is probably the best short-term and long-term investment for improving clinical practice and patient care. In studying mechanisms, it is critical to distinguish between cause and mechanisms of therapeutic change. By *cause*, I mean what led to change—a demonstration that some intervention led to some outcome. By *mechanisms*, I refer to those processes or events that account for the change.[3] A randomized controlled clinical trial (e.g., comparing treatment vs. no treatment) can establish a causal relation between an intervention and therapeutic change. However, demonstrating a causal relation does not necessarily explain *why* the relation was obtained. Thus, we may know *that* the intervention caused the change but not understand *why* (the basis for the cause or the mechanism) the intervention led to change.

As an example, consider cognitive therapy (CT) for the treatment of unipolar depression among adults. By all counts, this treatment is evidence-based and then some in light of the range of trials, replications, and comparisons (Hollon & Beck, 2004). Why does CT work—that is, through what mechanisms? In fact, little can be stated as to why treatment works. The conceptual model has emphasized changes in various cognitions. However, it is not obvious, clear, or established that changes in cognitions are the basis for therapeutic change. Indeed, suitable studies are rarely done. Designs are needed in which processes and symptom changes are evaluated at multiple points over the course of treatment (Kazdin, 2006). Some studies have demonstrated that changes in cognitions during treatment predict symptom change (DeRubeis et al., 1990; Kwon & Oei, 2003). Yet, it has not been clear in such studies whether symptom change *preceded* rather than followed changes in cognition. In general, there is a firm basis for stating that CT can change depression but little empirical basis for stating why.

Evaluating mechanisms of therapeutic change is important for several reasons:

1. There is an embarrassing wealth of treatments in use. I mentioned previously the 550+ therapies in use for children and adolescents. Among the subset of the 550+ treatments in use that do effect change, it is not likely that all treatments produce change for different reasons. Understanding the mechanisms of change can bring order and parsimony to the current status of multiple interventions.

2. Therapy can have quite broad outcome effects, beyond the familiar benefits of reducing social, emotional, behavioural, and psychiatric problems (e.g., suicidal ideation, depression, and panic attacks). In addition, therapy reduces physical ailments (e.g., pain, blood pressure), improves recovery from surgery or illness, and increases the quality of life (Kazdin, 2000b). Understanding how therapy produces change on such a diverse array of outcomes may clarify the connections between what is done (treatment) and what happens (outcomes).

3. An obvious goal of treatment is to optimize therapeutic change. By understanding the processes that account for therapeutic change, one ought to be better able to foster and maximize patient improvements. EBTs are often codified in manual form to provide explicit statements about what ought to be done in treatment. Most treatment manuals probably include the following components:

- practices (e.g., procedures, techniques) that genuinely make a difference to treatment outcome;
- practices that may not affect outcome but make the delivery more palatable and acceptable (e.g., the spoonful of sugar that makes the medicine go down);

- practices that reflect superstitious behaviour on the part of those of us who develop manuals (e.g., factors that we believe make a difference or that we like);
- practices that impede or merely fail to optimize therapeutic change.

The difficulty is that without understanding how treatment works, which element in a manual falls into which of these categories is a matter of surmise. If we wish to optimize therapeutic change, understanding the critical ingredients and processes through which they operate is essential.

4. Understanding how therapy works can help to identify moderators of treatment—that is, variables on which the effectiveness of a given treatment may depend. For example, if changes in cognitive processes account for therapeutic change, this finding might draw attention to characteristics of these processes or their underpinnings at pre-treatment. Pre-treatment status of cognitive processes (abstract reasoning, problem-solving, attributions), stages of cognitive development, and neurological or neuropsychological characteristics on which these cognitions might depend are just some of the moderators that might be especially worth studying. Other promising moderators that influence treatment might be proposed on theoretical grounds once the mechanisms of therapy are known.

5. Understanding the mechanisms through which change takes place is important beyond the context of psychotherapy. There are many interventions and experiences in everyday life that improve adjustment and adaptive functioning, ameliorate problems of mental and physical health, and help people to manage and cope with stress and crises and, more generally, navigate the shoals of life. As examples, participating in religion, chatting with friends, exercising, undergoing hypnosis, and writing about sources of stress all have evidence on their behalf. Therapy research is not merely about techniques but, rather, about the broader question—namely, how does one intervene to change affect, cognition, behaviour, experience, and functioning? Mechanisms that elaborate how therapy works might be useful for understanding human functioning more generally. Conversely, mechanisms that explain how other change methods work might well inform therapy. Basic psychological processes (e.g., learning, memory, perception, persuasion, social interaction) and their biological pathways (e.g., changes in neurotransmitters, brain activation

patterns) may be common to many types of interventions, including psychotherapy.

As I mentioned previously, a frequently identified priority of contemporary treatment research is to extend treatment to clinic settings (NAMHC, 1999, 2001). Diverse terms have been introduced to describe these extensions, including translational research, transportability, and tests of effectiveness. The terms refer to a common question—namely, will treatments work in "real-world" settings? We enter the clinical arena with one hand tied behind our back if we apply an unspecified and possibly low dose of a treatment that we do not understand. To optimize the generality of treatment effects, we want to know what is needed to make treatment work, what the essential conditions are, and what we ought to worry about, as some components get diluted when treatment moves from the lab to the clinic.

Weak treatments can be wonderful

Obviously, we wish to identify and develop strong treatments—that is, treatments that effect clinically significant change and do so with as high a proportion of cases as possible and with enduring effects. The search for EBTs is aimed at this lofty and important objective. There is an important role and place for weak treatments. By "weak", I mean interventions that may influence only a small proportion of individuals to which they are applied and/or might reduce but not eliminate the problem for those individuals or on a large scale (the larger group). Many interventions might be relatively weak but also require minimal effort or cost, and the benefits, relative to these costs, would be worth while.

One programme for cigarette smoking provides an example of what might be a weak treatment. In the United States and now worldwide there is an annual "smoke out day"[4] in which organizations at local and national levels delineate a day for people to stop smoking for the day. The delineation of the day publicly through the media is merely to make salient the need for people to stop smoking. Allegedly, more people give up smoking on that day—for one day or permanently—than on any other day. It is not likely that the intervention is very effective in terms of the proportion of smokers who completely stop smoking. On the other hand, this is a relatively low-cost intervention (e.g., advertising messages) that reaches millions of people worldwide. The percentage of smokers who quit permanently could be minute but still reflect a large number of people, given that there are many people (e.g., estimated 47 million in the United States alone) who smoke cigarettes. This is a very low-cost intervention, relative to some individual or group therapy.

EBTs as currently and narrowly defined ignore a pivotal question for public mental health. The issue is not merely what works (EBTs) but what works relative to their costs, scale of applicability, and prevalence of the problem. An intervention that can be implemented on a large scale and shown to have some impact might be quite worth while. There are therapies completed by self-help manuals, telephone, mail, Internet and computer, and videotapes. Not all the applications are effective using these media, but many of them are. For example, self-help manuals are a genre of do-it-yourself books that make extravagant claims, usually with no supportive evidence. However, many self-help manuals have been studied and are effective (Marrs, 1995).

Many other examples are available in controlled studies showing that other media can be quite effective for treating clinical disorders (e.g., anxiety, depression) and ameliorating stress (e.g., from divorce, death of a loved one). Under some circumstances writing about one's problems is special ways can effect therapeutic change (Smyth, 1998). Contact through the post (e.g., providing feedback and information) can reduce alcohol consumption among individuals with significant problems with alcohol (Sobell, Sobell, & Agrawal, 2002). I am not advocating any particular form of treatment or medium through which services are provided but, rather, conveying the importance of cost and disseminability of treatment as dimensions that complement the criteria used to identify EBTs.

The notion of *stepped care* has been introduced into psychotherapy to suggest that minimal treatments be used first before one moves to more intensive, time-consuming, and costly treatments (Haaga, 2000). In relation to EBT, minimal treatments ought to show evidence that they can effect change. Appeals through the post or self-help manuals are effective under many circumstances. Even if they are effective for only a small number of individuals, their ease of dissemination and relatively low cost may make them worth while. The focus on EBTs alone, as currently conceived, may miss critical facets of such treatments. We need a portfolio of interventions that vary in effectiveness, cost, and ease of dissemination.

Extending methods, not just treatments, to clinical work

The focus of much of research is on the treatments and their integration into clinical practice. Perhaps even more important than the interventions, some of the *methods of research* could be extended to clinical practice to enhance clinical care. EBTs, whether medical or psychological, are not likely to work for everyone. Many interventions might work or fail with a given patient. This makes all the more important the use of systematic assessment during the course of treatment. Decision making about continuing treatment, stopping, or shifting to another intervention could be aided by user-friendly assessments. Therapy that is not evaluated systematically is not likely to be in the patient's best interests, barring special circumstances where interventions need to be presented in the heat of the moment (e.g., on the battlefield, in response to trauma). More systematic assessment is available for use and could improve clinical care at least as much as using EBTs (Clement, 1999; Kazdin, 1993).

In considering the relevance of research methods for clinical practice, one might even wish to go further. For example, use of materials to aid therapists so they deliver treatment consistently (e.g., abbreviated manuals, CD-ROM guides to treatment) and ongoing treatment supervision may be critical to the effects of treatment obtained in research. Research may have to change to be more relevant to clinical practice, but there are parallel changes that clinical practice ought to make to improve patient care.

General comments

Identifying effective treatments is obviously a high priority. I have outlined a few critical issues, including weak criteria for deciding what is evidence-based (e.g., statistical significance), lack of attention to whether patients are palpably improved, and neglect of reasons why therapy is effective (e.g., mechanisms of change). Providing effective interventions will require much more than clinical trials to contrast treatment with various control and comparison groups. We do not yet understand processes involved in change so cannot optimize treatment effects. Also, disseminating treatment is an enormous task. Establishing more EBTs through research will do little to help children and families without developing the means to move these treatments into training programmes for mental health professionals and into clinics for service providers.

Because most children in need of treatment do not receive services, at least in the United States, more attention must be given to diverse models of delivery. At least some treatments must be deliverable on a wider scale than those that are currently investigated as evidence-based. Even if the results of controlled clinical trials (efficacy studies) generalize to clinical settings (effectiveness studies), the findings may remain academic if the treatment cannot be provided to those in need.

Psychoanalytic therapy: developing the research agenda

I have highlighted priorities and issues pertinent to child therapy research in general. I did not have in mind one model of psychotherapy more than another (e.g., psychodynamic, cognitive–behavioural, or family therapies). I would like to end with a discussion of possible lines of work that might be pursued in relation to child psychoanalytic therapy in particular. As child psychoanalytic therapy continues to pursue a research agenda, it is tempting to emphasize controlled trials to establish the treatment as evidence-based. No doubt controlled outcome studies across problem domains would be of great value. However, I believe that there are special opportunities for psychoanalysis that could advance child therapy research in a way that does more than add another set of outcome studies.

Focus on mechanisms in therapy

Perhaps more than other form of psychotherapy, psychoanalysis has given enormous conceptual attention to the processes of therapy. Facets of the relationship, emergent processes during therapy, and unproductive events that can thwart these processes are a few of the broad categories that have been elaborated. Among the questions that can be asked are: How do key processes emerge or unfold in treatment that affects the goals of treatment? What predicts and impedes their emergence (e.g., characteristics of therapist, patients, parents, family)? What interventions by the therapist—comments, techniques, foci—can change these processes (e.g., enhance or interfere with transference within a session)? A therapist who has practiced child analysis will have many ideas about each of these based on well-developed conceptualization treatment and clinical experience. Translating these ideas into questions and then specific research projects is, in my view, not that difficult.

The underpinnings of studying mechanisms of therapy might warrant conceptual clarification. Many therapies have blurred the distinction between theory of aetiology (how the current problem, condition, or state came about) and theory of change (what can be done at this point in time to effect change and what processes lead to change now). The distinction is easily illustrated in the context of medicine. Obviously, it is invariably useful to know aetiologies. For many problems (e.g., rabies, bacterial infection) knowing how the problem came about is pivotal for effective treatment. Yet there are many treatments (e.g., aspirin for headaches, chemotherapies for cancer) that are effective where aetiology is not clear.

In the context of psychotherapies, some treatments (e.g., for anxiety disorders such as panic attacks, agoraphobia) have been quite effective without understanding the aetiology of the problems to which they are effectively applied. Aetiology does not always inform treatment, but it can do so. For example, with children referred for aggressive and antisocial behaviour, inept and harsh child-rearing practices often play a pivotal role in developing the problem (aetiology) (Patterson, 1982; Patterson, Reid, & Dishion, 1992). Moreover, changing these parenting practices in treatment alters the problem. However, harsh punishing practices are not invariably the cause. Indeed, it is likely that conduct problems are multiply determined. From the standpoint of a theory of change, parent training focuses on learning and developing new repertoires in parents and children. As a model of change, the treatment is useful even when fundamental questions are raised about the multiple paths leading to the clinical problem.

Essential to treatment, and a priority for psychoanalytic treatment research, is to specify the model of change. The key questions are: What is therapy designed to change in the child? and What processes in the treatment sessions produce these changes? All sorts of options are available for answering these questions, even within a given approach. For example, within cognitively based therapies, there are quite different models of change. Cognitively based therapies share the view that an individual's thoughts, beliefs, and attributions play a central role in clinical problems and that changing these cognitions is essential for therapeutic change. A question is how one ought to change cognitions. One view is that one should focus on the cognitions themselves—that is, what the person believes—and try to change these by challenging them or having individuals practice alternative cognitions (e.g., self-statements). Another view is that the change process can focus on behaviour. That is one of the best ways to change cognitions (internal processes) is to have individuals engage in action. These examples convey that even with shared views on presumed—but not known—aetiology, different processes of change might be proposed.

Much of psychoanalysis focuses on the processes within the individual as the basis of the individual's current functioning and needing to be corrected or redressed. While there is general agreement that internal processes are pivotal, analytic therapy does not necessarily require a direct focus on these processes. One view that has been interesting historically comes from a practicing analyst (Herzberg, 1945) who believed that internal processes were key, but that the best way to change these processes was to have individuals behave quite differently in the world—that is, that engaging in activities, special assignments, tasks, and exercises in relation to one's clinical problems would lead to changes in critical internal states and processes.[5]

In relation to child analysis, it would be helpful to have a few articulated statements about how therapy leads to change. These processes could be readily evaluated to test directly whether the processes are related to and actually mediate change. This would be an enormous contribution not only to psychoanalytic therapy but to therapy more generally. Processes shown to operate in analytic therapy might well be evident in other treatments whether or not they explicitly engage the child in the same way.

Identifying psychoanalytically informed moderators of treatment

Moderators are those characteristics that influence the effect of other variables. In the context of psychotherapy, moderators might include characteristics of the child, parents, or family that influence therapeutic change (treatment outcome) or that influence processes in treatment (e.g., relationship). Moderators have been studied in child therapy, but typically they include various subject and demographic characteristics (e.g., socioeconomic disadvantage, marital status of the family, child age or sex, severity of dysfunction). I consider these to be *moderators of convenience* because they are usually based on information readily available (e.g., from intake information) and then are included in data analyses to determine whether they influence outcome. The moderators usually are conceptually bereft and rarely point to facets of the individual or treatment that will enhance understanding of treatment.

There are special opportunities for psychoanalysis in the study of moderators of therapy. Psychoanalysis has a great deal to say about who is likely to profit from treatment and the conditions that are likely to facilitate the treatment process. These characteristics are moderators. For example, are there characteristics in the family or child (e.g., attachment patterns, distorted cognitive analytic representational patterns) that might predict therapeutic change or influence whether one responds to child analysis at all? One way to generate the hypotheses on key moderators is to pose questions to experienced clinicians about what is involved in effective treatment. One merely asks, what are some of the reasons people do not get better with the treatment? Who does not get better? Why do you think that happens? Answers to these questions can move relatively easily to the study of moderators.

Moderators are not necessary restricted to the study of treatment outcome. Analytic therapies have views about critical processes that emerge in treatment. Understanding how these processes emerge and the role the processes play in therapy can be advanced by the study of moderators. The questions to guide research are similar to those noted in relation to outcome and perhaps share similar answers. What are the critical—ideal, necessary—processes that must emerge in treatment for treatment to proceed or be effective? What characteristics of the child or child–therapist interaction, clinical functioning, and so on are likely to influence the emergence of these processes? These latter characteristics are moderators.

The therapeutic alliance, infrequently studied in child therapy (Shirk & Karver, 2003), would be a good candidate for the study of moderators of treatment process. Who forms a good alliance? What factors are involved? Research that demonstrates factors that determine or influence a good alliance with the therapist would be a very important contribution to child therapy. Psychoanalysis has well-developed ideas on this front, and these could be readily translated to research.

Further method development

I have mentioned the focus on key constructs including mediators and moderators of child therapy. It is likely that more work is needed on method development to ensure that critical constructs can be reliably and validly assessed. For example, to examine the relation of process to outcome we would want psychoanalytically informed measures of each. There is already a model of the type of work that is needed in relation to therapy of adults. The well-known programme of research of Luborsky and his colleagues (e.g., Luborsky, Crits-Christoph,

Mintz, & Auerbach, 1988) provides a model of research on developing methods to test hypotheses about psychodynamic therapy. Substantive advances can be traced to several features of the programme. However, of special significance in relation to the present comments is the development of ways to operationalize key facets of the therapeutic relationship and treatment outcomes and to demonstrate their connection. The included observing many therapy sessions ("a review of miles of tapes of recorded sessions"; Luborsky et al., 1988, p. 150) and developing clinical rating scales that could more readily be used than direct observations. Development of clinically usable scales has permitted multiple studies to test predictions about both mediators and moderators of therapy.

Systematic efforts to develop and validate measures of processes in child therapy are needed. Measurement development is not daunting; the steps are relatively straightforward. The initial task is specifying the change processes that one wants to assess. Psychoanalytic therapy has completed this more difficult task. Moving to specific measures raises all sorts of assessment options that can vary as a function of age of the child and nature of the construct. Developing measures of the critical processes in child analysis will greatly augment empirical research and ought to be given special priority for research.

Multiple designs to evaluate treatment

The vast majority of contemporary psychotherapy research falls in the tradition of quantitative research that includes group comparisons and null hypothesis statistical testing. This is epitomized in the randomized controlled trials to evaluate treatment. There are ways in which these designs are without peer, even though they are not the only designs to experimentally demonstrate or establish intervention effects. From the standpoint of developing a research agenda for child therapy, and for psychoanalysis in particular, there are rich opportunities elsewhere.

Two methodological lines that are neglected in contemporary therapy research would be quite useful to exploit from an analytic perspective:

1. Qualitative research would be an excellent way to elaborate the experience of therapy of children of different ages, to chart the emergent processes in therapy, and to describe the course of experience and reflections on that experience. Qualitative research focuses on narrative accounts, description, interpretation, context, and meaning.

The goal is to describe, interpret, and understand the phenomena of interest. Through description and interpretation, our understanding of the phenomena can be deepened. The process of achieving this goal is to study in depth the experience of the participants, i.e., those who are studied, and to convey how that experience is felt, perceived, and the meaning it has.

I hasten to add that the term "qualitative research" has a history of misuse in the context of clinical work. Qualitative is sometimes used to refer to descriptive, anecdotal, and case study material or any narrative account. That is, the term has been inappropriately adopted to refer to any nonquantitative evaluation. This is a misuse—qualitative is not a synonym for loose, unsystematic "opinions" or for detailed and engaging case material. Indeed, it is an antonym for these characteristics. Anecdotal case studies and in-depth analyses of cases or use of case studies to support or illustrate conceptual points are not examples of qualitative research. Qualitative research is rigorous, scientific, disciplined, and replicable. The usual scientific tenets and practices (e.g., operationalization of terms, confirmation and replication, check on reliability of the data) are pivotal (e.g., Berg, 2001; Denzin & Lincoln, 2000).

Psychoanalytic work could profit enormously from rigorous qualitative research that would permit systematic documentation and elaboration of the therapeutic processes. The methodology provides the means for evaluating broad themes in therapy. Among the many advantages of the methodology is the ability to capture experiences in the contexts in which they emerge. The research could at once test as well as generate hypotheses about therapy and developmental issues in relation to critical processes.

2. Another method that could elaborate psychoanalytic therapy would be empirical case studies. There is a rigorous methodology referred to as single-case experimental designs in which cases are studied and strong inferences can be drawn. An excellent example this methodology in psychoanalytic work is the study by Fonagy and Moran (1990) on the effects of therapy on brittle diabetes. Single-case experiments are excellent for rigorous demonstration but depart from the suggestion here. Advances have been made in elaborating the methods of conducting and evaluating case studies that do not require the rigorous controls of single-case experimental designs. Use of case methods with systematic assessment can yield inferences about treatments and their effects (Clement, 1999; Kazdin, 1981, 1993; Sechrest, Stewart, Stickle, & Sidani, 1996).

There are different facets of case evaluation that can be distinguished. One is using the case to draw inferences about processes, outcomes, and their interrelations and to inform therapy more generally. Another is to evaluate treatment in a way that helps the clinician make decisions that guide and improve treatment for a particular patient. They are related but can differ slightly in the extent to which therapeutic change in this patient at this time is the primary goal versus drawing broader inferences about therapy. Both foci require some systematic evaluation and that assessment could draw on the methods of quantitative or qualitative research.

General comments

Research on child analysis could pursue multiple lines of inquiry that would contribute to its own empirical base as well as to child therapy more generally. The most obvious lines to pursue would be to fall in line with existing research priorities in child therapy research. These include establishing that treatment is evidence-based and seeing whether treatment can be applied in clinical practice. To be sure, these are important questions and at some point cannot be avoided. However, for my part, these ought to be given a lower priority than they are accorded in current work. Advances in treatment and care of patients are likely to come from other quarters.

Another approach to the research agenda would be to lead with the strengths of psychoanalysis. These include theoretical work about processes in development and in the therapeutic relationship that will influence adjustment and functioning. It would not be difficult to delineate a set of hypotheses about key mediators and moderators of psychoanalytic treatment and then to begin the work to test these. A potential gain is to elaborate processes of inner experience in new ways and to elaborate interpersonal interactions in ways that extend well beyond the confines of therapy.

In suggesting lines of research, I have restricted my comments largely to the context of child therapy. The focus of the chapter ignores the fact that psychoanalysis has much to say about human functioning and interpersonal interaction more generally. Support for tenets of psychoanalysis and advances in understanding human functioning can come from many additional lines of work. Two examples convey the point:

1. Neuroimaging of psychological states and processes of analytic significance would be a natural focus. Methodologies and tantalizing

results are available showing the underpinnings of cognitive and emotional states such as regret and pain and as well as language meaning (e.g., Camille et al., 2004; Hagoort, Hald, Bastiaansen, & Petersson, 2004; Singer et al., 2004). Drawing on techniques such as neuroimaging and electroencephalogram to understand subjective states and inner experience provides enormous opportunities for evaluating psychoanalytic constructs.

2. Animal cognition might be connected to tenets of analysis. At first blush, animal analytic research may sound like either a wild idea or simply an insult. Actually, a great deal of attention has been given to animal cognition, including language, planning, understanding, and novelty in responding (e.g., Rumbaugh & Washburn, 2003). It has been surprising to many how "human-like" animals are (the reverse phrasing of this apparently is less appealing). Any facets of psychoanalytic thinking that could weave into this literature and lead to experimental tests would be of a very high priority. Of course, there is precedent such as research on experimental neuroses and conflict, which used animal laboratory research and drew on psychoanalytic concepts (e.g., Masserman, 1943). I mean something different and indeed better—namely, to draw hypotheses from psychoanalysis and see whether these fit within paradigms for studying planning, communication, and social interaction among animals.

Psychoanalysis connects with human functioning in many ways beyond therapy. The future agenda for research can be expanded to make connections with advances in basic research on the brain, attachment, and other areas (Mayes, 2003). There are enormous opportunities to bring together sophisticated methodologies to address sophisticated conceptual views of inner experience. Advances in child therapy will come in part from connecting treatment to other areas of work. Psychoanalysis can take a leadership role in making these connections.

Conclusions

Child psychotherapy research has advanced considerably. The emphasis on EBTs is significant. The emphasis on evidence moves us away from the recent past in which therapeutic approaches, schools, and orientations were the way of presenting child therapy to professionals, trainees, and the public at large. Approaches towards treatment (e.g., family-based, psychoanalytic, behavioural) are useful in order to conceptualize problems, but both the conceptualization and the treatments are the basis for research and not ends in themselves.

I have raised issues and concerns about EBTs, what they mean, and how treatments are established as evidence-based. Let me close by underscoring a few key points.

1. There are now several interventions identified as being evidence-based. This is a decided advance in research in part because in the not-too-distant past it was unclear whether treatments had any solid evidence on their behalf.

2. The criteria for establishing treatment as evidence-based are probably too lenient. Merely showing a statistically significant difference in group comparisons of treatment versus some other condition is not very demanding. In clinical work, we care about patient change—that is, genuine changes in adaptive functioning, symptoms, and participation in life. More work is needed to identify whether treatment and which treatments have palpable impact on people's lives.

3. A high priority for professional organizations and funding agencies is extending treatment from controlled settings to clinical services. This is obviously worth while but has enormous challenges for the training of therapists, supervising ongoing treatment, and demonstrating effects.

4. Research attention is needed on why treatment works. Understanding how treatment works is the best investment in extending treatment to clinical practice. The reasons why a given treatment works are often discussed but rarely evaluated empirically.

5. An important focus will be to move EBTs into training programmes for residents, fellows, interns, and graduate students in the mental health professions. This is not easy to do. Those involved in supervision of trainees are usually from a generation in which EBTs were not trained. Supervisors would need to learn EBTs—not a minor challenge.

I have expressed misgivings about the EBT movement, research, and findings. That said, there is a message that ought to be stated clearly. For any clinician in practice, it would be difficult to justify using a non-EBT as the first line of attack if there is an available EBT. If the EBT treatment fails, switching to another treatment ought to be noncontroversial. Clearly, an EBT treatment is the place to begin. It is one thing to say that the strong evidence from controlled trials *may* not apply to clinical settings. However, it is quite a leap to use this as a justification for applying an alternative with no evidence on its behalf if an EBT is available.

My comments ended with a focus on psychoanalytic research and areas that I consider to be remarkable opportunities for advances. A natural temptation would be to devote most resources to the current child therapy research agenda: to wit, establish treatment as evidence-based for various clinical problems and test treatment in clinical service settings. Clearly, more attention is needed to establish the efficacy of treatment across the range of problems to which the treatments are applied. However, I recommend complementary priorities for research on child analysis.

The strengths of psychoanalysis include the attention to conceptual issues and processes in treatment and human functioning more generally. The strengths can be translated to hypotheses about mediators and moderators of treatment. I do not see the challenges as particularly daunting. Further measurement development of key constructs—a precondition for advances—would not be that difficult. In addition, testing of key concepts outside the context of therapy could provide a solid base understanding how processes influence human interaction more generally.

NOTE

This work was supported, in part, by grants from the William T. Grant Foundation (98-1872-98) and the National Institute of Mental Health (MH59029).

1. I use the term children to represent both children and adolescents, unless the distinction is pertinent to a particular point or discussion.

2. These efforts have used different terms to delineate such treatments including "empirically validated treatment", "empirically supported treatments", "evidence-based practice", and "treatments that work". The term "evidence-based treatment" (EBT) is used in this chapter in keeping with a tradition already established in several other areas (e.g., dentistry, nursing, health care, social work, education, psychiatry, and mental health) where interventions are used to produce change in a particular clientele.

3. *Mediator* is often used as the term intended to signify a cause or mechanism of change and distinguished from *moderator* (Baron & Kenny, 1986). For this discussion, I retain "mechanism as the term". Mediator analyses raise multiple issues and may identify factors that do not explain why treatment works, a topic beyond the scope of this chapter (Kraemer, Stice, Kazdin, Offord, & Kupfer, 2001; Kraemer, Wilson, Fairburn, & Agras, 2002).

4. www.quit-smoking.net/greatamericansmokeout.html
www.cdc.gov/tobacco/research_data/mm4219

5. Interestingly, Herzberg anticipated graduated exposure, currently an effective intervention for the treatment of anxiety. Herzberg found the treatment to be quite effective with his cases in scores of applications, observations that later were supported empirically with contemporary versions of the technique.

Commentary

Jonathan Hill

It seems highly appropriate that this chapter, written for the inaugural book of the new Anna Freud Centre, should raise conceptual and perhaps also philosophical issues alongside the empirical. Alan Kazdin points out how the proliferation of the RCT "evidence base" has not been accompanied by a comparable level of understanding of the way treatments work. This leads to many practical and empirical questions to which I return, but also underscores how we have to pay attention to differences in underlying ways of thinking that are rarely articulated.

There is a general assumption that a "scientific" approach to the evaluation of treatments for children is needed. This may be a useful idea, but only if the concept of science is relatively straightforward and is used uniformly within the field. However there is by no means unanimity regarding the meaning of the term. A distinction that may be rather crudely characterized in a contrast between ancient Egyptian and Greek traditions is still with us (Toulmin & Goodfield, 1961). The Egyptian tradition emphasized observation and prediction. By accumulating evidence and identifying regularities and patterns, one is able to predict the future. The Greek tradition, by contrast, was concerned primarily with understanding the underlying causal principles. The key in Greek science was the use of mathematics to model the physical world, and this remains the dominant tradition in the physical sciences. Observation is of use only inasmuch as it informs the quality of the causal theory. Echoes of this contrast could be seen in the stand-off during the second half of the twentieth century in the United Kingdom between scientists and psychoanalysts regarding psychopathology. In most instances, with perhaps the exception of the radical behaviourists and the reductionist psychophysiologists, the scientists took a predominantly Egyptian stance. The key to the science of psychopathology was thought to be classification. Meanwhile, standing firmly in the Greek tradition, the analysts pursued the holy grail of a unifying theory of psychopathology. The first was sterile and the second reckless! Although each of these untenable positions persists to a certain degree, there has been a major, and highly productive, rapprochement, as evidenced in this volume. However, the underlying tension remains important and should fostered! The search for the "evidence base" through the new holy grail of the randomized controlled trial (RCT) has to be tempered by an enquiry into underlying processes and a willingness to propose theory that goes beyond current evidence, and these in turn must influence empirical studies.

Kazdin's chapter tackles this head-on. His analysis shows that work in the Egyptian tradition, accumulating more facts regarding treatment outcomes, has run well ahead of the search for causal mechanisms, characteristic of Greek science. Furthermore, as he says: "In studying mechanisms, it is critical to distinguish cause and mechanisms of therapeutic change." He is drawing the contrast between the conditions that have to be satisfied for factor A to be a cause of outcome B, laid down in Mill's methods of agreement and difference (Bolton, 2002; Mill, 1843), and the question of mechanism, which remains unaddressed even after these causal conditions have been satisfied. He highlights some of the reasons this is problematic, including that we have no basis for rational choice among hundreds of "effective" treatments, we do not know whether different treatments work because of common underlying similarities or via different mechanisms, we do not know how to weight the value of contrasting outcomes, and in the absence of an understanding of the key ingredients, we do not know where to give emphasis in seeking to optimize therapeutic impacts.

The key, I will argue, is to reconnect the traditions, and in doing that also to state in even more stark terms the assumptions that need to be examined when doing this. In brief these include that (a) individuals with the symptoms are the appropriate target of the intervention—and, crucially, those without, are not; (b) individuals with similar symptoms are sufficiently similar in underlying processes and mechanisms that the treatment can be thought of as appropriate to most or all, and similarly the measured outcome; (c) the remission of symptoms is an adequate index of therapeutic efficacy; (d) the timescale for the evaluation of change is a relatively minor issue.

The crude characterizations of the targets of intervention as symptoms or "diagnoses" (enough symptoms!) highlights how far our field is from much of evidence-based practice in medicine. We can learn from that paradigm without having to sign up to the medicalization of psychotherapy research. The key points are that in medicine the *presence* of symptoms is generally an effective signal that something is wrong, the *patterning* of the symptoms may help in determining what that is but is rarely definitive, and the *absence* of symptoms cannot be taken as showing that the person is healthy. In medicine the key to making progress beyond the symptomatic presentation is the "differential diagnosis", meaning: Given a set of symptoms, what are the (often many) alternative explanations? In other words, there is an assumption that behind the commonality of symptoms there is generally considerable heterogeneity of process and mechanism. Choosing a treatment based on symptoms would constitute medical malpractice, as would relying on the remission of symptoms as an indicator of treatment success.

Thus, paradoxically, when it comes to the evaluation of treatment efficacy, the behavioural sciences are closer to the Egyptian tradition, while medicine appeals more to the Greek! How, then, might more of the Greek be brought to bear on the Egyptian in psychotherapy research? Recent advances in technology, such as DNA analysis and functional imaging, have tremendous potential to illuminate process and mechanism. Equally, just as in medicine, such techniques are impotent unless coupled with theory. And currently we do not have a settled view of "good theory". The problem is not so much which theory, but how much do we expect theory to do? Some theories—notably various forms of psychoanalytic theory—aim to cover most or all of normal psychology and psychopathology. Others, for example making simple distinctions between types of childhood antisocial disorder, have modest but specific aims. The history of attachment theory illustrates how there can be fluctuations in the scope even of the same theory. In its original formulation, expressed in Bowlby's three volumes, *Attachment* (1969), *Separation* (1973), and *Loss* (1980), attachment theory shares ambitions with psychoanalytic theory to show how development proceeds normally and how perturbations in that process lead to psychopathology in childhood and adult life. Empirical studies have brought into question some of the central tenets of the theory—for example, that there is substantial continuity of attachment security over development (e.g., Weinfield, Whaley, & Egeland, 2004), and that attachment insecurity is fundamental to psychopathology (Dozier, Stovall, & Albus, 1999). Once the smoke has cleared, the extent to which this or that part of the theory is correct will probably be less important than its capacity to continue to inform the design of productive studies. In particular, it shares with psychoanalysis a developmental perspective that has tremendous potential to illuminate psychopathology and hence RCTs.

The value of a developmental perspective is amply illustrated through further reference to cognitive therapy for unipolar depression in adults. Kazdin comments that "By all accounts this treatment is evidence-based . . ." and then points out that very little is known about the mechanisms involved. He makes the case for studies of mediators of change in order to understand mechanisms. This will work if the mechanisms of change are sufficiently uniform across samples of depressed individuals. However, it may be undermined if the underlying mechanisms involved in the origins and maintenance of the disorder vary across subgroups with similar symptoms. There is emergent evidence that this is indeed the case. Reduced hippocampal volumes have been reported in adults with depression, and it has been suggested that this is a consequence of disrupted regulation of corticosteroids. However the findings have been inconsistent. Vythilingam and colleagues (2002) reported that reduced hippocampal volumes were confined to a subgroup of referred depressed adults who had experienced childhood maltreatment. This would suggest that the mechanisms in depression are quite different, depending on childhood experiences. The relevance of this finding for psychotherapy is further illustrated in a study conducted by the same group (Nemeroff et al., 2003). Patients with chronic forms of major depression were randomized to treatment with an antidepressant, psychotherapy (Cognitive Behavioural Analysis System of Psychotherapy: CBASP), or the combination. The findings were quite different depending on whether account was taken of a childhood history of maltreatment. Overall, the effects of the antidepressant alone and psychotherapy alone were equal and significantly less effective than combination treatment. However, in the maltreated subgroup psychotherapy alone was superior to antidepressant, and there was little advantage in the addition of medication to psychotherapy for those maltreated in childhood.

Age of onset of depression may also reflect different pathways and hence mechanisms. Jaffee and colleagues (2002) and Hill, Pickles, Byatt, and Rollinson (2004) found that there were markedly different developmental pathways to major depression in young adult life depending on age of first episode. Adults who had first been depressed before the age of 16 came from families with multiple adversities, and as children they had increased hyperactivity and disruptive behaviour problems and peer relationship difficulties. By contrast, adults with later onset had, when they were young, differed very little from other children in their behaviours and social functioning, and they came from families with few psychosocial risks, but they did report more child sexual abuse than non-depressed adults. These multiple and marked differences in pathways to adult depression may indicate the need for different treatments for subgroups defined in terms of age of first episode.

At worst judging the efficacy of a treatment from the reduction of symptoms may be no better than concluding that Paracetamol is an effective treatment for a brain tumour because it reduces headache. Equally, pointers to more appropriate treatment outcomes can be found by examining symptoms in relation to processes. Teasdale and colleagues (2002) found that residual symptoms of depression were associated with decreased "metacognitive awareness"—a cognitive set in which negative thoughts/feelings are experienced as mental events rather than as self. Among patients with residual depression following treatment, reduced accessibility of metacognitive interpretations of negative thoughts or feelings predicted relapse. These findings suggest both that metacognitive awareness may be an important target for treatment because it represents a mechanism in relapse, and that measurement of residual symptoms of depression may be appropriate inasmuch as it provides an index of underlying processes and mechanisms.

Developmental theory would also suggest that treatments should target life-stage-dependent outcomes. For example, teenage pregnancy in vulnerable girls adds to risk for subsequent episodes of depression (Maughan & Lindelow, 1997). However, risk for teenage pregnancy is likely to be linked to previous depression. Episodes of depression in adolescence, themselves, have an effect on psychosocial functioning—for example, increasing emotional reliance on others (Rohde, Lewinsohn, & Seeley, 1994)—and hence may increase the risk for teenage pregnancy. Vulnerability factors for depression, such as helplessness (Harris, Brown, & Bifulco, 1990), may also increase risk for teenage pregnancy, in addition to any effects of episodes. Thus the case for teenage pregnancy as a treatment outcome is based on consideration of risk mechanisms for depression, those arising from depression in early adolescence, and those for recurrence in late adolescence and into adult life.

Once vulnerability is a target for treatment, the presence or absence of symptoms becomes a weaker indicator of who needs treatment. Young people with low metacognitive awareness or those who are at risk for teenage pregnancy but who do not have symptoms of depression may be as much at risk for subsequent depression as those who are symptomatic. In that case, there is the possibility that depression can be prevented by treating vulnerable, but asymptomatic, groups. Equally, it cannot be assumed that vulnerabilities operate uniformly over development, and only longitudinal studies can tell us whether and at what ages apparent vulnerabilities that have not yet been expressed symptomatically are still associated with risk for later psychopathology. Longitudinal studies, coupled with treatment studies with long-term outcomes, are also needed if the relative merits of different indices of efficacy are to be evaluated. In relation to depression, which frequently takes a relapsing or chronic course, the resolution of symptoms over months is relatively uninformative. Equally, outcomes such as metacognitive awareness will be of interest only if they can be shown to relate to relapse and persistence in the long term.

The obstacles to implementing programmes informed by issues raised by Kazdin and picked up in this commentary are formidable. As he points out, many of these considerations imply a study of moderators of treatment. Statistically these are evident as interactions between the treatment variable and one or more other predictor variables (Baron & Kenny, 1986), and that implies even bigger sample sizes! And that means larger grants, which are not commonly available for psychotherapy research. Equally, as Kazdin's chapter shows, the mere application of the RCT methodology does not provide an adequate agenda for child psychotherapy research. He has highlighted the need to understand psychotherapy and how it produces change, and I have added a plea for good theory and a developmental perspective.

CHAPTER EIGHT

Effectiveness of psychotherapy in the "real world": the case of youth depression

V. Robin Weersing

In 1957 Eugene Levitt published a devastating review of the child and adolescent psychotherapy literature. The Levitt paper followed on the heels of the more famous Eysenck review (1952) of adult therapy and drew similar conclusions—there was little to no empirical evidence to suggest that psychotherapy was, in fact, beneficial. Across 18 studies, youths who received therapy recovered from their "neuroses" no faster than did untreated youths, and, in a follow-up paper, Levitt (1963) reported that the recovery rate for child and adolescent psychotherapy might be marginally worse than the mere improvement associated with the passage of time.

Fast-forward three decades. A new crop of review papers has been published on the effects of psychotherapy, using the still-novel method of "meta-analysis". In these new meta-analyses, quantitative data from individual therapy studies are coded, placed upon a common effect-size metric, and statistically examined, giving an estimate of treatment effects across the entire psychotherapy literature, which, by the mid-1980s, had grown to hundreds of studies. Results of these meta-analyses appear to be good news. Psychotherapy for adults and for youth produces medium-to-large effects when therapy is compared to no treatment or a waiting-list control group (e.g., Casey & Berman, 1985; Smith, Glass, & Miller, 1980; Weisz, Weiss, Alicke, & Klotz, 1987). On average, the symptom levels of treated youths are close to a standard deviation lower than the symptoms of control youths (*ES* = .79; see Weisz et al., 1987). Therapy may work better for some problems, age groups, and treatment types than for others, but in many minds psychotherapy is saved.

However, the story is not yet finished. In the three decades separating the work of Eugene Levitt (1957) from that of John Weisz and colleagues (1987), how psychotherapy was studied underwent a methodological revolution. The Levitt and Eysenck reviews produced intense debate, with much of the criticism focused on the methodological weaknesses of the psychotherapy studies that served as a basis for the authors' negative conclusions. Early treatment studies were guilty of a litany of design sins, including: (a) failure to randomly assign youths to treatment and control conditions; (b) using therapy drop-outs as a comparison group; (c) failure to specify what therapy procedures were used in the intervention; (d) allowing therapists or other non-blind raters to assess outcome; (e) enrolling very heterogeneous samples of youth in terms of diagnoses and developmental level; and (f) failing to assess for important moderators of treatment outcome within these mixed samples (for review see Kazdin, 1978). To give psychotherapy a fair and rigorous test, modern clinical trial methods were developed, with clear inclusion and exclusion criteria, random assignment, blinded and standardized diagnostic assessment, and manualized treatments. At the same time as these method developments, the type of therapy studied also shifted from less structured, insight-oriented, and client-centred models to cognitive and behavioural skill-building approaches, although disagreement exists on whether the constraints of clinical trial methods forced this change (Westen, Novotny, & Thompson-Brenner, 2004) or whether the researchers who stepped forward to submit their treatments to experimental test hailed from behavioural backgrounds (cf. Weisz, Weersing, & Henggeler, 2005). In any case, by 1987, the how and what of psychotherapy research was almost entirely different from what it had been three decades earlier.

Given these developments, it is perhaps not surprising that the conclusions Levitt and Eysenck reached about the effects of psychotherapy were different from those of the meta-analysts of the 1980s. In many respects, they were no longer studying the same thing. Perhaps more importantly, in recent years it has become increasingly apparent that while therapy *research* had changed dramatically between 1957 and 1987, the *practice* of psychotherapy in the real world may not have. Therapists in everyday practice report using eclectic, predominantly insight-oriented therapy techniques (Weersing, Weisz, & Donenberg,

2002), rather than the manualized cognitive–behavioural protocols that have been tested in clinical trials (Addis & Krasnow, 2000). Diagnostic assessments, presumably the basis of treatment planning, are not standardized, and available data suggest that clinician diagnoses many be unreliable and do not concur with the results of research diagnostic procedures (Jensen & Weisz, 2002). Clinicians and practices accept heterogeneous samples of youths for treatment, most of whom suffer in all likelihood from multiple comorbid problems rather than a single "inclusion" diagnosis (e.g., Hammen, Rudolph, Weisz, Rao, & Burge, 1999). Along these and many other dimensions, the clinical practice of psychotherapy bears little resemblance to psychotherapy delivered in research studies, raising a fundamental question: is the *effectiveness* of therapy in practice equivalent to the *efficacy* of therapy in clinical trials? In other words, can we generalize from the results of the psychotherapy clinical trials literature to the likely effects of real-world clinical interventions?

This distinction between efficacy in research and effectiveness in practice was highlighted in the 1990s by Weisz, Weiss, and Donenberg (1992), and the pursuit of an answer to the generalizability question has driven a large potion of the psychotherapy research agenda since that time. Work has begun to rigorously assess the effects of community "treatment-as-usual" (TAU), using methods drawn from clinical trials (e.g., blinded and standardized assessment). Initial results have not been encouraging (see, e.g., Bickman, 1996; Weiss, Catron, Harris, & Phung, 1999), leading many researchers and professional organizations to suggest that community TAU might be improved if practitioners adopted the (primarily) cognitive–behavioural treatments identified as efficacious in clinical trials (e.g., Task Force on Promotion and Dissemination of Psychological Procedures, 1995). However, most of these therapy protocols have never been tested in the heterogeneous samples of clinical practice, and it is unclear whether the interventions shown to be efficacious in controlled clinical trials would be effective in the real world. The generalizability question becomes, thus, more complex.

The remainder of this chapter wrestles with the question of generalizability, using our programme of research into the treatment of depressed youths as an example. We present data on: (a) the efficacy of cognitive–behavioural therapy (CBT) for youth depression in clinical trials; (b) the effectiveness of eclectic, community TAU for depressed youths; and (c) preliminary data on the effectiveness of CBT for depressed teens, when CBT is transported to real-world practice environments. This review is designed to be illustrative rather than comprehensive and to provoke consideration of the issues involved in examining the effectiveness of youth psychotherapy in the real world.

Efficacy of cognitive–behavioural therapy for depression in youth

We begin with a brief review of the efficacy of cognitive–behavioural treatments (CBT) for mood disorders in children and adolescents. As many as 1 in 5 youths will suffer a significant episode of depression before the end of puberty (Lewinsohn, Hops, Roberts, Seeley, & Andrews, 1993), and early onset of mood symptoms is associated with impairments in current social and educational roles and with deficits in later adult functioning (e.g., Rohde, Lewinsohn, & Seeley, 1994). Although youth depression is a significant mental health problem, psychopathology research with this population is of recent origin, and there are no published clinical trials of psychotherapeutic interventions before 1980. Perhaps unsurprisingly, the clinical trial literature is relatively small. At last review, there were only 21 controlled studies of psychotherapy (Weersing & Brent, 2006), with 86% of these assessing the efficacy of the dominant therapy model: cognitive–behavioural therapy (CBT).

Cognitive–behavioural theory. CBT techniques for treating depression are based on two complementary views of the origin and maintenance of depressive symptoms. Cognitive theories postulate that the syndrome is the result of inaccurate, overly negative views of the self, the world, and expectations for the future (Beck, Rush, Shaw, & Emery, 1979; cf. Abramson, Metalsky, & Alloy, 1989; Abramson, Seligman, & Teasdale, 1978). When individuals are faced with daily disappointments and serious life events, this negative cognitive set is hypothesized to interfere with accurate information processing, lead individuals to feel dysphoric, and contribute to worsening mood symptoms over time. Behavioural theories of depression, such as social learning theory (Lewinsohn, Gotlib, & Hautzinger, 1998), also place stress at the centre of their models but emphasize the negative mood consequences brought about by the disruption in adaptive behaviour patterns caused by stressful events. This disruption is more severe for individuals with weak mood regulation skills (e.g., those unskilled in how to use pleasant activities to raise mood). Behavioural theory is not incompatible with cognitive models: indeed, in social learning models, depression may emerge from several possible diatheses (stressful events, maladaptive cognitions, behavioural withdrawal) that interact with other risk factors to disrupt adaptive behaviours and spiral mood downward.

CBT clinical trials. CBT for youth depression seeks to alleviate symptoms by addressing the core cognitive and behavioural factors implicated in these etiological models. Common treatment techniques in CBT protocols include: (a) teaching youths to monitor their moods and observe what makes them feel both happy and depressed (mood monitoring); (b) helping youths to examine their thoughts and assumptions and assess the accuracy and affective consequences of their views (cognitive restructuring); (c) promoting engagement in meaningful and pleasant activities (behavioural activation); (d) teaching youths relaxation techniques to cope with continuing environmental stressors; (e) providing social skills and conflict resolution training; and (f) teaching general problem-solving skills (Kaslow & Thompson, 1998; Kazdin & Weisz, 1998). Different CBT manuals employ various combinations of these techniques, but, across these studies, CBT has shown positive effects. In research settings, CBT for youth depression reliably outperforms waiting-list and attention placebo control conditions, and meta-analyses of CBT outcomes yield medium- to large effect sizes (Compton et al., 2004; Lewinsohn & Clarke, 1999; Reinecke, Ryan, & DuBois, 1998). For adolescents suffering from depression, CBT also may be superior to family and supportive therapies (Brent et al., 1997) and relaxation alone (Wood, Harrington, & Moore, 1996).

CBT for youths with depression appears to be an efficacious treatment. Intervention effects are stronger at post-treatment than over follow-up, and by two years post-therapy the majority of treated youths will have experienced a recurrence of disorder (Birmaher et al., 2000). Despite these limitations, CBT is clearly the research "gold standard" therapy in terms of empirical support (Compton et al., 2004). How do the effects of current community models of care for depressed youths compare to the results of these CBT efficacy studies?

Effectiveness of community treatment-as-usual

To answer this query, we conducted a naturalistic investigation of community TAU in six Los Angeles-area community mental health centres (CMHCs). In this study (Weersing & Weisz, 2002), we did not manipulate treatment, and therapists were free to use whatever eclectic combination of therapy techniques they thought would be of greatest value in the conduct of their cases. For the purposes of the research evaluation, we identified youths with depression at CMHC intake, verifying diagnoses of Major Depressive and/or Dysthymic Disorder with an independent, structured research interview. These youths were then followed over a period of two years, tracking the services received and clinical outcomes achieved, using well-validated symptom measures, such as the *Children's Depression Inventory* (Kovacs, 1992)

On initial examination, the data told a simple story. At the time of intake into the CMHCs, youths' depression symptoms were, on average, at the 95th percentile, compared to a normative sample of healthy peers. By one year later, these symptom scores were well within the normal range. During treatment, depressed youths got better. However, there were several alternative interpretations of these results. Our naturalistic investigation was designed to be minimally invasive to the regular operation of the clinics, and, as such, there was no random assignment to community TAU versus a control condition. Depressed youths improved during therapy, but did they improve because of therapy? Natural remission is always a potential confound in uncontrolled designs; this is even more the case in an investigation of depression, given the episodic nature of the disorder. In order to place the CMHC results in a meaningful context, we turned to the efficacy literature and used the outcomes of CBT in clinical trials as a "benchmark" against which the results of community TAU could be measured.

Benchmarks have been broadly useful in our work, well beyond this first study of community TAU, and we refer back to them throughout the remainder of this chapter. Accordingly, in the following section, information on the creation and calculation of benchmarks is provided in some detail.

Creation of the benchmarks. Benchmarking, as a method of programme evaluation, first appeared in the treatment outcome literature in 1998 (see Weersing, 2005). Traditionally, the method has been used to assess the effects of a known intervention, such as CBT, in a new context. For example, Wade, Treat, and Stuart (1998) trained community therapists in CBT for adults with panic disorder, a treatment with a very strong efficacy literature. Outcomes for CBT in the community were assessed using the same methods and measures as in two seminal clinical trials for panic. At the end of the study, the effects of CBT in practice were compared point-by-point to the results of the CBT conditions in these "gold standard" studies. In practice, the CBT response rate and effects on dimensional measures were almost identical to clinical trial results, supporting the effectiveness of the intervention in the new context of community practice.

Our use of benchmarking was somewhat different. We were not seeking to assess the effects of a known intervention. Other than our own results, there were little available in terms of data on the effects of community TAU for depressed youths and no single seminal study that could clearly serve as a point of comparison for the results in our sample. Under these circumstances, we turned to the entire CBT efficacy literature to construct composite benchmarks of "best-case" and "worst-case" outcomes for youth depression. The best-case benchmark was created using data from the active CBT treatment conditions, across all published CBT clinical trials for youth. The worst-case benchmark was calculated from data on the control conditions (attention-placebo, waiting list, no treatment) in these same studies.

These composite benchmarks were constructed drawing methods from meta-analysis. The CBT clinical trials used a range of outcome measures, and the first step was to place these measures on a common effect-size metric. For each CBT clinical trial, we identified the primary dimensional depression outcome measure, and we obtained published normative data for the measure in non-clinical community samples of youth (see Weersing & Weisz, 2002). Next, we used the mean and standard deviation of the measure in the normal sample of youth to compute normative z scores for CBT (z_{nt}) and control (z_{nc}) groups in each study at each assessment point. These computations took the form $z_{nt} = (\bar{x}_t - \mu)/(\sigma)$ and $z_{nc} = (\bar{x}_c - \mu)/(\sigma)$, where $\bar{x}_t$ was the CBT group mean, $\bar{x}_c$ was the control group mean, μ was the normal population mean, and σ was the normal population standard deviation for the depression measure (Kendall & Grove, 1988). The normative z scores were then aggregated within condition (CBT and control) across studies at each available assessment point. Studies typically assessed outcomes at three-month intervals, giving us aggregate benchmark means for intake, post-treatment, 1- to 3-month follow-up, 4- to 6-month follow-up, 7- to 9-month follow-up, and 10- to 12-month follow-up. As the final step in the creation of the two composite benchmarks, 95% confidence intervals were calculated for each benchmark, at each time point, in order to capture the variability in outcomes across studies.

Note that the control group benchmark had fewer data available at long-term follow-up than did the CBT composite benchmark, as many of the clinical trials used short wait-list control conditions.

Effects of community therapy. Figure 8.1 displays the symptom trajectory for depressed youths treated in the CMHCs, plotted against our two composite benchmarks. As can been seen in the figure, the results do not appear to be good news for community treatment. At intake, CMHC youth exhibited depression symptoms as severe as youth in clinical trials. Yet, despite this similarity in starting point, there were substantial differences in depression recovery. Youth treated in CBT conditions of clinical trials showed steep improvements in their depression symptoms within three months, and these improvements were maintained over follow-up. Overall, depressed youth treated in the CMHC had much shallower symptom trajectories than youth in CBT, and the CMHC means clearly fall outside the confidence intervals of the CBT benchmark, until 12 months after intake. Indeed, the mean symptom slope for community treatment more closely resembled the clinical trial control condition benchmark than the CBT benchmark.

Why did youth in the CMHC fare so poorly? Clinical differences between samples did not appear to be a viable explanation. Youth had similarly severe depression at intake, and, although CMHC youth had higher rates of comorbid disorders, comorbidity did not pre-

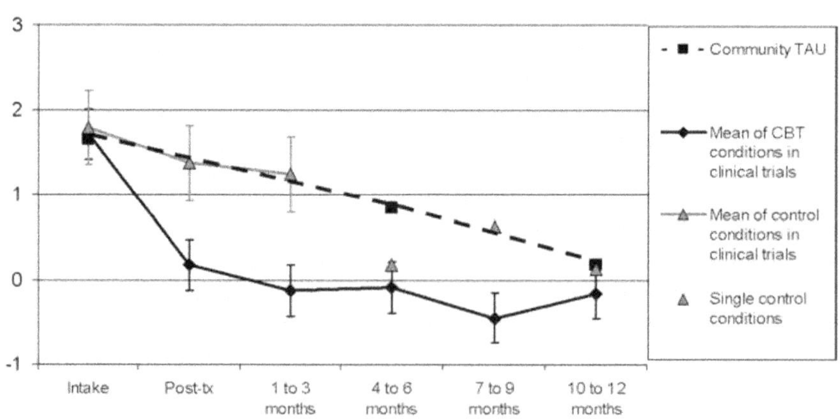

Figure 8.1. Comparison of community treatment as usual (Community TAU) with CBT clinical trials and with clinical trial control conditions (Weersing & Weisz, 2002).

dict symptom slope within the community sample. It is possible that demographic and contextual differences may have played a role in producing worse CMHC outcomes. Ethnic minority youth (52% of cases) and youth receiving a very low dose of therapy (less than eight sessions) appeared to receive very little benefit from CMHC treatment; however, even when examining only Caucasian youth and high-dose youth, the CMHC sample still performed more poorly than did clinical trial participants.

While this investigation did not compare CMHC therapy and CBT head-on in a randomized trial, differences in therapy type did appear to be a compelling explanation for differences in outcome: CMHC therapist reported using eclectic, unstructured sets of techniques, with a heavy emphasis on insight-oriented therapy, whereas therapists in clinical trials provided a pure dose of CBT. Interestingly, the CMHC results bear a strong resemblance to the pattern seen in studies of the natural course of untreated youth depression. In youth, the median length of an episode of major depression has been estimated to be nine months (Kovacs, 1996), with a 94% cumulative probability of recovery by one year after the onset of the episode (Kovacs, Obrosky, Gatsonis, & Richards, 1997).

Generalizability of cognitive–behavioural therapy in the "real world"

It appears that there may be room for improvement in community psychotherapy for depressed youth. While data on the effects of usual clinical care are still thin, accumulating evidence suggests that there may be value in directly assessing the effects of CBT under the conditions and in the populations of real-world clinical care. Should CBT prove as effective as it is efficacious, there may be a valid argument for improving clinical practice by changing the type of therapy provided in community settings.

To date, there are no published investigations of this type of dissemination research—where CBT for youth depression has been transported to an active practice environment and the effectiveness of the intervention assessed. The most relevant published data on the "robustness" of CBT in practice may come from studies examining predictors of clinical trial treatment response. Unfortunately, findings in these investigations have been somewhat contradictory (cf. Brent et al., 1998; Clarke et al., 1992; Jayson, Wood, Kroll, Fraser, & Harrington, 1998; Rohde, Clarke, Lewinsohn, Seeley, & Kaufman, 2001). For example, in the Brent clinical trial comparing the efficacy of CBT, family, and supportive therapy, subject referral source was found to be a significant predictor of treatment outcome. Compared to youth who were recruited into the trial via newspaper advertisement, "real-world" youth who were referred to the study from clinical settings were significantly more likely to still meet criteria for major depression at the end of treatment (Brent et al., 1998). However, in the same clinical trial, Brent and colleagues found that CBT was significantly more robust than were alternate psychosocial interventions (family or supportive therapies) *even* for youths who had been clinically referred (Brent et al., 1998). In addition, CBT was significantly more efficacious than the other two treatments in the face of clinically complicating subject characteristics, such as psychiatric comorbidity and high levels of suicidality (Barbe, Bridge, Birmaher, Kolko, & Brent, 2001; Brent et al., 1998).

To add to this sparse knowledge base, we have followed up our naturalistic investigation of community TAU with two similar investigations of "real world" CBT for adolescents with major depressive disorder. In the first study, we examined the effects of CBT in a speciality clinic serving youths with serious depression and suicidality—a clinically important population that has frequently been excluded from clinical trials. In our second study, still in progress, we moved even farther into the realm of clinical practice, assessing the effects of CBT in the general outpatient service of a large managed care organization. Neither of these investigations provides a definitive test of the effectiveness of CBT in practice; however, the results may provide an initial estimate of the generalizability of the intervention and illuminate practice variables that may impact CBT outcomes in the real world.

Effectiveness of CBT in a depression speciality clinic. Data for our first project were collected from a depression speciality clinic, the Services for Teens at Risk (STAR) Center. The STAR Center is a working outpatient service based at Western Psychiatric Institute and Clinic that serves youths with serious depression and at high risk for suicide. While the STAR Center functions as an active clinic, it does share many features with clinical trials. As in most clinical trials, the STAR Center concentrates on the treatment of a focused clinical problem—depression. The Center uses CBT as its psychosocial intervention model, and, upon joining the Center, therapists are extensively trained and supervised in CBT techniques. Treatment at STAR is fully funded by the state and is free to teens and their families, similar to therapy research studies. Furthermore, STAR has a direct tie to a depression clinical trial in that the Center served as a referral source for the Brent (1997) investigation comparing CBT, family, and supportive therapy for adolescents with major depression.

In a number of other respects, however, therapy at STAR is representative of real-world clinical care. While therapists are trained in CBT at the beginning of their employment, they operate autonomously once they are senior clinicians. The length and session-by-session content of treatment is not fixed across patients, and psychotropic medication may be used as deemed medically necessary (Birmaher & Brent, 1998; Hughes et al., 1999). Teens and families come to the STAR Center via clinical referral routes, including direct referral from inpatient units in the psychiatric hospital. Finally, unlike the Brent clinical trial, the STAR Center does not exclude youth from treatment if they meet criteria for serious comorbid diagnoses (e.g., substance abuse) in addition to their primary diagnosis of depression.

Given this blend of clinical trial and clinical practice characteristics, we viewed the STAR Center as a natural laboratory in which to begin examining the effectiveness of CBT under clinically representative conditions. As a part of the STAR Center's operation as a CBT clinic, standardized assessments are administered to teens and their parents at intake and during therapy. Historically, these data have been used to guide treatment planning and provide youths and their families with feedback about treatment progress. In the current investigation, these data allowed us to model improvement in depression symptoms over the course of treatment, using multilevel modelling techniques. To anchor the magnitude of these effects, we then compared the STAR symptom trajectory to a specific, and very relevant, efficacy benchmark, the results of the Brent et al. (1997) CBT clinical trial.

As can be seen in Figure 8.2, youth ($N = 80$) provided CBT in STAR experienced significant improvement in depression symptoms approximately six months after intake (Weersing, Iyengar, Birmaher, Kolko, & Brent, 2006). This time to recovery was almost twice as long as in the Brent CBT clinical trial (1997). However, results of STAR CBT may compare favourably to outcomes achieved by community TAU. Recall that in our previous work, we found that depressed youth treated with community TAU did not experience significant symptom reduction until one year after intake. Data from these depressed adolescents also are included in Figure 8.2, as a point of comparison. The

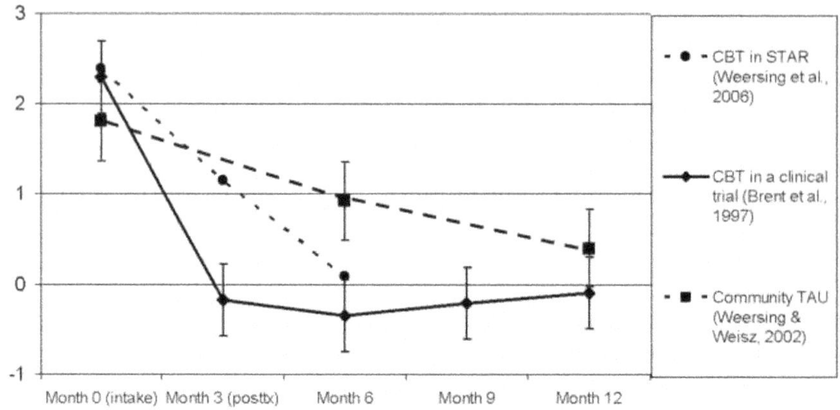

Figure 8.2. Comparison of CBT in a clinically representative speciality clinic (STAR) with the Brent CBT clinical trial and with community treatment-as-usual.

effects of CBT in STAR appear to split the difference between these two benchmarks.

As with our community study, we next sought to unpack these data and understand why youths in STAR did not have outcomes as favourable as youths in the CBT benchmark (Brent et al., 1997). STAR served as a referral source for the Brent trial, and, unsurprisingly, the demographic characteristics and level of depression symptoms in the two samples were virtually identical. Of STAR youths, 20% did meet criteria for at least one comorbid psychiatric diagnosis that would have resulted in exclusion from the clinical trial. However, within the STAR sample, comorbidity did not significantly predict outcome, suggesting that the overall differences in trajectories were not likely to be due to this factor. The Brent study and usual care in STAR did differ in terms of therapist supervision and monitoring, but there were no measured variables available to model the possible effects of therapist factors.

Within the Brent sample, referral source had emerged as a significant predictor of treatment outcome (Brent et al., 1998). Youths who came to the study through clinical referral routes (including referral from STAR) has significantly worse outcomes than did teens whose families had heard about the investigation through advertisements. In a set of exploratory analyses, we merged the raw data from the Brent clinical trial and our STAR investigation and modelled outcome for the combined sample, using clinical referral source as a key predictor variable. This analysis revealed a clear ordering of outcomes: youths who came to the clinical trial via advertisement had the best outcomes, followed by clinically referred youths in the clinical trial, followed by youths seen for CBT in STAR itself. All pairwise comparisons were statistically significant, although the difference between the STAR group and the clinically referred study group was very small and not clinically meaningful (less than a one-point difference on the *Beck Depression Inventory*, over six months). In the Brent sample, referral source was associated with high levels of hopelessness. Hopelessness was not assessed in STAR, but it is certainly possible that the STAR sample was feeling quite hopeless—for example, 50% of the sample had a history of suicide attempts, and many youths had a history of unsuccessful treatment prior to finding their way to the speciality clinic.

Taken together, the results of the STAR project suggest that (a) CBT may be able to exceed the poor effects of therapy seen in community care, but (b) that outcomes may well be attenuated from those seen in clinical research. It is possible that the source of this CBT–CBT outcome gap may be therapist factors, but some variance seems attached to qualities of youths and families associated with "referral status".

Effectiveness of CBT in a large managed care organization. In our most recent project, we have been working with colleagues at a large managed care organization (MCO) to examine the outcome of a completed in-house CBT dissemination project. Five years ago, therapists at multiple sites within the MCO were trained in the *Coping With Depression (CWD-A)* programme for adolescents (Lewinsohn, Clarke, Rohde, Hops, & Seeley, 1996). The *CWD-A* programme is the most studied CBT protocol for adolescents with depression (Clarke et al., 1995; Clarke, Lewinsohn, Rohde, Hops, & Seeley, 1999; Clarke et al., 2001; Clarke et al., 2002; Lewinsohn, Clarke, Hops, & Andrews, 1990), and the *CDW-A* manual has served as the base for a variety of other "independent" CBT treatment programmes (e.g., TADS Team, 2004). At the MCO, clinicians were provided with a short initial didactic training and the complete CBT treatment manuals. Therapists were instructed to use the manual to treat groups of depressed teenagers, although no additional supervision or case consultation was scheduled. Participating youths' depression symptoms were systematically assessed at intake and at six-month follow-up assessment.

Perhaps unsurprisingly, under these conditions, CBT does not appear to have been particularly effective (Weersing, Hamilton, & Warnick, 2006). As can be seen in Figure 8.3, the mean trajectory of youths

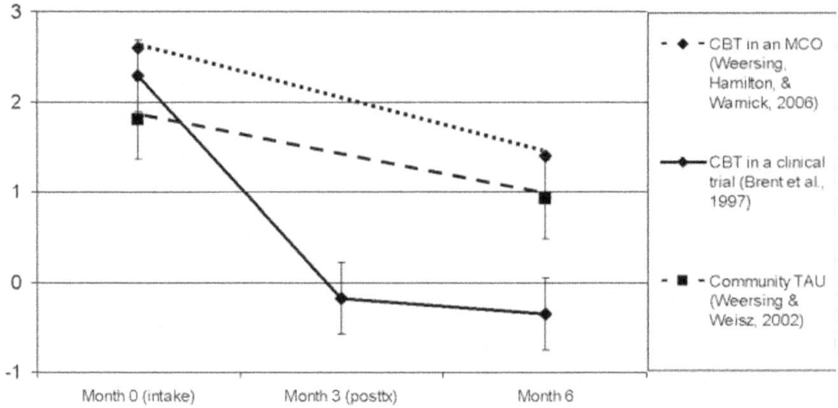

Figure 8.3. Comparison of CBT in a large managed care organization (CBT in an MCO) with the Brent CBT clinical trial and with community treatment-as-usual.

treated with CBT in the MCO ($N = 76$) parallels the poor outcome of youths seen in community clinics in Weersing and Weisz (2002). The results of the Brent et al. (1997) clinical trial are also included in the figure, for contrast. Limited data on teen characteristics or therapist behaviour are available to unpack these effects. This investigation is still in progress; however, based on interviews with therapists and reviews of medical records, one notable factor emerges: the CBT treatment was substantially modified from the original protocol described in the manual. Session length was shortened from 90 to 45 minutes; teens attended for fewer than half of the sessions called for in the protocol, and therapists reported adding non-CBT techniques to sessions.

Conclusions and future directions

In this chapter we have sought to highlight some of the issues involved in conducting real world treatment effectiveness research. Drawing from our own nascent work on youth depression, we (a) reviewed the clinical trial literature supporting the use of cognitive–behavioural procedures; (b) detailed a recent investigation of community care for depressed youths; and (c) described two initial studies designed to shed light on the likely effects of CBT in practice. In sum, the conclusion echoes Levitt (1957), it appears that CBT for youth *can* work well, and community care in all likelihood does not. However, this blanket statement obscures a number of critical variables that may define the conditions under which CBT for youth depression will be of benefit.

In our dissemination studies, CBT for youth did appear to be robust to the presence of many other comorbid psychiatric conditions—a substantial bit of good news for those who hope to improve community therapy outcomes by exporting CBT protocols to the more clinically complicated samples of community care. Looking within the STAR and Brent et al. (1997) samples, however, it appears that CBT may be of greatest help to the motivated youths and families who seek out care. In the Brent clinical trial, CBT was most efficacious for youths who came to the study via advertisement. Youths who were clinically referred to the investigation achieved remission of depression symptoms at a substantially slower rate—at a rate almost identical to the steady, but modest, recovery of youths seen in the CBT STAR speciality clinic. Referral status (clinical vs. advertisement) may be a proxy for a range of true psychological processes—from differences in motivation to the structure of pathology (i.e., hopelessness depression).

Preliminary data from a study of CBT in managed care highlights the importance of another set of real world moderators—variables associated with treatment adherence, quality of implementation, therapist training, and dose. These treatment parameters are set at the highest-possible-quality level in clinical trials. Maintaining quality assurance procedures, such as frequent therapist supervision and feedback, may be integral components of the large effect sizes seen in CBT efficacy studies (for discussion, see Kendall & Southam-Gerow, 1995). The economic cost involved with these procedures is quite high, and additional work defining the "what" and "how much" of clinical trial therapy structure and support would be of both scientific and practical import.

There are many additional areas of worthwhile generalizability research that have not been a focus of the discussion in this chapter (e.g., generalizability of effects across cultures). It is our hope that the brief overview provided in this chapter has proved convincing, not in its specific findings, but in the overall message that research to understand the effectiveness of therapy in practice is a worthy goal to pursue in our next 50 years of child therapy research.

NOTE

Preparation of this manuscript was facilitated by support from the Klingenstein Third Generation Foundation, the William T. Grant Foundation, and Robert Wood Johnson Foundation, and the National Institute of Mental Health (MH064503–01A1 and MH066371–01).

Commentary

Mary Target

Robin Weersing, in an elegant and deceptively straightforward presentation of the currently most challenging issue in psychotherapy research, offers a worrying portrayal of psychological therapy services. Can therapies, shown to be efficacious in research studies, remain effective in the real world? She shows that, notwithstanding the strong evidence base of cognitive behaviour therapy (CBT) in comparison with those of other approaches, when offered in the context of a community mental health service, CBT does not show comparable effectiveness. As one of the most original and open-minded researchers currently at work, attempting to address the so-called efficacy versus effectiveness issue (the difference between research treatment outcomes and those seen in routine clinical practice), any data presented by Weersing will command attention. These data are at once intriguing and challenging. In my commentary on her views I discuss the general problems of research on psychotherapy for depression in young people and then consider ways in which psychoanalytic clinical work might benefit from Weersing's analysis, as well as perhaps casting some further light on the findings she reports.

The psychological treatment of depression in children and young people

While most of the lessons from the chapter are applicable to the psychological treatment literature in general and the treatment of children and young people in particular, it should be noted that all Weersing's conclusions rely on data from childhood depression. While it may be appropriate to talk of adults as "having depression", it is perhaps more appropriate for us to think of children with depression as confronted by a complex set of behavioural, emotional, learning, relationship, and family problems that are best addressed together, even in children where depression is the primary concern. A fundamental difference is that, whereas adults with depression mostly recognize that they have a problem, children and young people generally experience depression as if "*they were* the problem".

This is, of course, very relevant in the evaluation of treatments for depression in this group, as most young people who might benefit from psychological therapies neither seek them nor welcome them when offered. Thus any treatment trial, other than those focused on the small proportion of depressed young people who are so severely self-harming or incapacitated that they are admitted to inpatient units, is likely to concern itself with a somewhat atypical group—those who are recognized as depressed and referred for help. Research so far has major limitations, as Weersing points out. The vast majority of studies are confined to community samples of young people with subclinical levels of depression or groups meeting clinical criteria but recruited through advertising. Young people in both of these groups are likely to have fewer of the entrenched problems and associated disorders that a clinician is expected to address together.

Through the influence of the work of Weersing and others, there has been a move among outcomes researchers—in this problem area as well as in others—to recruit increasingly realistic clinical samples. In an unpublished survey of the samples of outcome trials for childhood depression, Cotgrove and colleagues (2004) found the samples unrepresentative in terms of age, exclusion criteria (particularly comorbidity), recruitment, and the treatments offered. The figures on comorbidity are particularly striking, as noted by Weersing. Goodyer's work (e.g., Goodyer & Cooper, 1993), in common with reports from many other studies, has shown that the vast majority of cases referred to an outpatient clinic for depression have a comorbid diagnosis. Yet the largest trial of CBT so far, the Treatment for Adolescents With Depression Study (TADS Team, 2004), excluded patients whose depression was comorbid with conduct disorder.

Notwithstanding the fair wind behind controlled trials, the efficacy they demonstrate—taken as a whole—is modest. For example, no psychological therapies have been shown to maintain significant superiority even to non-active control treatments at one year or more follow-up. Weersing's research makes it clear that while a range of therapies produce gain during treatment that is well-maintained at follow-up, even minimal treatment comparison groups appear to catch up over the 6–12 months post-treatment period. The adult literature (Roth & Fonagy, 2005) implies that, for a proportion of patients at least, psychological treatments or indeed pharmacological treatments offer little. The pattern is that some people seem to get better, and for these psychosocial treatments accelerate the process, but some are "resistant" to any kind of intervention. Our review (NICE, 2005) suggested that group CBT, individual CBT, Interpersonal Therapy, non-directive supportive therapy, family therapy, and individual psychoanalytic psychotherapy all had some RCT evidence base. The strength of the current evidence is approximately in the order listed. Differences in effectiveness between therapies account for far less of the variance than do service user characteristics such as comorbidity, severity, chronicity, family dysfunction and the presence of abuse or trauma, and the absence of social support. All these points bear strongly on Weersing's conclusions concerning the relatively poor outcome of clinic-based treatments, where patients with these characteristics are more common. None of these factors on its own is likely to be definitive. For example, Weersing tells us that in the study of CBT as delivered in a university-based clinic (STAR), comorbidity did not predict worse outcome.

Implications for the practice of psychoanalytic psychotherapy

Stepping beyond the specific problem of childhood and adolescent depression, Weersing's chapter is rich with implications for the practice of psychological therapy, and not least for psychoanalytic psychotherapy. Her comparison of CMHC therapy and CBT, in randomized trials, shows CBT to be substantially more effective, and the course of those treated in CMHC therapy follows closely the course of no treatment control cases. As CMHC therapists report using more insight-oriented, unstructured psychodynamic/eclectic techniques, an uncharitable reader of the data might assume that these techniques, rather than differences in client groups or other aspects of the treatment setting, account for the inferior performance of CMHC therapy. This is not the claim that Weersing is making. The more constructive suggestion by Weersing is that there may be "room for improvement" in how psychotherapy is delivered (as opposed to what type of therapy is delivered) in the community.

The treatment given by the specialized depression clinic at the Western Psychiatric Institute and Clinic (WPIC) is almost as effective as laboratory-based studies. The treatment offered is likely to be close to standard CBT, as that is the training of the clinicians and the orientation of the clinic. But does this suggest that for psychoanalytic clinicians to be effective they should abandon their insight-oriented approach and start working in a cognitive–behavioural way? In my view this would be a premature conclusion, and it is not what Weersing proposes: (a) The university-based clinic offers a far better structured context for offering treatment than may generally be the case. (b) It is attended by less complex cases (20% as opposed to 93% comorbidity); on the other hand, they are more complex than patients in RCTs that rely on recruitment through advertisement or that exclude comorbidity. They are comparable to the genuine clinic-referred cases in some other RCTs. (c) There is a significant difference between CBT delivered in the community and CBT delivered in research studies or even in the routine work of a university clinic. When clinicians working for a managed care organization were trained in a specific CBT protocol, CBT did not emerge as being particularly effective. The reason for this is probably complex, but the fact that both the number and length of sessions offered in the community context were half those prescribed in the original protocol may have important implications.

The differences between these treatment settings may have less to do with the specific treatment approach offered, since the differences between treatment outcomes in RCTs are small, and more to do with the offering of a highly integrated model of care characterized by an institutional environment that is relatively structured, and a treatment that aims to offer consistent, coherent, and thoughtful psychological care. These are to be thought of less as non-specific aspects of psychotherapy, such as therapeutic alliance, and more as aspects of effective treatment delivery. In order for any psychological treatment to be effective, it must be delivered in a medium that permits its effective components to have their impact. I would argue, given the clear evidence that manualization of treatment and close supervision of therapy process improve outcomes (e.g., Addis, Wade, & Hatgis, 1999), that the relative ineffectiveness of psychodynamic therapies in some of the routine treatment-monitoring studies may not be to do with an inherent lack of effectiveness of that kind of treatment, but more with delivery in an inconsistent or intuitive way that has drifted away from the rigorous model that may have been the original training. The short usual duration of treatment also strongly suggests that the insight-oriented approach was being adapted to brief work in a way that might have been rather *ad hoc*. The evidence from the recent European multi-site study of Trowell and colleagues (Trowell et al., in press) demonstrates that when manualized and supervised, psychodynamic psychotherapy is very effective with complex and severe clinical cases. Why should this be the case?

Implications of psychoanalytic theory for the routine practice of psychological therapies

Work to identify generic features of psychotherapy has tended to concern itself with the attempt to find common mutative components across psychosocial treatments, such as creating hope, offering a secure attachment relationship, enhancing interpersonal understanding, and so on. Equally important are counter-therapeutic components that therapies share, which we know far less about and which include confusion in either the therapist or the client, aimlessness, unexplained changes in focus, lack of competence in the required techniques, using interventions that are theoretically contraindicated, associated guilt and rationalization on the part of the therapist, incoherent explanatory frameworks, inattentiveness by the therapist, and not having effective strategies to deal with commonly encountered barriers. These types of phenomena are known to all of us regardless of orientation. They are, however, most easily *understood* within a psychoanalytic framework that sees clients invariably as unconsciously resistant to therapeutic help, with gains of symptom removal often unconsciously outweighed by loss of hidden previous gains, or by the loss of repetition of the familiar (Freud, 1937c). This powerful but unacknowledged resistance to change creates an inevitable pressure on the therapist unconsciously to collude with the client's sabotage of his or her own conscious efforts to change. (In the case of children and adolescents it is, in any case, often a desire and effort more driven by the family than by the young person—an important point to keep in mind.)

Only a clear and coherent framework of theory and technique can help the therapist to withstand the pressures inevitably generated in any consulting-room. Most of us need more than training to maintain this framework: we also need active support to keep us on the straight and narrow. In structured, symptom-focused therapies, therapists benefit from a manual (divisions between phases, labels for particular skills to be learned, etc.) structure to the course of therapy and for each session. For those working in longer-term, unstructured therapies that aim to address personality and relationships as well as symptoms, manuals are more difficult to write and to apply in routine practice, and training thus needs to be very extensive, because the theoretical model and technical principles need to be heavily internalized. However, for all types of therapy, regular supervision and perhaps other assessments of adherence (e.g., taping of sessions and use of process measures) are vital to ensure that therapy remains coherent and true to the theoretical model being practised.

Much work remains to be done in evaluating the results of good-quality delivery of the range of treatment models we now have available. Once it is clearer which models offer most to which kinds of patients, then we need to evaluate how these approaches can be "rolled out" to the community settings (clinics, schools, home, and other) in which the young people struggling with mental health problems—and of course the social and educational problems that accompany them—are to be found. Weersing's work has been from the beginning, and promises to remain, a shining example of most intelligent, careful work in this area, being at once pragmatic, theoretically well informed, and willing to engage with the full complexity of these issues.

CHAPTER NINE

Controlling the random, or who controls whom in the randomized controlled trial?

Anthony W. Bateman

The randomized controlled trial (RCT) is revered by researchers and has become the gold standard by which treatments are assessed. In effect, most people believe that the RCT and high-quality evidence go hand in hand. Of course this is perfectly true if there is no deviation from protocol and minimal difference between contrasting groups other than the intervention under study. But life is rarely so simple. The application of the RCT in a clinical context and to psychotherapy outcome research is not so straightforward, especially in the study of personality disorder. The aim of this chapter is to consider some of the problems of implementing RCTs within a routine clinical service and to identify some ways of addressing the difficulties.

RCTs and psychotherapy research

The application of the RCT to psychotherapy research is deceptively simple. A homogeneous group of patients with a specific problem are allocated randomly to different treatments. Skilled therapists deliver interventions in a pure and measurable form and in a specific dose—such as 16 sessions—and outcome is reliably measured. But there are a number of problems in actual practice.

(a) Randomization of patients to different therapies does not represent normal patient entry into and continuation with treatment. Strict randomization may lead to patients being allocated to treatments they would otherwise not normally accept or be offered. Patients with personality disorder are not known for their consistency and, having accepted randomization, may not accept their allocated group and either drop out of the trial at this point or demand the alternative treatment. At the first hurdle a non-random sample is emerging. I will return to this later because it is, I believe, a problem that is underestimated in the study of personality disorder. In addition, therapists attempt to circumvent the randomization process, believing that their clinical assessment has identified that one of the contrasting treatments holds the best chance of good outcome—despite the extremely limited empirical evidence for this clinical view. (b) There is increasing evidence that patient expectation of therapy is important for outcome (Horowitz, Rosenberg & Bartholomew, 1993), and so offering patients a treatment that they have no belief in is hardly likely to help them to remain in treatment over the long term or to optimize outcome. RCTs favour short-term treatments, since they are difficult to maintain over a prolonged period. In long-term treatment patients tend to drop out, seek additional treatments, or begin to resent the repetitive intrusion of data collection and decline to take part. This disadvantages research in longer-term therapy, which has, until recently, been underrepresented in the literature other than through the "open trial" or cohort study. (c) Sample size is often small, and attrition of patients may be significant, leading to a situation in which patients remaining in a trial are far from random. Those patients may also respond differently to the same treatment, leading to variation in outcome within the same group, which may distort the outcome. (d) The "named" treatment is often delivered by different therapists, so, even if a manual is followed, patients may well be getting treatment that differs in significant respects. Therapists show considerable flexibility in interpreting manuals even after training (Gibbons, Crits-Christoph, Levinson, & Barber, 2003). Fidelity of application is commonly measured by recording sessions, although few studies record all sessions and randomly transcribe them to ensure therapists keep to the model of therapy. Manualization of therapies has, in any case, been found wanting empirically. Henry and colleagues (1993) demonstrated that adherence to treatment protocols obtained by additional training results in decreases in the quality of generic therapist functioning. This may either reduce the effectiveness of a therapy or, at least, not improve it (Bein et al., 2000). (e) Therapists themselves are rarely matched to patients, even though patient–therapist fit may influence outcome (for review see Lambert, 2004; Rubino et al., 2000). (f) Non-specific factors powerfully influence outcome, and blind evaluations are hard to achieve. (g) Possibly most importantly, investigator allegiance affects outcome (Gaffan, Tsaousis, & Kemp-Wheeler, 1995). In randomization, the ideal control group may be no treatment at all, but this is rarely ethically or practically possible and does not control for the effect of attention. A placebo treatment is also impossible because it is inconceivable that any activity between two people would have no positive or negative therapeutic effect. Researchers have therefore tended to restrict themselves to comparison of an active treatment either with treatment as usual in the case of longer-term therapies or with another active therapy in the case of short-term therapies. Tellingly, they most often provide the control therapy themselves, even though professionals heavily identified with a therapy are more likely to show a better outcome for that therapy than would an alternative control. Luborsky and colleagues (1999) suggest that the allegiance of the researcher accounts for 70% of the variance in outcome studies, suggesting that most of the time we can predict which treatment is likely to be most effective merely on the loyalty of the researcher.

Of course many of these difficulties are not specific to psychotherapy, and it is to the credit of psychotherapy researchers that they take the problems more seriously than do most other research groups. Research into the effectiveness of medication is beset with similar problems (Moncrieff, 2002). (a) Outcomes of treatment with medication are better in trials conducted by pharmaceutical companies than those that are independently funded and conducted by autonomous investigators (Freemantle, Anderson, & Young, 2000) (b) Trials are rarely performed using an active placebo, which means that "blindness" of participants and researchers becomes highly unlikely. Most medication has unwanted effects that are obvious to patient and researcher, and this aspect of "unblinding" is rarely measured (Even, Siobud-Dorocant, & Dardennes, 2000).

Complex interventions and abandoning the RCT?

Given all these problems, it is not surprising that some people are abandoning the RCT altogether. But who are these brave people? They are primarily those who are involved in the study of complex interventions (Hawe, Shiell, & Riley, 2004), such as implementation of health promotion schemes or community service re-organization and its effect on long-term outcomes; as yet it is not psychotherapy researchers, although many psychotherapy interventions for personality disorder are clearly "complex interventions". These courageous few are turning away from the RCT in spite of the opinion of lead thinkers and funding bodies. The United Kingdom's Medical Research Council (MRC) continues to insist that trials of complex interventions should "consistently provide as close to the same intervention as possible" by "standardising the content and delivery of the intervention" and do not see the difficulty in doing this with a complex intervention as a reason to abandon the RCT as the primary research method. Yet the more complex an intervention becomes, so it becomes increasingly difficult to standardize. Of course, the acceptability of the MRC statement may depend on careful definition of a complex intervention. But they have come up with a vague definition arguing that "the greater the difficulty in defining precisely what exactly are the active ingredients of an intervention and how they relate to each other, the greater the likelihood that you are dealing with a complex intervention". In other words, from a cynical perspective, if you don't really know what is happening within an intervention or you haven't thought through your intervention carefully enough, then it is a complex intervention!

In truth, a complex intervention is more likely to be one that cannot easily be decomposed into its constituent parts. Any attempt to do so loses the essence of the intervention itself. The intervention may be built from a number of different components, but the whole is more than the sum of the parts, and the whole itself and its effects cannot be defined through its different elements. Thus the intervention will display phenomena or have results that are inexplicable by any conventional analysis of the constituent parts. This level of complexity will result in difficulties in standardization across settings and between practitioners and problems of replication within health systems simply because a complex intervention needs adaptation to local circumstances, and practitioners are likely to implement it in an idiosyncratic manner.

Take therapeutic communities as an example—attempts to define exactly what they are and to replicate them successfully have proved impossible for research purposes, although the opinion of their effectiveness is, rightly or wrongly, relatively favourable. Their defining characteristic involves

> communalism in sharing tasks, responsibilities and rewards; permissiveness to act in accord with one's feelings without accustomed

> social inhibitions; democratic decision making; reality confrontation of the subject with what they are doing in the here-and-now; as well as social analysis or Main' s culture of enquiry. [Norton, 1992]

But this type of definition is so broad that it becomes impossible to standardize across settings or even for the practitioners themselves to agree on what they are doing (Haigh, 2002). Demonstrable effectiveness on one site cannot be assumed to mean that a similarly named treatment elsewhere implemented by other practitioners would be equally effective. This is important, because it becomes impossible to provide effective and equable health care unless we can ensure standardization of treatments.

This difficulty with complex interventions does not mean that we should abandon process research the aim of which is to understand the change process, but that we need to be careful when reducing interventions to discrete elements. The key is to ensure that complex interventions are defined according to principle, form, process, and function and not solely compositionally.

Complex psychotherapeutic interventions and MBT

If we accept a definition of a complex intervention as one that cannot easily be dismantled to meaningful components, most psychotherapeutic treatments for personality disorder are likely to fall within this category. The names that some of them have been given—transference-focused psychotherapy (TFP) (Clarkin, Kernberg & Yeomans, 1999), dialectical behaviour therapy (DBT) (Linehan, 1993), schema-focused psychotherapy (SFT) (Young, 1990)—are full of complexity, and the long trainings that have been suggested imply an intricacy and attention to subtle detail that militate against generalization to health-service settings. In addition, all these treatments have arisen within the context of a "laboratory" and have been implemented by highly trained mental health practitioners. This research process of testing a treatment within "ideal" conditions has much merit but has recently been challenged, and increasing importance is being given to "real-world" studies.

Implementing treatment within a routine clinical service is, of course, not new. But it challenges the current situation in which most trials take place within the "laboratory" and then have to be translated into routine practice. It is now well known that this method of moving from efficacy to effectiveness research is flawed: treatments that work well in the "laboratory" rarely lead to equally effective interventions in clinical practice. The success of family interventions in reducing relapse in schizophrenia in carefully controlled trials has not been matched in clinical practice (Andersen & Adams, 1996); research outcomes using CBT for depression do not equate with those found in everyday clinical settings. Perhaps it is better to move from effectiveness to efficacy or even to start in the "real" world and to remain there. Of course, the reasonable and balanced person will, rightly, say that there is a place for both. Yet the problems of starting in the "real" world and remaining there are formidable, although not insuperable.

There are a number of clinical problems that need to be addressed by the clinician researcher when working in the "real" world. (a) There is the implementation of a RCT itself within a clinical service. I have previously mentioned that practitioners in services not used to research are likely to oppose implementation of randomized treatments, believing that they have a special knowledge of what is best for "their" patient and therefore resisting their random allocation. Many specify one of the available treatments, justifying their opinion using specious arguments. This problem is best addressed through a seminar on evidence. But we have also implemented a scheme in which the assessors note their treatment recommendation. The outcomes for those patients with concordant allocation are then compared with those whose placement was discordant, and the results are fed back to the assessors. So far, no assessor is better than chance! (b) The aims of treatment have to be clearly defined and matched to specific outcome measures. (c) The patient population to be studied needs careful characterization, particularly in terms of severity. (d) The treatment method must be manualized, so that it is defined adequately, is practical within the confines of a service, and can be learned by practitioners without extensive training. (e) There may be problems with maintaining patients within treatment and ensuring that the control within the system does not get out of control.

While these are only a few of the problems that beset randomized clinical trials, they are of particular importance in the study of personality disorder. The aim of the final part of this chapter is to consider some of them in the context of mentalization-based treatment (MBT) (Bateman & Fonagy, 2004a, 2004b) and to discuss ways in which they may be overcome.

Problems, problems, problems

Aims of treatment and meaningful outcomes

In the study of personality disorder, there is no agreed outcome battery, although it seems likely that in the United States the NIMH will agree core measures at some point. Until then, researchers have to decide what are the best measures available and tailor those to their treatment. There is a hierarchy of aims in MBT each of which is matched to outcome measures.

1. There is a need to engage the patient in therapy and to reduce any actions or social disadvantage that might impede access to treatment. This is monitored through assiduously checking drop-out rates, attending to social problems such as unstable accommodation, and addressing self-destructive behaviours. The latter are measured according to a suicide and self-harm inventory, which is used to collect data in an organized manner. The criteria for suicidal acts are: (a) deliberate; (b) life threatening; (c) result in medical intervention; (d) medical assessment is consistent with a suicide attempt. Criteria for acts of self-mutilation are: (a) deliberate; (b) resulting in visible tissue damage; (c) nursing or medical intervention required. The interview asks specific questions not only about numbers of acts but also about dangerousness of acts—that is, presence or absence of another person, likelihood of being found, preparation, and lethality. Multiple acts over a short period of time, for example a frenzied self-cutting, are counted as a single act.

2. The second aim is to reduce severity of symptoms and to improve social and interpersonal function. These are monitored using a symptom battery. Patients' subjective experience of symptoms is measured using the SCL-90-R; depression and anxiety using the Beck Depression Inventory (BDI) and the Spielberger State/Trait anxiety scale, respectively. In order to assess areas targeted by psychoanalytic therapy, social adjustment and interpersonal function are measured pre- and post-trial using the modified Social Adjustment Scale-self-report (SAS-M) and the Inventory of Interpersonal problems–Circumflex version (IIP). The SAS-M and the IIP provide an assessment of an individual's work, spare-time activities, and family life and difficulties with interpersonal function. The reliability and validity of all these instruments is well established.

Monitoring of symptoms during treatment is one area in which the randomized controlled trial can easily become an uncontrolled and random trial. Reproduced below is a sample of a fully annotated version of the SCL-90 and the BDI by a patient who had developed "instrument fatigue" and complained that the questionnaires were not meaningful to her problems.

SCL 90-R

Question: Tick anyone box for each problem and do not skip any item. If you have by mistake ticked the wrong box please strike it out and tick the right one.

Answer: Why can't I skip? It is not a test, can't it be a game? This is threatening. You should reassure people if you don't want them to get exam nerves. But then therapy is more threatening than exams. Anyway, this clearly isn't adult learning for that might involve games, and if it is not a test either, it must be therapy or research.

I prefer to cross them out, not strike them out, because I'm cross here. There is no right answer. Actually, I prefer to scribble because I want to be a creative writer, not a researcher.

BDI

Question: I am critical of myself for my weaknesses or mistakes.

Answer: This is a good one if being critical is a process "like running or walking along by a river you can't be very" critical. As in you can't be a very running although you can't be running very easily with those shoes on makes sense. However, if being critical means being skilful at or engaged in criticism then you can be very critical. People tend to think of criticism as a negative word. Positive and negatives are extremes. Therefore to be very critical implies an extremely negative attitude. Processes on the other hand do not have such extremes. Therefore, to be critical does not in itself imply a negative, so fuck off.

Question: I am completely absorbed in what I feel.

Answer: It wouldn't be good to be completely absorbed into anything because this suggests total stasis. Absorption is a more active frame of reference. Therefore, "I feel complete absorption in what I am doing" does not have the same overly negative undertones or something. I can't be bothered with it any more. Are you lot trying to do my head in or something.

3. It is important to reduce hospital admissions. Hospital admission is costly and of little benefit to patients with personality disorder. For all patients, a search of the hospital inpatient database is made to obtain the number of hospital admissions and the length of stay both before a trial, during the trial, and during follow-up.

It is clearly inappropriate solely to have primary outcome measures of symptom or behavioural change when the aim of treatment is to change the psychological capacity to mentalize. To this end we have used the Adult Attachment Interview in order to rate reflective capacity before and after treatment and in addition developed a questionnaire measuring relevant personality dimensions. This data awaits analysis.

Despite the fast growth of the number of diagnostic instruments, and despite the availability of tests to measure personality traits in the normal population, the clinical field still lacks a diagnostic tool specifically designed to evaluate the severity of personality pathology in patients. Because of this, the research field lacks a reliable instrument for measuring structural changes in personality functioning as a result of psychotherapeutic intervention. Thus, there is a clear need for the development of an instrument with these capacities, and the Zanarini BPD scale has gone some way to address this (Zanarini et al., 2003). However we have developed an instrument that is potentially meaningful in terms of the aims of MBT, and we constructed a new 100-item questionnaire, the Severity Index of Personality Pathology (SIPP-100), jointly with a research group in Holland.

The questionnaire was constructed in English and Dutch, using a formal translation procedure. Item generation was based on the idea that personality disorder is a malfunctioning of adaptive capacities (both positive and negative). A four-dimensional model of personality traits was constructed, with each dimension having both self- and relational traits: regulation, reflection, actualization, and responsibility. The resulting 8 dimensions were each operationalized by 3 small groups of items: the facets. The item generation was checked by asking a group of clinicians to match the items with the dimensions in the model. After pilot testing in patients ($N = 100$), items with low variance were deleted. The conceptual model was further tested with the use of a confirmative factor analysis in a larger group of patients. Norm scores were derived from a sample of the normal population. This instrument remains in development, and the data are now being analysed.

Data collection and loss of control

Most patients with personality disorder, especially borderline patients, do not easily accept randomization. For BPD the search is for stability and control; for antisocial and narcissistic patients the need is for exploitation of others and self-gratification rather than acceptance of authority or recognition of a "greater good" and participation in research to further the treatment of future patients (Lapsley, 2004). Offering them referral into a research project in which their allocation appears to be dependent on the toss of a coin confronts them with loss of control and threatens tenuous stability. This can translate into refusal to participate in research, criticism of the research instruments, and angry complaint about exploitation. Randomization out of the treatment into a control group can similarly lead to refusal to cooperate. Some patients may even take pleasure in ensuring that researchers do not get the information they ask for at the time that it is needed, leading to further sampling problems. Given the relatively small cell sizes of RCTs of treatment for personality disorder, attrition represents a serious threat to internal validity.

The issue for research is how to maintain patients in a trial lasting for one year or longer. Our practice now is to involve patients at the outset of a trial, to provide regular feedback of results, and to personalize some of the instruments. For example, the circumplex version of the Inventory of Interpersonal Problems allows a circumplex diagram to be developed of personality characteristics. We allow the patients to do this for themselves and to plot their own changes, and this informs the therapy sessions.

Mentalization-based treatment and manualization

In many ways our own treatment, mentalization-based treatment (MBT), suffers from problems of complexity. So, what was a complex intervention had to be simplified, not only by disaggregating its component parts, but by defining principles of intervention, process, and function in a manner that was understandable to both patients and practitioners. We had in mind the need for relatively straightforward training, replication, and generalization. As a result we were able to implement treatment using generic mental health nurses working in a routine clinical service rather than highly skilled doctoral students, trained psychotherapists, or senior practitioners.

Principle of intervention

The guiding principle of MBT is that psychotherapy with borderline patients should focus on the capacity for mentalization, by which is meant the implicit or explicit perception or interpretation of the actions of others or oneself as intentional—that is, mediated by mental states or mental processes. An important common factor in many psychotherapeutic approaches is the shared potential to recreate an interactional matrix of attachment in which mentalization develops and sometimes flourishes. The therapist mentalizes the patient in a way that fosters the patient's mentalizing, which is a key facet of the relationship. The crux of the value of psychotherapy with BPD is the experience of another human being having the patient's mind in mind. It should be clear from this that, unlike a number of the approaches in MBT, *the process* of interpretation is at the heart of the therapy, rather than *the content* of the interpretations or the non-specific supportive aspects of therapy. The explicit content of interpreting is merely the vehicle for the implicit process that has therapeutic value.

This is highly significant. For practitioners there is no longer anxiety about getting the "correct" interpretation, but a concern that the patient's mental state remains at the core of the therapeutic process. There is no right and wrong in, say, an interpretation, as long as it forms part of a process in which the therapist demonstrates to the patient that his primary concern is the patient's mind and how s/he experiences the world. The therapist is continually constructing and reconstructing an image of the patient, to help the patient to understand what s/he feels. Mentalizing in psychotherapy is a process of joint attention in which the patient's mental states are the object of attention. Neither therapist nor patient experiences these interactions other than impressionistically.

Training practitioners to develop and to maintain this process is a simpler task than trying to ensure that they say the "right" thing all the time. The complexity of patient–therapist interaction prevents the latter strategy, even though there are those who still think that if only the "right" interpretation had been given, all would have been well. For MBT, the practitioner maintains a mentalizing stance—why is the patient saying this now? why is the patient behaving like this? what might I have done that explains the patient's state? why am I feeling as I do now? what has happened recently in the therapy or in our relationship that may justify the current state?—and is perfectly at liberty to ask such questions aloud in a spirit of enquiry. Thus there are many roads to a mentalizing stance, and each therapist has to find her/his own route.

Form of intervention

In MBT the form of the intervention is individual plus group psychotherapy. It is not enough to prescribe one or the other. Both are probably required for optimal outcomes, although we do not yet have any data to confirm this, so it remains an empirical question. The simultaneous provision of group and individual therapy is an ideal arrangement within which to encourage mentalization. Thus the form the intervention takes complements the principle of treatment. A patient who is excessively anxious and aroused in group therapy will be unable to explore his problems within that context, and so the individual therapy session becomes the place of safety where he can reflect critically and thoughtfully about himself in the group. At these times the individual therapist ensures that the patient concentrates on his problems within the group and the interpersonal context in the group that may be driving the anxiety and how his fears relate to current and past aspects of his life. This requires careful coordination between the individual and group therapists to minimize adverse consequences of splitting of the transference and to make certain the patient moves towards mental balance rather than continuing to manage anxiety through splitting, idealization, denigration, and withdrawal.

The danger of patient and therapist unwittingly slipping into a closed therapeutic world within individual therapy in which both of them believe that they, and only they, understand the problems is avoided by the simultaneous provision of group therapy. This patient/individual therapist "enclave" results from a move in the patient, often unrecognized by the therapist, into pretend mode. Patients who take psychological refuge within individual therapy continue to be confronted within the group by other patients who rapidly detect pretence and tackle anyone who hides behind intellectual defences and false understanding.

Taking the principle and form together, it should be possible to implement MBT within clinical services without complex changes to service organization. Most services for PD offer group and individual psychotherapy, but in order to implement MBT, what is important is the interrelationship between the two, the constructive interactions of professionals offering each component and, above all, providing an experience for a patient of being the subject of reliable, coherent, and rational thinking. Too frequently, components of a treatment package for BPD are fragmented, unreliable, and erratic, with limited coordination between practitioners. This is not MBT.

The final component of a complex intervention has to be its core elements, even though some may argue that it is not possible to analyse a complex treatment into meaningful parts.

Core elements

We have defined a number of core elements to treatment. These include (a) bridging the gap between affects and their representation; (b) working mostly with current mental states; and (c) keeping in mind the patient's deficits.

Bridging the gap. There is a gap between the primary affective experience of the borderline patient and its symbolic representation. This gap has to be bridged in therapy if the reflective process is to develop with a view to strengthening the secondary representational system. This is done by making identification of affects a key feature of the therapeutic process. Each feeling and its interpersonal context has to be recognized and explored as it arises. This may sound laborious, and indeed it is, because it must be done in detail. Cursory, sweeping approximation of emotional states will not suffice.

Retaining mental closeness and working with current mental states. Retaining mental closeness is akin to the process by which the caregiver's empathic response provides the infant with feedback on his or her emotional state to enable developmental progress. However, it is more than empathy, although the task of the therapist is to represent accurately the feeling state of the patient and its accompanying internal representations. Interventions by the therapist must be phrased in such a way that they represent the perspective of the patient and a heavily abstracted understanding that the therapist has of the patient's state. Let us take a patient who is angry with the therapist at lack of progress in treatment. From an empathic point of view the therapist would solely identify the anger. Retaining mental closeness requires the therapist to add the most immediate consequence of the anger for the patient: "I can understand that you are angry (empathically identifies the immediate affect), and that must make it hard for you to keep coming to sessions to see someone whom you find of no help at the moment." This therapeutic style of mental closeness allows treatment to focus on the interaction between patient and therapist and therefore for work to be done within the transference relationship.

Many patients dwell on their past lives and their manifest ill-treatment. Embittered and resentful, they harbour hostile grievances that prevent progress. While it is important to recognize these serious environmental insults and traumatic experiences, there can be little therapeutic gain from continually focusing in the past. The focus needs to be on the present state and how it remains influenced by events of the past rather than on the past itself. If the patient persistently returns to the past, the therapist needs to link back to the present, move the therapy into the "here and now", and consider the present experience.

Keeping in mind the patient's deficits. Borderline patients may appear to be capable, thoughtful, sophisticated, and accomplished, and yet it is well known that their unemployment rate is similar to that seen in schizophrenia (Gunderson, Carpenter, & Strauss, 1975). While it is important to recognize the strengths of all patients, it is equally vital to understand their deficits, otherwise therapists develop unrealistic expectations, anticipate rapid improvement, and set inappropriate goals.

Deficit in the capacity for mentalization can be masked by an apparent intellectual ability that lures therapists into believing that borderline patients understand the complexity of alternative perspectives, accept uncertainty, and can consider difference. In fact, at one moment a borderline patient may hold a particular view and yet at another time maintain the opposite is true; in one therapy session a patient may describe a feeling that holds special significance but is later denied as being relevant, and continuity of feeling, belief, wish, and desire may be lost between therapeutic sessions. Constancy of belief and consistent experience of others elude the borderline patient, resulting in idealization at one moment and denigration the next. The task of the therapist is to establish continuity between sessions, to link different aspects of a multi-component therapy, to help the patient recognize the discontinuity, and to scaffold the sessions without holding the patient to account for sudden switches in belief, feeling, and desire.

Conclusions

A randomized controlled trial can easily become out of control when implemented within clinical services. Variables that require special attention include the randomization procedure itself, the assessors and their preconceptions, therapist competence and trainability, clarity of interventions, and—of particular importance in personality disorder—the constructive cooperation of the patient. None of these problems is insuperable if researchers work closely with both patients and therapists while bearing in mind the system within which the clinical service operates. What is necessary is for a trial to become a joint endeavour, in which the concerns of the patient are meaningfully incorporated into the method itself, the contribution of the patient is recognized through feedback, complex treatments are defined not only according to their constituent parts but also their form and function, and therapists are trained to implement a treatment with reasonable fidelity. Only then will a trial remain in control.

Commentary

Steven R. Marans

One of the greatest strengths of the Anna Freud Centre has been the long tradition of demonstrating a deeply held appreciation for the complexity of human development and functioning in its approaches to research and clinical care. Throughout the history of the Centre, the recognition that careful observation leads to a breadth of data has also led to multiple approaches to organizing complex naturalistic and clinical data in ways that inform and define all areas of the Centre's approach to psychoanalytic work. The guiding principle in each of these areas has been that careful observation and detailed methods for recording empirical data are the strongest basis for developing questions and hypotheses that inform training, research, and clinical care.

For years the requirement for AFC trainees to observe normally developing infants, toddlers, and young children in a variety of settings as well as those involved in paediatric hospital or residential care or in schools underscored the emphasis placed on learning how to observe as a crucial prerequisite to learning how to engage in psychoanalytic clinical and research activities. The development of the Hampstead Provisional Diagnostic Profile and the Index were attempts to arrive at detailed assays of clinical and treatment phenomena while they strove to help clarify, operationalize, and demonstrate theoretical constructs. These central goals would be equally applied to treatment-based research activities involving a range of clinical populations, including children with physical handicaps, chronic medical conditions, and severe personality disorders, to name a few. During the past two decades, the ground-breaking work of Moran and Fonagy (Moran, 1984; Moran & Fonagy, 1987) and Fonagy and Target (Fonagy, Target, Cottrell, Philips, & Kurtz, 2002) have bridged earlier case-based psychoanalytic approaches to research to contemporary approaches of the broader behavioural sciences. These newer approaches in which the Centre has engaged have been applied to both systematic and controlled studies of constituent aspects of normal development as well as to studies of treatment outcome and efficacy. It is within this context and rich tradition of integrating close clinical observation, elaboration of clinical constructs, and development of rigorous research methodology that Anthony Bateman's work is embedded.

In this chapter Bateman describes the development of research approaches to the treatment of individuals with borderline personality disorder. In a clear and thoughtful way, he lays out some of the inherent dilemmas in developing rigorous research methods because of the very nature of the disorder itself and describes solutions that have been developed to address these challenges. It is his observations of, and attention to, clinical phenomenology that forms the basis of new approaches to treatment outcome in the difficult area of borderline psychopathology.

Bateman points out that even though it is a gold standard of research designs, the use of randomized controlled treatment presents immediate challenges based on the realities of severe borderline psychopathology itself. This, Bateman points out, may be especially significant with regard to patients' capacity to comply with, adhere to, and follow through with the research protocol precisely because of the general disorganization, affective dysregulation, unstable relationships, and views of self and others that are characteristic of the borderline personality disorder. As a result, problems with attrition are serious rate-limiting factors in successfully carrying out such studies. In Bateman's work, as a result of the recognition that the same vulnerable areas that were target areas of treatment would also interfere with attempts to carry out research, much greater attention has been paid to potential stumbling blocks to participation and follow-through. Far more than is typical in similar treatment studies, patients were engaged in the development of the assessment protocol—modifications of questionnaires were made on the basis of patients' review and critiques—and prepared for their participation in the study. Bateman's work demonstrates that this kind of participation, closer fit between clinical characteristics and assessment tools, as well as a considerable preparation for involvement in the study itself were all important contributions to decreasing the kind of attrition that is typical in studies of patients with this kind of personality disorder: no patient who completed the partial hospitalization intervention was lost to follow-up. While not part of his discussion, Bateman's approach raises the question about the extent to which engaging patients as partners in the research process may in fact call upon and perhaps increase higher-order levels of functioning while decreasing reality bases for patients to experience treater/researchers as controlling, exploitative "bad objects".

Again drawing on a wealth of clinical experience, Bateman addresses another issue that complicates attempts to develop randomized controlled studies with borderline patients—ensuring that the population involved in the study is as homogeneous as possible. Bateman points out that this issue is especially significant in research involving BPD, as the diagnosis covers such a broad range of clinical presentations that, while sharing a common underlying pathology of personality organization, may vary enormously in severity of symptoms and impact on adaptive functioning. While other studies have employed measures of symptom severity, Bateman developed measures that combine assessment of behaviour, symptoms, as well as dynamically relevant domains involving characteristics of the underlying personality pathology itself. In the Severity Index for Personality Pathology, Bateman operationalized areas crucial to dynamic consideration and comprehensive clinical observation that offer reliable and valid measures of areas of crucial interest to analytic and non-analytic investigators and clinicians alike. Additionally, operationalizing theoretical and empirically based constructs informs not only evaluation and outcome measures—self-report and treater observations—but also the manualization of core treatment strategies that offers the opportunity for randomization of treaters.

If the best psychoanalytic traditions are defined by the extent to which we are able to remain open to questions and hypotheses that fit our clinical observations and to scepticism/openness to competing hypotheses and then further questioning, then Bateman's work more than fulfils these traditions. In raising questions about the success of his approaches to randomization, the benefits and risks of manualization, the validity of approaches to assessment, and outcome measurement, Bateman provides a model of psychoanalytic inquiry and sets the stage for collaborative consideration and exchange of ideas about diagnostic, clinical, and research issues.

This chapter successfully stimulates questions about additional research questions that may further clarify issues that impact various aspects of clinical care. For example, one of the questions raised is whether it would be useful to include a greater research focus on the relationship between the nature and level of consistency of daily programme structures—such as consistency of care with regard to scheduling of activities; providers; degree of team-based, coordinated individualized and group treatment approaches; sharing of clinical information; and so on—and treatment outcome and follow-up in both experimental and control treatment groups/settings.

Additionally, Bateman's work raises critical questions about the implications of research findings for policies that dictate the types of resources and clinical services that are available for patients with well-defined disorders. When able to advance our science, improve clinical cares *and* demonstrate that proper care is also cost-effective, clinical research of the kind that Bateman describes is most likely to benefit the broadest number of patients and ensure the continued availability of treatment models with established clinical efficacy. For example, Bateman's report that in the follow-up to the partial hospital programme there was considerably greater service utilization has important implications both clinically and financially. If patients in the experimental treatment group make fewer visits to the emergency/casualty department in local hospitals, the implication could be that they have achieved greater relative psychological stability, as indicated by fewer severe crises of the kind that warrant emergency care. An increase in personal stability and a decrease in severity of crises may be reflected not only in a decrease in emergency/casualty department visits, but in other areas as well: other acute urgent care provision (e.g., police, social service, emergency first response) or frequency of visits to GPs (for disorder-inspired complaints/symptomatology). Decreases in any of these areas translate into enormous savings that might then be diverted into a range of more effective treatment strategies that address the psychopathology of such costly symptomatology. Exploring these areas would perhaps be a fruitful extension of Bateman's research efforts. These crucial issues, and the initial success of the approaches developed by Bateman and Fonagy (2004), also raise the question about the extent to which the current treatment strategies have been replicated in other parts of the National Health Service and whether or not the research protocol is a standard part of implementation in similar psychoanalytic partial hospital programmes.

Bateman continues a psychoanalytic approach to clinical research in the long tradition of the Anna Freud Centre as he and his colleagues have been able to translate what is learned in the consulting-room and other clinical settings to inform the development of interventions that have the broadest impact on the lives of children and adults. The work of the Anna Freud Centre and of the Yale Child Study Center has long had an enormous impact on our understanding of normal development, psychopathology, clinical care, and social policy. The work of Bateman and his colleagues in the area of BPD also embodies this tradition of integrating observation, theory, research and clinical practice. If psychoanalysis is to have a voice and place in the scientific field and if it is to have any influence on the nature of treatment available to children and adults, the work described in this chapter is precisely the kind of work in which we need to be engaged.

CHAPTER TEN

Psychoanalytic responses to violent trauma: the Child Development–Community Policing partnership

Steven R. Marans

Although circumstances have shifted—from the consulting room, to the Hampstead War Nurseries, to paediatric wards, to the care of Holocaust survivors, to the best interests of children in custody and placement disputes—child psychoanalytic inquiry and practice have always been based on, first, taking the perspective of the child. At its best, the field of child psychoanalysis has developed theories that articulate clinical and naturalistic findings that derive from multiple points of observation. Direct clinical work has not been the only beneficiary of the decades of this work. In addition to developing the conceptual tools for conducting the psychoanalytic treatment of children, child analysts like Donald Cohen, Anna Freud, Hansi Kennedy, George Moran, Sally Provence, John Schowalter, Al Solnit, Stuart Twemlow, and others have devoted much of their work to conveying a psychoanalytic appreciation of children's experiences to those other professionals whose work affects the care of children and the course of the children's development.

The task of child analysts has been to bring complex formulations about the inner and outer life of children into a language of observations that can be recognized by anyone who can bear to see and revisit life through the eyes of a child. Anna Freud (1968) set the standard for the child analyst's role of consultant/collaborator with two essential goals: (a) to appreciate the complexity of children's experience of their lives, and (b) to describe the implications of that experience in ways that are accessible to those professionals whose handling and decisions have a potential bearing on the trajectory of a child's development. Anna Freud taught her students to attend, to listen, to observe, and to apply a psychoanalytic perspective to the clinical and extraclinical interventions that aim to maximize developmental potential.

Since Freud's (1926d [1925]) earliest work, trauma has been a central and enduring concern of psychoanalytic inquiry. In recent years, the problems of childhood have gained increased clinical and conceptual focus while the general public has become more aware of the vast numbers of children who are exposed to the violence associated with war and domestic and neighbourhood disputes. Children living in urban centres afflicted with high rates of violence are especially vulnerable to the psychic trauma that occurs when the "actual danger" (Freud, 1926d [1925]) is in the form of gunfire, wounding, or death. Traditional clinical services alone are unequal to the task of responding to the numbers of children whose development may be compromised as a result of their acute and chronic experiences of violence in their homes, on the streets of their neighbourhoods, and at school.

In Anna Freud's tradition of involving ourselves with other professionals concerned about children (child-care workers, teachers, paediatricians, social workers, and lawyers), under the leadership of Donald J. Cohen, a child analyst and the director of the Child Study Center until his death in October 2001, child analysts and analytically oriented faculty members at the Child Study Center recognized the central role played by a group whose professional relationship with children has not always been appreciated: the police. As the profession with the most immediate and frequent contact with children and families exposed to and involved in violence, police officers can have a profound impact on the ways children experience their increasingly unsafe, disorganized world.

The collaboration between child analysts and police, the Yale Child Development–Community Policing (CD–CP) programme,[1] is based on the application of psychoanalytic concepts that provide a frame of reference for extending the observations and interventions of police officers and analytically informed clinicians in responding to the needs of children who have been exposed to, or involved in, violent events. Prior to the inception of the CD–CP programme, police contact with mental health professionals generally was limited to delivering psychotic or suicidal patients to the hospital emergency service. Similarly, official responsibilities and options regarding children were restricted to such acts as arresting juvenile offenders and referring abused and neglected children to social services. Police did not refer for clinical services the numerous children they encountered on the scenes of violent crimes or exposed to family violence. The goal of the CD–CP programme is to expand the role and options available to police officers through training and consultation and to introduce a new partnership in which psychoanalytic principles are conveyed and applied.

A major result of the New Haven Department of Police Service–Child Study Center collaboration is the expansion of our clinical field of observation. Since 1991, clinical contact has been initiated on the scene by officers and child analysts and analytically oriented clinicians, sometimes only moments after shootings, stabbings, beatings, and other scenes involving the potential for psychological trauma. As a result, we have had an opportunity to learn more about a child's experience of violence and overwhelming danger. In addition, this close and immediate contact has afforded us the chance to respond to the various reactions of parents, professionals, and the larger community in ways that help to mediate the overwhelming anxiety/trauma that often accompanies involvement in such events. While the core of the CD–CP programme remains the police–mental health partnership, domestic violence advocates, juvenile probation officers, child protective services, and education personnel have become part of the work that has developed in New Haven and elsewhere during the past decade. In this time period, the CD–CP programme has been implemented in numerous communities around the country, and the number is growing. Current CD–CP sites include Chelsea, Massachusetts; Madison, Guilford, Stamford, and Bridgeport, Connecticut; Baltimore, Maryland; Charlotte, North Carolina; Nashville, Tennessee; Pinellas County, Florida; and Spokane, Washington.

In 1998, President Bill Clinton, Attorney General Janet Reno, and Deputy Attorney General Eric Holder established the National Center for Children Exposed to Violence (NCCEV) at the Yale Child Study Center. Based on the CD–CP model of collaborative responses to violent traumatization, the NCCEV was charged with providing (a) consultation, training, and technical assistance to other communities implementing similar models of response; (b) increased public and professional awareness about issues of childhood trauma and violence exposure; and (c) a web-based resource centre for information regarding diagnostic, treatment, and systemic issues related to childhood trauma and violence exposure.

The context of community policing

Until the last decade, standard police practice in the United States could be characterized as primarily reactive. Officers patrolled in squad cars and were dispatched by central headquarters to one complaint or crime scene after another. They were generally not known by members of the communities in which they worked. In the absence of establishing a continuous, personal presence in the neighbourhoods, police were often viewed as ineffective or as intruders in the neighbourhoods where they responded to criminal activity. They frequently arrived too late and left too soon. Within this system, police themselves often felt dissatisfied. In spite of their difficult and often dangerous work, they felt that there was little they could do to make a lasting difference. They repeatedly came back to the same neighbourhoods, hangouts, and homes to deal with recurrent illegal activities and the tragic aftermaths.

Criminal justice experts have recognized the limitations of the standard model (Brown, 1990; Bureau of Justice Assistance, 1994; Goldstein, 1977; Kelling & Moore, 1989). In many cities in the United States and around the world, police practices are being reorganized around an innovative philosophy, often referred to as community-based or problem-oriented policing. Community-based policing puts officers in neighbourhoods where they walk beats, develop relationships, and try to prevent rather than simply respond to one crisis after another. In the New Haven model of community policing, police have increasingly been recruited from the racially and ethnically diverse communities they patrol. When these officers are placed in neighbourhoods and work from small substations rather than central headquarters, they observe and experience the lives of children and families much more acutely. They learn who is involved in criminal activities, where and with whom trouble is likely to occur, and why things are heating up. They see and often know the many victims of violence—not only those who have been shot, stabbed, or beaten and their assailants, but the many child witnesses who observe the events in horror or run for safety. As they have become a more established and personal presence, the police place greater emphasis on devising strategies to prevent or interrupt crime and on developing problem-solving relationships with members of the neighbourhoods in which they work. Officers who walk the beat understand the rhythms and underlying dynamics within their communities. This day-by-day engagement brings with it additional personal burdens. As officers become closer to and invested in the people who either ask for or require their interventions, they also run an increased risk of being overwhelmed by the problems they confront.

This vulnerability to seeing and feeling too much is especially pronounced in officers' engagements with children at risk. They find it particularly difficult to see children caught in the spiral of inner-city violence, the children who are witnesses to family battles and street crime and who then move from being victim to being active perpetrator. On the beat, police officers begin to feel the pain and frustration that go with a sense of impotence, and they naturally wish to have the competence and authority to intervene more effectively.

Police and the psychoanalytic perspective on children

In contrast to police officers, mental health professionals are equipped to respond to children's psychological distress. However, the acutely traumatized children who are most in need of clinical service are rarely seen in existing outpatient clinics until months or years later—if at all—when chronic symptoms or maladaptive behaviour brings them to the attention of parents, teachers, or the juvenile courts. Lost are valuable opportunities to intervene at the moment when professional contact could provide both immediate stabilization and bridges to a variety of ongoing services. To be effective in their new roles within communities, officers need to be provided with a framework for understanding children and families, and they need new partners who can help them deal with the challenges and tragedies they encounter.

In the CD–CP programme, psychoanalytic theories about development—the ego and superego mediation of instinctual life; the interaction between conflict and defence; the concept of developmental lines and phases; the interaction between significant environmental factors and psychic reality (A. Freud, 1936, 1965)—provide a shared frame of reference. Similarly, the programme follows a model of consultation pioneered by Anna Freud and adapted by Al Solnit and others, that relies on a process of learning about the perspectives and experiences of the other professional with whom one is working to consider the developmental implications of shared observations and actions. Psychoanalytic clinicians in the CD–CP programme have learned that, to be useful to police officers, they first must see the clinical phenomena from the officers' point of view. They have been able to do so through the institution of fellowships for clinicians and supervisory officers.

In the Police Fellowship, clinicians move into police settings—in ride-alongs in squad cars, joining police at crime scenes, or sitting in on discussions of case investigations—and learning about their tasks, demands, and professional needs. At the same time, through the Clinical Fellowship, officers become familiar with mental health settings and psychoanalytic perspectives by observing clinical activities and consultations. Also, a 24-hour consultation service and weekly case conference provide ongoing opportunities for applying developmental concepts in the field. Where each of these components serves as a basis for the continued development of the collaboration, the seminars attended by senior police officers, Child Study Center analysts, and analytically informed clinicians provide the shared conceptual framework that guides observations, discussions, and interventions.

Seminars on child development, human functioning, and policing

The central task of the seminars is to engage officers in the examination of (a) basic human needs; (b) capacities for self-regulation and mastery; (c) phase-specific sources of danger/anxiety; (d) the link between behaviour and underlying psychic processes (i.e., the relationship between anxiety and defences); and (e) individual variation in potential life adaptations. Proceeding along a developmental sequence, the seminars also highlight the ways in which phenomena originating in an earlier phase of development may be observed in various forms throughout the life cycle. Seminar leaders use scenarios encountered in police work, films, and videotapes about children and cases initiated through the Consultation Service to demonstrate that a greater understanding of human functioning does not mean inaction or decreased vigilance with regard to personal safety. Rather, by helping the informed officers understand the complexities of human development, the goal of the seminars is to help the police to discover new ways of observing and formulating responses to children. In addition, the officers have the opportunity to establish a realistic appreciation of the impact they can have on the lives of children and families with whom they interact.

Typically, at the first meeting, in which seminar members introduce themselves and talk about their expectations of the course, discussions begin about early development. The topic of infancy is introduced by the supervisory officer, who co-leads the seminar with an analyst, who describes the following scene: "You have responded to a complaint of breach of the peace and arrive at an apartment where music is blaring. You are greeted by an angry young mother, an apartment that is disordered and dirty, and three children under the age of four in similar disarray. Diaper changes for two of the children appear long overdue. What is your reaction?" The officers often begin the discussion by expressing their feelings of despair and anger about a scene that is all too familiar.

As the instructors probe the nature of these reactions, the class begins to identify concerns about the babies, who are unable to fend for themselves; about the children's physical discomfort; and about the notion that the mother is overwhelmed. What emerges from the discussion is the group's awareness of an infant's physical and emotional needs and the role of the mother in mediating and responding to those needs. The seminar leaders ask, "And what happens to the infant if those basic needs aren't met?" The answer is usually that the baby will be overwhelmed with pain, discomfort, and despair, because it is not yet equipped to feed, clothe, or comfort itself or to satisfy the demands of its feelings on its own. The leaders ask for more details, and the class responds by identifying the child's lack of abilities—the absence of verbal language, motoric maturation, and coordination; underdeveloped cognitive processes for problem solving; and, finally, the utter reliance of the infant on the mother for the experience of physical and emotional well-being. Attention then turns to the young mother. "How", the leaders ask, "do we understand her apparent insensitivity or incompetence?" The discussion must first address her surly response to the officers and their consequent indignation. Here the concepts of displacement and externalization are introduced. The seminar leaders expand the discussion to a young woman apparently unable to look after her children, let alone herself. They ask, "How might she feel about herself?" The answers vary: "Like a failure?" "Maybe she just doesn't care!" The seminar leaders ask, "Given either of those possibilities, how might she feel when two police officers come to her door?" "Like we're going to tell her off, tell her what she should be doing, how she should behave." "And who are you to her at that moment? Who tells you you're not getting it right, messing up? Parents? teachers? a critical boss or colleague?" In one session, an officer jumped in and offered, "Right, and then when she feels criticized, she takes on an obnoxious attitude and treats us like dirt." Another officer added, "As though she already knows you are." In this particular discussion, the clinical co-leader suggested that perhaps from the moment of their arrival, the officers represent something very familiar to the young woman: "Before you open your mouth, you may be the critical voice, the presentation of authority, the voice that agrees with her own self-criticism and assessment of incompetence. How does it feel to be criticized? What is it like to feel inadequate and to have someone, by their very presence on your doorstep, point it out to you? Is it possible that her surly and combative response serves a defensive function that is triggered by you but is not about you personally?" The discussion goes on, often ending with some greater appreciation for the complexity of the scene and the interaction but with the residual wish to do something concrete for the babies. That wish is either to implore the woman to be a more attentive mother or to remove the children so that they can have a better home.

The Robertsons' film *John* (Robertson & Robertson, 1969) is shown in the following session. In the discussion that follows, seminar members describe the 17-month-old's efforts to soothe himself in the midst of a nine-day separation from his parents. They note John's attempts to reach out to the child-care nurses, cuddly toys, and the observer—and his utter despair when these efforts fail. The discussion also compares John to the other children who have spent their entire lives in the residential nursery. Seminar members often observe that, while seeming unfazed by the limited attention and multiple changes of nursing staff, in contrast to John, these children appear dominated by aggressive, driven, and need-satisfying behaviour. Slowly, and often painfully, as the discussion continues, the simple solution of removal from care when parenting seems inadequate fades. The idea that removal always represents rescue is replaced by a growing appreciation for the complexity of the child–parent relationship. There is a recognition of the developmental significance of continuity of care and the impact of disrupting it. In addition, seminar members have a fuller understanding of the balance between the child's needs and capacities as well as the distress that follows when needs are not met.

The link between these processes and overt behaviour *and* the observer's responses and overt behaviour is pursued as the seminar moves into the next session, in which the hallmarks of the toddler phase are introduced. Using videotapes of normal children engaged in imaginative play, officers are able to consider children's use of fantasy, identifications, and burgeoning cognitive and physical resources to achieve aim-inhibited sources of pleasure and mastery. Failures to negotiate oedipal conflicts over competition, envy, love, and hate, along with the often unstable, overstimulating home situations, are explored in discussions of latency-age children who come to the attention of police because of their antisocial activities. Similarly, puberty is discussed in the context of the intensification of struggles over sexual and aggressive urges.

Seminar leaders introduce phases of development by asking officers to describe the most salient aspects—either observed or assumed to play a part—of a given period of life. As the discussion evolves, officers often invoke their own memories as a vehicle for understanding the behaviours they observe and encounter on the street and as a way of becoming conscious of the complicated identifications that these interactions may evoke. For example, when discussing puberty and early adolescence, officers initially describe their concerns about the provocative, tough, drug-involved, pregnant youngsters and the frustration the officers experience when logic and warnings about consequences seem to have no impact on behaviour. As they begin to talk about their own experiences of this phase of development, however, the frustration and angry dismissal of these children is substantially altered. Officers often describe memories from their own lives or recollections of children whom they have met over the course of their work, whom they have not been able to forget. The accounts speak to the vulnerability, anxiety, and loneliness so common in this period of development and the various means used to defend against these feelings. Stories of fighting, social isolation, school difficulties, and losses alternate with the ones about best friends, first girlfriends and boyfriends, team sports, and the like. Each of the discussions inevitably focuses on concern about body image, group acceptance, struggles with parents, losses, and the overreaching experience of embarrassment and urgency in the competing wishes for competent, independent functioning and feelings of utter inadequacy and the embarrassing wish to remain a small child.

John Singleton's film, *Boyz n the Hood* (1991), and Michael King's Emmy award-winning film, *Bangin'* (1998), are used as the text for the seminars that deal with adolescence. Both films provide rich opportunities for seminar participants to discuss the challenges, hopes, and dilemmas inherent in adolescence. In the discussion of Singleton's film, issues of race and the socioeconomics of the inner city are interwoven with perspectives on the internal and external worlds of two brothers in the film: one becomes a gun-toting drug dealer, the other a high school football star bound for college until he is shot dead by gang members. King's documentary looks at the impact of violence on young people as both victims and perpetrators. Through interviews with incarcerated adolescent violent offenders, officers and clinicians are afforded insight into the experiences and thoughts of children with whom contact would typically have been limited to times of arrest or brief emergency-room or court-ordered evaluations.

As the seminars come to an end, officers increasingly refer to their responses to the scenes of violence and suffering they confront on a daily basis. Sealing over, "getting used to it", and distancing themselves as best they can, or displacing their frustration onto citizens or their own family members, viewing the world dichotomously—"us versus them"—and heightening their sense of vigilance to danger are all themes that commonly emerge in the discussions. These responses are discussed in terms of the defensive functions they serve against unwanted feelings of fear, inadequacy, sadness, despair, and anger. As a result of these discussions, officers become more aware that the nature of their work makes it especially difficult, but absolutely necessary, for them to be able to recognize and distinguish between internal responses and external reactions.

Changes in police responses

Regardless of the setting, the aim of the discussions for officers and clinicians alike is to "place ourselves in the position of children of different ages, of different developmental phases, and of different backgrounds" (Goldstein, Freud, & Solnit, 1979, p. 137). For the officers, the opportunity to reflect on what they observe, to have a framework for ordering what might otherwise have been too overwhelming to notice, and to have colleagues with whom to share the burden of responding—at any hour—has led to dramatic changes in police practices regarding children. These changes are reflected in the officers' regularly referring children who have witnessed and experienced violence as well as, increasingly, children who have committed serious violent offences.

Incorporating developmental perspectives, the changes are also apparent in standards of police practice that go beyond making referrals for children victimized or involved in violence. These standards include, for example, consideration of how parents are treated when issued a warrant or put under arrest. In one typical seminar discussion, an officer described a high-speed chase involving a man and a 5-year-old boy on a motorcycle. When he finally stopped the man, the officer began screaming at him about his endangering the young boy. In reporting the scene, the officer described the panic he felt that accompanied his fantasy of the motorcycle crashing and killing the boy. What bothered him the most after this incident, however, was that, as he yelled at the man, the boy began to cry and shouted at him to stop being mean to his father. The officer pointed out that, while he had justified his tirade as being in the boy's best interest, he had completely left out any consideration of the boy's identification with or admiration of the father, regardless of whatever anxiety he might have felt about father's reckless behaviour. In addition, the officer's wish for the boy to view the police in a positive light had, in fact, been undermined by his own intense emotional reaction of fear followed by anger. In retrospect, the officer decided that taking the father aside and discussing the danger and his concerns for the boy's safety, in addition to issuing a ticket, might have served the boy's and his own professional interests far more effectively.

Similarly, officers have become more attentive to the humiliation and potential for dangerous confrontation when they deal with adolescents—especially juvenile offenders—in a harsh manner. As officers have become regular fixtures in the neighbourhoods, they have replaced anonymous responses to the groups of kids on the streets with interactions that are informed by familiarity and relationships with individuals. From the seminars to the streets, this contact is enhanced by officers' increased appreciation of the upheaval of adolescent development, often compounded by the despair and feelings of impotence associated with severe social adversity. As a result, wholesale condemnation, frustration, and anger are no longer the only responses to the provocative—and, at times, illegal—behaviour with which adolescents confront the police. The recognition of displacements and counterreactions that are so often associated with police–adolescent interactions on the street has also led to a more judicious and strategic use of authority when it is based on new relationships that replace stereotypic responses of the past. In turn, police imposition of authority (e.g., clearing a street corner known for drug activity, keeping public noise down, picking up truant students, etc.) is more frequently now met with compliance rather than an immediate escalation to violent confrontation and arrest.

Where the application of developmental principles has affected police approaches to typical interactions with youth on the streets and in schools, it has also led to interventions that are anything but standard in the traditional approach to law enforcement. Following the shooting death of a 17-year-old gang member, there was good reason for concern about retaliation and further bloodshed. In the days that followed the death, grieving gang members congregated on the corner where the shooting had taken place. Efforts at increased presence and containment took the form of police, neighbourhood-based probation officers, and clinicians spending time on the corner listening to gang members express their grief.

As one senior police officer put it, "We could show our concern for their trauma by being with them, lending an adult ear to their misery. Alternatively, we could put more officers on the street, show them who's boss, and, with a show of force, sweep them off the corner as often as necessary. We could then offer them an additional enemy and wait for them to explode." At that crucial moment, however, the police did not assume the role of enemy. They did not serve as the target for displaced rage or, in confrontation, offer an easy antidote to sadness and helplessness. Rather than turning passive into active "payback" in blood, gang members became active, discreetly assisting the police to make a swift arrest in the shooting. As one gang member, the brother of the victim, put it to a neighbourhood officer, "You were there for us. That helped—and we were there for you."

Where arrests continue to be an essential tool for police, a new look at the range of prevention measures has been added to the repertoire of law enforcement. In New Haven, arrests of juvenile offenders involved in drug dealing, assault, or murder are often accompanied by requests for consultation from psychoanalytically: oriented clinicians. In many situations, the officer's concern about the psychological status of a young offender may lead to questions about whether jail or hospitalization is the more appropriate, immediate disposition. In the context of collaboration, questions about what the child needs have expanded to what the officer has to offer the child, the family, and the community beyond the arrest and detention.

Since 1995, juvenile probation officers and corrections personnel in the juvenile detention centre have been trained as part of the CD–CP programme. Juvenile offenders are now provided a continuity of interventions from arrest, to detention, to adjudication, to treatment planning and implementation that had never previously existed. The programme provides child psychiatric coverage for the detention centre and makes available on-call clinical services for youngsters involved in the probation programmes.

CD–CP responses to trauma

As police officers and others have found a forum for reflecting on what they had observed and as they have found partners in responding, they have no longer needed simply to turn away from the traumatogenic events they were unable to prevent. Instead, the police are able to consider the children's unfolding experiences and needs long after they have left the crime scene. While officers have an opportunity to expand their knowledge and repertoire of interventions, the collaboration with the police provides clinicians with a new setting to increase their understanding of the impact of violence and trauma. Discussions about referrals from the CD–CP Consultation Service frequently emphasize the extent to which children describe the violent events they have witnessed in terms of developmental phase-specific anxieties that are aroused. By following the unfolding stories of the children exposed to violence, clinicians in the programme are able to see more clearly what constitutes the specific dangers that overwhelm the individual child, which aspects and meanings of the event are experienced as "traumatizing". Clinicians, generally, assume that traumatization is related to the "facts" about violence that has been witnessed. These assumptions may have little to do with the child's actual experience of the event or the meaning that is attributed by the child in its aftermath. And little attention may be paid to learning about the child so as to begin to appreciate what an experience of violence might be for the child in the context of his or her life-history, family constellation, developmental phase, defence configuration, and the like, and therefore which interventions might be most useful. As Anna Freud pointed out:

> Traumatic events should not be taken at their face value but should be translated into their specific meaning for the given child. Attributes such as heroism or cowardice, generosity or greed, rationality or irrationality have to be understood differently in different individuals, and judged in the light of their genetic roots, their phase and age-adequateness, etc. [A. Freud, 1965, p. 139]

Consideration of the child's perspective has led to a lessening of the additionally traumatizing effects of how the police react to a child's situation in the wake of exposure to violence. Sgt. G described Lisa, a seven-year-old girl who had witnessed a beloved neighbour bleed to death after being fatally stabbed by another woman living nearby. Believing he was protecting her from the gore of the crime scene, Sgt. G had Lisa wait on the porch while officers conducted their investigation inside the house. Haunted by the intent gaze, a mixture of despair and rage, that Lisa fixed on him, he finally invited her into the apartment as the officers were leaving. The next day Sgt. G returned to the house and spoke with Lisa and her grandmother. He realized that his attempt at being helpful had backfired because he had not considered what Lisa was experiencing and what she needed and from whom.

As Sgt. G explained in the case conference, "Especially in the midst of so much blood and terror, what she needed was to be close to her grandmother, the most stable figure in her life, not to be stranded alone with images of the scene." Both Lisa and her grandmother eagerly accepted his offer of a referral for clinical services. Lisa's treatment revealed the extent to which frightening themes and fantasies involving extremes in love and hate dominated her inner life. Her ambivalence and uncertainty about relationships were heightened by her experience of growing up with a heroin-addicted mother, who dropped in and out of her life, and by concerns about her aging grandmother's fragile health. Internalized as well as external conflicts were boldly underlined by her confusion of loyalties in the stabbing. While she mourned the death of one beloved and idealized maternal substitute, she anxiously told her therapist about the love letters she was writing to the assailant, now in jail on murder charges. Even this dangerous woman seemed safer and more available than her inconsistent but absent mother.

Nine-year-old Mike witnessed the shooting death of an idolized teenage neighbour, John. The older boy had squarely beaten an opponent in a game of one-on-one basketball and was then accused of cheating. The two teenagers got into a shoving match that culminated in John's challenger pulling out a gun and shooting John twice in the chest. John died almost immediately. Mike was the only witness to the murder, and the police needed to interview him. Mike was understandably distressed by the death of his friend, and the police decided to interview him later that day. Rather than see him at police headquarters downtown, the investigating officer asked the boy and his mother where they would be most comfortable, and if they would like a referral to a CD–CP therapist. At their request, Mike and his mother were seen by the therapist immediately after the police interview.

In the acute phase of the intervention, the therapist invited the boy to draw pictures. He drew picture after picture in which the shooter and gun grew larger and larger while the boy and his teenage friend shrank to mere dots on the page. Over the next days, Mike had recurring nightmares and was irritable at home and school; he fought with his younger brother and peers. Despite Mike's father having abandoned them when Mike was three years old, mother described an unremarkable developmental history prior to the shooting. He did fairly well in school. His mother's only concern was that Mike spent too much time away from home, hours on his own or watching the older boys play basketball on the courts where the shooting had taken place. She worried that Mike would fall under the influence of the drug dealers who were part of their public housing landscape.

During the course of the twice-weekly psychotherapy that continued for eight months after the shooting, Mike's drawings and accompanying narratives grew more elaborate. In them he revealed the central role that John had played in his inner life as a realization of a dimly remembered and highly idealized father—strong, competent, and interested in Mike. Mike described how John's attention—letting him hang out at the basketball court and occasionally teaching him some shots—had been an important contrast to his mother's nagging and worries about his safety, which made him feel like a baby. In this context, as Mike repeatedly returned to depicting the moment that John was shot, his sense of disbelief turning to grief and then to rage and guilt. As he described the enduring image of watching John fall to the ground with an expression of surprise, Mike could now put into words what constituted the essence of his traumatic moment. The figure of strength and competence with whom he so desperately identified now seemed like a helpless baby. Mike again felt abandoned and helpless. Recognizing the link between the past and the present, associated with his longings for a father and friend who had abandoned him, Mike and his therapist could begin to make sense of the irritability and fighting that enabled Mike to re-establish power, express rage, and defend against "babyish" feelings and connect with longings for a father and friend who had abandoned him. Increasingly, Mike was alerted to those situations in which his sense of competence felt under attack—whether the joking of friends, teasing of a younger brother, or the concerns and expectations of his mother—and gave rise to angry counterattacks. His irritability and fighting diminished and eventually stopped, as did the nightmares that captured his terror and robbed him of the safety of sleep. While Mike ended his treatment with a good resolution of his posttraumatic adaptation, both his life setting and his history make Mike vulnerable to a dangerous future. How will the shooting and all its meanings be organized and represented in the developmental phases to come?

Children referred to the CD–CP programme by police give child analysts the opportunity to learn more about the ways trauma is defined for each child by a convergence of current and past experience. A child's experience of overwhelming anxiety derives from the realization of nodal, phase-specific fantasies, concerns, and conflicts regarding aggressive and sadistic wishes, fears of object loss, invasion of bodily integrity and damage, or guilt and shame associated with loss of control and infantile feelings of helplessness (Marans, 1994; Marans & Adelman, 1997; Marans, Berkman, & Cohen, 1996). Moreover, the psychoanalytic understanding of development and psychic functioning guide the process of appreciating the child's and family's experience of potentially traumatic events.

Psychoanalytic perspectives on violence and trauma

The psychoanalytic understanding of trauma in families, of the impact of witnessing violence in the inner city, and of the multiple pathways that can lead children from being traumatized into becoming aggressive is an important complement to other approaches to understanding children in this era of violence (Marans, Berkman, & Cohen, 1996; Marans & Cohen, 1993; Murphy, 2002). Psychoanalytic theories stand alongside sociological, political, economic, and other "explanatory" systems. In this area of research, contemporary psychoanalysts play a special role in underlining the complexity of these various relationships, the role of individual differences among children and families, and the distance between outer displays and internal experiences.

Anna Freud and Dorothy Burlingham (1943) demonstrated that during the Blitz children responded as much to their parents' affects and to disruptions in parenting as to the actual dangers of bombing (Hellman, 1962, 1983). These observations have been repeated wherever children are studied during warfare—for instance, in Israel during the missile attacks in the Gulf War, when child analysts worked with children and families evacuated from their homes, and in the midst of natural catastrophes (Laor, Wolmer, & Cohen, 2001; Laor et al., 1996, 2002). When children are provided an interpretive frame, when they and their families can see their exposure and suffering within a community and a shared set of beliefs, the experience of trauma is given a context and is transmuted. However, unlike British families during World War II or Israeli families that endured a series of wars since the founding of the nation, children exposed to violence in the inner cities of the United States often have little in the way of community, ideology, or, sometimes, cohesive family structure on which to rely for mutative support and amelioration of trauma. It is in those circumstances that police officers, properly equipped and supported by acute clinical intervention, may be the first best source of stability and containment available to children and their families. Psychoanalytic understanding of the nature of trauma and of the importance of intellectual, interpretive, and psychosocial mediation of experiences guides all efforts to help children caught in war and otherwise experiencing or witnessing violence.

Through acute and long-term involvement with children overwhelmed by their exposure to violence, child analysts have an opportunity to extend the field of observation and inquiry into the long-term impact of trauma. Here there is an important convergence of psychoanalytic understanding of individual differences in the processing and meaning of events, biological theories of brain functioning, and developmental theories about critical stages in development. There is thus a confluence between what the brain perceives and what the mind understands. That which is traumatic represents the conspiracy of both when the protective barriers give away; presumably psychological structures as well as biological structures are overwhelmed (Burges Watson, Hoffman, & Wilson, 1988; Pynoos & Nader, 1989; Pynoos, Steinberg, & Wraith, 1995; van der Kolk, Greenberg, Boyd, & Krystal, 1985). One model of the neurophysiological mediation of stress and trauma proposes that, when an individual is unable to anticipate or defend against an experience of overwhelming danger, the central regulation of the noradrenergic system—which mediates heart rate, respiration, and startle reflexes—is compromised (Perry, 1994; Southwick et al., 1993; Yehuda, 2002; Yehuda, McFarlane, & Shalev, 1998).

In the work with the New Haven Department of Police Service, child analysts have had the advantage of observing children and adults within minutes of exposure to acute episodes of violence. This proximity and timing of involvement has allowed these clinicians to follow patients' responses from their acute to longer-term adaptations. Regardless of their pre-morbid or pre-violence-exposure functioning, each child and adult seen has presented with a range of acute symptoms involving dysregulation of affect, attention, memory, and such bodily functions as sleep. Subsequently, each has shown a marked exacerbation or introduction of increased anxiety and new symptomatic behaviour.

Integrating physiologic and psychoanalytic models is extremely useful for understanding the acute presentation of trauma. In the acute phase, a person's attempts to process, anticipate, and regulate levels of excitation through typical patterns of mentation and defence may be seen in increased motor agitation at one end of the spectrum, and withdrawal, isolation, and numbing at the other end. Subsequent hypervigilance, symptom formation, and a propensity for dysregulation of basic ego functions—generalized or restimulated by traumatic reminders—may thus reflect alterations in central neuroregulatory capacities as well as attempts to mediate somatopsychic experiences through the reintroduction of ideational representation, signal anxiety, and subsequent defensive responses in the service of restitution and ego reorganization.

Short-term distress, as in brief separations, leads to adaptive coping, structure formation, and healthy defences. These reactions prime a child's psychological "immune" system, allowing him or her to accommodate to the experiential "viruses" of the real world. Persistent distress, as in repeated exposure to violence in the home, in school, or on the streets, predispose the child to fail to develop the ability to feel safe and secure with others or when alone; to enjoy reciprocity, and to be able to tolerate normal frustrations. What constitutes a normal, "immunizing dose" and what overwhelms the mental adaptive immune system remain crucial questions for those studying children living in psychosocial adversity. These questions represent potential areas of collaboration among child psychoanalysts, child psychiatrists, social workers, and developmental psychologists. The Child Development–Community Policing programme offers a vantage point for addressing these questions.

Post 9/11

In the midst of its ongoing activities, the National Center for Children Exposed to Violence (NCCEV) was mobilized within moments after the news of the attacks on the World Trade Center and the Pentagon. In the hours, days, and weeks that followed, psychoanalysts and analytically informed faculty members responded immediately to requests for consultations with colleagues in New York and lower Fairfield County, CT, as well as providing direct services to children and families in affected neighbourhoods in New York City. In addition, NCCEV faculty met with members of Congress and their families, as well as advising members of the U.S. Departments of Justice and Education in addressing the psychological needs of children and families directly affected by the attacks and those affected across the country. Interviews with print and broadcast media were another outlet for disseminating psychoanalytically informed views about the psychological effects of the terrorist attacks on children and families and ways of ameliorating their impact.

In the aftermath of 9/11, the NCCEV published guidelines for parents, mental health professionals, primary healthcare providers, and clergy about how to understand stress, trauma, and bereavement and about how to talk with children about their concerns about the attacks and subsequent threats. They also wrote guides for mental health workers, primary health care providers, and clergy about stress, trauma, and bereavement in the aftermath of 9/11. These materials were posted on the NCCEV website (http://www.nccev.org) and disseminated on linked websites around the country. They were also distributed by the U.S. Departments of Justice and Defense, through all members of the U.S. Senate and House of Representatives, and through a range of professional organizations, including the Academy of Pediatrics. The NCCEV, in conjunction with the Departments of Psychiatry at Yale and the University of Connecticut, have delivered training and direct services throughout the state of Connecticut and are working with the governor's office and commissioner of mental health to develop comprehensive mental responses to possible subsequent crises.

On behalf of the U.S. Department of Education and the New York City Board of Education, I, along with child analyst Robert Pynoos and his colleague from Los Angeles, Marlene Wong, consulted with school, mental health, and disaster officials about coordinated responses to children throughout the New York City school system. In collaboration with the Mental Health Partnership in New York City, the NCCEV has continued to consult with and provide school system-wide training for developing school-based crisis response and mental health service delivery approaches. All this work has derived from the extensive experience gained in New Haven and around the country, in responding collaboratively to thousands of children who were affected by violence and disaster during the past decade, whether at home, in their neighbourhoods, or in school.

Conclusions

Regardless of the setting, child analysts have been most successful in applying psychoanalytic knowledge when they have invited collaborators to observe the world first of all from the perspective of children. Similarly, when analysts have been able to provide a common language and a conceptual framework that helps collaborators from other fields to organize and increase their range of observations, partnerships between analysts and others grow. Anna Freud exemplified these approaches to applied psychoanalysis. She was not content simply to observe and learn about the inner workings of children's minds or about the paths of children's development. What, she might have asked, can we learn about the unfolding lives of children so that we can support their optimal development and do the least amount of harm to them? And who must see what we have learned? And with whom must we work to apply what we have learned and intervene when children's development is threatened by environmental factors that may all too often reach traumatic proportions?

Anna Freud and later child analysts have been devoted to the notion that a greater understanding of development and of children's perspectives can inform the ways in which children are treated—in a psychoanalytic treatment, a custody dispute, a hospitalization, a routine paediatric exam, the classroom, and the home. Both in and out of the consulting-room, their work reflects an interest in the special populations of children who have endured special, significant environmental factors that shaped internal experience and adaptations in daily life. In considering the role of the environment in children's development Anna Freud suggested

> that every single aspect of the child's personality is affected adversely unless definite sources of supply and support are made available to him has been proved beyond doubt by analytic work carried with the children of severely disturbed parents, concentration camp and disinstitutionalized children, orphaned children, handicapped children, etc. [A. Freud, 1968, p. 116]

She discussed the dilemma that often confronts analysts when their assessment indicates that the damage to a child's development is "caused and maintained by active, ongoing influences lodged in the environment" (p. 115). She pointed out that whether these negative influences disregard and frustrate or actively oppose the normal course of development, the child victim is in need of therapeutic help. However, "in neither case is the type of help clearly indicated, nor the therapist's role in the process clearly circumscribed" (p. 115).

Our ability to make psychoanalytic findings about the inner lives of children accessible to non-analysts has determined the extent to which psychoanalytic ideas have helped to shape policies and practices that affect the lives of children in many circumstances and settings. The pioneering work of Anna Freud and those who would follow introduced a model for the roles played by child analysts outside clinical hours—as consultants, teachers, and partners—translating and applying psychoanalytic principles of development to a variety of settings. These roles have been an especially important complement to direct clinical work, particularly in those cases and situations in which the type of therapeutic help, the role of the therapist, or the needs of the child could not be adequately defined or addressed in the consulting room alone. Without the opportunity to learn from children in the clinical setting, we would have few opportunities to help others consider what children need. Without venturing beyond the consulting-room, child analysts might have few occasions to be heard or to learn more about those exigent circumstances in children's lives that so often undermine developmental potential and immobilize the efforts of adult caregivers to intervene on their behalf.

In the Child Development–Community Policing programme and in the work of the National Center for Children Exposed to Violence, child analysts and analytically informed colleagues have found a new setting in which psychoanalytic principles of development can be applied, explored, and expanded. Through these programmes, the fields of observation have been increased by collaborations requiring the development of a common language in which to extend the observations, concerns, and approaches of disparate professionals who deal with the children at greatest risk for developmental psychopathology.

For many of the children and families seen through the CD–CP services, the chronic symptoms and adaptations that immobilize progressive development may, fortuitously, no longer be the only outcome of their exposure to violence. When the significance of their exposure is first recognized by police officers, children and families no longer need to be alone in their struggle with the immediate effects of trauma. When partners from various social services share a developmental perspective, interventions can be comprehensive and driven by the specific needs of the children and families they serve. For the professionals involved, the availability of immediate consultation, access to acute situations, and a broader scope of information and intervention options have decreased their burdens. Police officers and mental health professionals in particular are able to become active in the immediate aftermath of violence and tragedy rather than being overwhelmed by it. For so many of the children and families seen, the police and mental health response may offer a rare experience of feeling regarded and feeling that one's experiences of tragedy, fear, and trauma are recognized as exceptional no matter how frequently they may be part of one's life. In many of the situations requiring acute response, police, seen as representatives of the larger social order, are viewed not simply as providing too little too late but as benign figures of authority who are able to play a role in re-establishing a semblance of stability in the midst of the emotional chaos.

In weekly case conferences, child analysts and other analytically informed investigators and clinicians, police, and other partners are able to explore the effects of exposure to violence on children, their families, and the professionals who become involved with them. In turn, all involved are in a better position to assess short- and longer-term psychotherapeutic, policing, social service, probation, medical, and educational interventions that may offer the best hope for ameliorating the impact of violence and trauma. To help children and their families return to the optimal paths of development and functioning, CD–CP partners continuously attempt to learn more about the implications of our respective interventions, as well as the potential benefits and limitations of our coordinated efforts. Whether responding to children who have witnessed the deadly outcome of a domestic dispute between parents, or to a neighbourhood that has seen young men die in a shootout, or to a school community that has witnessed the death of classmates and teachers at the hands of fellow students, or to a city and country stunned by the destruction and loss of life resulting from a terrorist attack—a mutual psychoanalytic stance is mobilized and informs the background for response.

NOTES

Reprinted from: B. Skalrew, S. W. Tremlow, & S. M. Wilkinson (Eds.), *Analysts in the Trenches: Streets, Schools, War Zones* (pp. 211–236). Hillsdale, NJ: The Analytic Press, 2004.

This work is supported by the U.S. Department of Justice, which established the National Center for Children Exposed to Violence at the Yale Child Study Center in 1999.

1. The Child Development Community Policing model, developed at the Yale Study Center, is being replicated around the United States under the auspices of the United States Department of Justice.

Commentary

Efrain Bleiberg

The collaboration and the appreciation of different perspectives and approaches—between psychoanalysis and developmental research; the Anna Freud Centre and The Yale Child Study Center (a collaboration that Menninger and The Menninger Department of Psychiatry at Baylor College of Medicine is happily joining); and, in Steve Marans' timely, eloquent, and compelling description, between psychoanalytically informed mental health clinicians and law enforcement personnel—aims to achieve innovation and advances in scientific understanding and clinical effectiveness.

The great civil rights leader Martin Luther King, Jr, stated almost four decades ago that "the choice today is not between violence and non-violence, but between violence and non-existence". The Child Development–Community Policing Partnership (CD–CP) organized by Marans at the Yale Child Study Center in collaboration with the New Haven Police Department and the basis of The National Center for Children Exposed to Violence created by President Clinton is an affirmation that the key to understanding and collaboration between individuals, organizations, or cultures and, arguably, to the capacity to respond effectively to violence and it's maladaptive aftermath, lies in the very mechanism underlying the human capacity to conceive of our own and others' humanity and existence as human beings—that is, *mentalizing*.

Mentalizing is the genetically prepared disposition to largely spontaneously and procedurally read, interpret, and predict human behaviour—that of ourselves as well as that of others—based on mental states, such as thoughts, feelings, beliefs, goals, attitudes, and values. This largely intuitive recognition of one's mind and the minds of others leads to an appreciation that mental states are *subjective representations* of reality rather than reality itself. This appreciation is crucial for the development of symbolic processing, for the achievement of a sense of "ownership" of our own behaviour, and for the possibility of understanding the other's perspective—even when it is different from our own (Allen, 2003; Fonagy, Gergely, et al., 2002).

Marans points out that the collaboration between mental health clinicians and law enforcement personnel, in response to children and families exposure to violence, is rooted in the work of Anna Freud's tradition of the involvement of psychoanalytic clinicians with other professionals concerned with children, such as teachers, paediatricians, social workers and lawyers. According to Marans, Anna Freud (1968) aimed to invite other professionals, regardless of the setting, to reflect on what they saw *from the perspective of the child,* in order for them to appreciate the complexity of children's experience and the implications of that experience to the children's development. One of Marans's crucial insights in developing the consultation model pioneered by Anna Freud and Solnit is that, in order for this "invitation" to result in the genuine collaboration that can lead to developmentally informed interventions requires, first, a process designed to promote the ability of mental health practitioners and of police officers to "put themselves in each other's shoes" in order to learn and appreciate the perspective and framework of the other profession and to consider the developmental implications of shared observations and actions. In so doing, Marans brilliantly puts in practice a basic lesson of developmental research: mentalization develops in the context of secure attachments, in interactions with caregivers attuned and responsive to the children's internal states. Caregivers optimally promote mentalizing in their children when their responses convey their own grasp of their children's internal states and intentionality (Fonagy & Target, 1997). This lesson from early development appears just as relevant to adults engaged in the complex tasks of law enforcement or the provision of mental health services: to feel and understand someone else's perspective begins with the experience of "feeling felt" and understood (Allen, 2003). This experience is particularly crucial when the task at hand involves putting ourselves in the shoes of children whose bodies and minds have been exposed to the destructive intrusions of abuse and violence, the very experiences that normally trigger the inhibition of mentalizing.

The Yale Child Development–Community Policing Program (CD–CP), which is being replicated across the United States, embodies a programme to restore inhibited mentalizing by promoting two fundamental processes that are crucial for adaptation and resilience in the face of adversity and trauma (Terr, 1991; van der Kolk, Burbridge, & Suzuki, 1997; van der Kolk & Fisler, 1994):

1. The CD–CP recognizes that trauma and exposure to violence disrupt the brain–mind disposition to seek and identify contingencies, coherence, and organization (Terr, 1991; van der Kolk, Burbridge & Suzuki, 1997, van der Kolk & Fisler, 1994), a disposition from which we derive a sense of anticipation, activity, control, and agency—the agentive self (Fonagy, Gergely, et al., 2002). It is from this vantage point that the CD–CP aims to create a collaboration between police officers and mental health practitioners that can help children transmute personal trauma—and the resulting sense of passivity, helplessness, and disorganization—by providing them with what Marans calls "an interpretive frame".

2. The CD–CP appreciates that we develop "interpretive frames" in the context of intersubjective two-way exchanges with others—that is, when we exercise the capacity to mentalize. It is quite plausible that one of the evolutionary functions of mentalizing is to protect us from our own destructiveness. Given our evolutionary selection as beings whose survival and adaptation is predicated on a brain "designed" to be organized by social experience and to function in a human, interactive context, a key function of our ability to read internal states is the decision between when it is safe and adaptive to go into an attachment mode and when to go into fight-or-flight. Functional neuroimaging research is beginning to document how the "intention to trust" correlates with brain activity changes that result from experience with an interactive partner (King-Casas et al., 2005). Neuroimaging studies such as these are laying the foundation to test the hypothesis that under ordinary mind–brain activity, when the mentalizing mechanism is operational, it is extremely difficult for human beings to kill, maim, or otherwise torture and violate another human being. Such actions are feasible only when mentalizing and attachment are inhibited and the fight-or-flight system is activated—a point at which we can no longer interpret and experience the "other" as a human being but more as an object whose removal or destruction may be necessary for our own survival.

One critical aspect of psychoanalytic and psychotherapeutic training is to learn, indeed, to "manage" our countertransference—that is, first and foremost, to avoid losing a mentalizing perspective when subjected to the emotional barrages of patients' transferential and nonspecific, non-mentalizing approaches.

Combat training, by contrast, strives to achieve the opposite goal: to prepare soldiers to "turn-off" mentalizing and empathy in order to overcome the normal inclination to see the "other" as a human being, rather than "the enemy".

Police officers live on the edge of both: needing to preserve a mentalizing perspective to prevent exacerbating situations in which their survival or the survival of the citizens they protect may indeed require a temporary turning-off of mentalizing.

The CD–CP Program promotes mentalizing in police officers with exercises designed to appreciate the different perspectives of those involved in a violent incident—including their own. They become attentive, for example, to the humiliation that may be experienced by a juvenile offender approached in a harsh or threatening manner. They learn to recognize the anguish and despair behind a parent's apparent indifference or incompetence.

The outcome of those therapeutic interventions is suggested by moving and compelling anecdotes, yet lacks empirical evidence. It is compelling, however, to wonder whether the more fundamental question lies in the potential to develop therapeutic interventions as focused, systematic, and clearly defined as the CD–CP Program, designed to more specifically assist children exposed to violence—as well as rekindling in their families the very capacity to create mind and mindfulness. In so doing, treatment can aim to restore the natural healing and protective mechanisms that allow not only individuals and families but also, as Marans's work suggests, entire communities to become more able to sustain effective and adaptive social interactions.

CHAPTER ELEVEN

Multi-contextual multiple family therapy

Eia Asen

Context reading, context making, context managing

Family therapy—now more accurately named systemic therapy—has developed over the past five decades and has now come of age. Different schools and approaches have evolved over the years, reflecting changing societal, cultural, and political priorities and landscapes. We have seen the emergence of strategic and structural family therapy models, followed by Milan, post-Milan, and social constructionist schools, as well as behavioural, psycho-educational, solution-focused, and narrative approaches. Nowadays it is fairly rare for allegedly "pure" models to be practiced, as the huge cultural variety of our clients and their families, as well as their presenting problems and the contexts within which systemic work is carried out, all require diverse and flexible responses. Postmodern systemic therapists tend to be multi-modal practitioners, working in many different settings, both public and private. In the public domain, systemic practitioners tend to be part of multidisciplinary teams, and their interventions need to be part of the overall framework and approach of the team. Some once precious if not self-congratulatory interventions, designed behind one-way screens by teams of four, now tend to be a thing of the past. Systemic practitioners find themselves, instead, employing "swampy lowland principles" (Rycroft, 2004) and often have to become "context chameleons" (Asen, 2004) to remain engaged and effective. They require three distinct skills: context reading, context making, and context managing.

Understanding the request for help and the nature of the referral is usually the first step for most clinicians—whatever their theoretical orientation. The questions: "Who wants help for whom (or what), and Why now?" help to read the context of the referral and presenting problem. Problems can be contextualized at various different levels—the individual level, the level of the family or other significant relationships, the immediate social and cultural setting, the level of the professional network that is generated around the problem (and often inadvertently "helps" to maintain it)—and the wider political context. Such multi-level context reading permits clinicians to position themselves, and helps them to consider how and with whom to start—be that the individual patient, members of the family, referring agencies, or various combinations thereof. Context reading should not be a one-off activity but an ongoing process throughout the course of therapeutic work with patients and their families. The CMM (Coordinated Management of Meaning) model provides a complementary map for understanding context: in therapy, speech acts and nonverbal communications are given meaning by viewing them in the context of emerging interaction sequences and episodes, which, in turn, reflect a relationship context, itself informed and shaped by life scripts that can be seen through the lens of yet another "higher" level of context: the cultural patterns (Pearce & Cronen, 1980).

However, clinicians are not employed to merely read layers of context and consider how these seem to explain the presenting problem(s): clinicians are meant to translate their understanding into action, so that distress can be relieved and mental health promoted. To do this, clinicians search for and create therapeutic settings—in short, they make contexts for change. A basic question can help clinicians to achieve this: "what are the contexts that I need to use—or make—to address the presenting problems and issues?" This question opens up a multiverse of possibilities, particularly when de-constructing the notion of "context". From a pragmatic point of view it may be helpful to consider five types of "context": different "person contexts", a variety of "time" and "place" contexts, as well as a whole range of "activity" and "modality" contexts.

The question of *who* (the "person context") should be present for therapy "sessions" (an unfortunate term that seems to fix what goes on) opens up many possibilities: it could be "just" and individual, it could be partners, a group of families, religious figures, neighbours, other clinicians, ex-service users, maybe even managers or politicians—or any combination of the above. When considering *where* (the "place context") the therapeutic work is carried out, there are also a number of options: in the clinic setting, the home, school, hospital ward, supermarket, court, mosque, temple, church, community centre, town hall, car—the list would seem endless. Working in a naturalistic setting, a setting where the problem manifests itself concretely, can be more effective for some families than to confine all clinical work to neutral if not sterile clinic settings. The "time context" (*when?*) can be defined in terms of length, frequency, and duration of the therapeutic work: 10–20 minutes may be an appropriate time frame for carrying out preventive work in general practice, as this is an accepted time slot and thus fits the primary care context. At the other end of the spectrum we have "multi-problem families" with chronic histories and entrenched interactions with multiple agencies: it is unlikely that they will respond to 60- or 90-minute sessions at monthly intervals. Here time frames for sessional work may have to be much longer, perhaps whole days, with a frequency of possibly four or five days a week and a duration of two or three months, if not longer. Clinicians need continuously to think—and re-think—together with their clients whether the time structures created—or imposed—are still helpful. It is the joint process of continuous co-construction, evaluation, and revalidation of this process that itself can contribute to healing. *What* (the "activity context") we do in our clinical work is clearly of major importance. Psychotherapeutic encounters generally tend to be primarily word-focused, with the various participants firmly placed in chairs (if not on a couch), engaging in "narratives" and "conversations". Yet it is also possible to work therapeutically in non- or para-verbal ways—from ordinary play to psychodrama, from making collages to making music, from "in vivo" exposure to "real-life issues" to staged multiple family events, from cultural encounters to working with local networks. *How* (the "modality context") clinicians do what they do depends on their training, personal experiences, and their "self". It has already been mentioned that in the systemic field there are now many diverse schools and orientations. All these approaches have developed at particular times and in highly specific contexts—as have other non-systemic approaches, be they psychodynamic, behavioural, or somatic. It would seem limited and limiting for clinicians to remain insecurely attached to just one "religion" and proudly label themselves as a "narrative" or "structural" or "solution-focused" or "post-Milan" therapist. Surely different presentations and problems, different cultural and social contexts, require different responses from clinicians. Furthermore, the problems and preoccupations of our patient shift—we, the clinicians, also need to shift to keep up with their changing focus. A therapeutic modality, appropriate at the outset of a piece of clinical work, may not be appropriate or effective a few weeks or months later.

The multi-contextual approach opens up new perspectives and provides choices for the clinician as well as for clients. If the contextualizing questions ("who?", "where?", "when?", "what?" and "how?") are asked throughout the course of therapeutic work, then our approach is not at risk of becoming stale and irrelevant. By involving our clients in this questioning process, we hope to co-construct relevant contexts for change, opening up, for them and us, a multiverse of new ways of seeing and experiencing. Furthermore, if clinicians are able to entertain multiple models—systemic and non-systemic ones—simultaneously, then a multi-modal approach can emerge, based on what the patients and their various systems require, rather than what a particular dogma requires. Multi-contextual work implies that a number of different interventions are simultaneously addressed to different levels of the system: this may include work with the individual, in parallel with work with the family, as well as work with the professional network and the neighbourhood. Involving families with other families with similar presentations is another useful context for change.

The evolution of multiple family group work

It is more than four decades ago that a group of clinicians, working with hospitalized patients with schizophrenia in New York, first experimented with treating a number of families together (Laqueur, La Burt, & Morong, 1964). They invited the patients' relatives into the hospital milieu and involved them directly in discussions about home life and treatment issues, with the aim of improving inter- and intra-family communication. With several families being seen together in one large group, it soon became apparent that family members developed ideas of how to address chronically stuck issues. By not only focusing on their own ill relative but also on one another, family members increasingly became aware of their own roles and began to examine their interactions with the ill person from multiple perspectives. The early multi-family groups were appropriately described as "sheltered workshops in family communication" (Laqueur, La Burt, & Morong,

1964), taking place on a fortnightly basis for a few hours. By exchanging ideas and experiences with members of other families, it seemed possible to compare notes and to learn from one another. Furthermore, it seemed that the presence of other families allowed the patient—and other family members—to struggle towards increasing independence and self-differentiation, for example by identifying with members of other families and learning by analogy (Laqueur, 1973). This approach inspired other clinicians working with psychotic patients and they also included relatives in their family group work (Anderson, 1983; Kuipers, Leff, & Lam, 1992; Leichter & Schulman, 1974; McFarlane, 1982). McFarlane and his group (McFarlane, 1993) developed a manualized version of a well-structured multi-family therapy programme and argued that families found it helpful to see some of their interaction and communication patterns in others—including their own seemingly "dysfunctional" behaviours. The approach emphasizes modulated dis-enmeshment, communication normalization, concrete crisis management, re-socialization, and stigma reversal.

Much of this type of multiple family group work takes place at weekly or monthly intervals, usually in sessions lasting a few hours at a time. Sometimes families participate in such work without the index patients being present, at other times the patients are part of the multiple family groups. A major aim of multiple family group work is to reduce the levels of Expressed Emotion (EE), above all the critical comments and over-involvement, in line with the well documented research findings of significantly reduced relapse rates if EE in key relatives is lowered (Vaughn & Leff, 1976). Over time it has been shown that the frequency, duration, and focus of this approach are appropriate, and multiple family group work has established itself as an effective supplementary treatment for families that include a psychotic patient. However, with other client groups a more intensive approach appears to be indicated.

Current models of intensive multiple family group work

There are families—and individuals within these families—with serious mental health issues and other problems that seem resistant to change. One such example are so-called "multi-problem families" who present with psychological problems and symptoms simultaneously in more than one person, with co-existing violence and abuse, as well as with educational failure and social marginalization. These families attract multiple helpers, who often provide contradictory input, leading frequently to highly complex "problem-generated" systems. The families' seeming helplessness soon paralyses the professionals, with "chronic" and entrenched relationships developing all around. It was the encounter with such seemingly "chaotic" and "treatment-resistant" families with dependent children that led to an intensive form of multiple family group work for multi-problem and multi-agency families. This approach was developed by Alan Cooklin and his team at the Marlborough Family Service in London (Asen et al., 1982; Cooklin, 1982), and it consisted of putting 6–8 "impossible" families together under one roof, for prolonged periods of time, as a kind if "therapeutic community" of dysfunctional families. A highly structured daily programme with deliberately built-in "controlled" crisis situations—similar to those they might encounter in their every-day life in their homes—forced them to address daily living issues in a therapeutic context. The aim was to enable these families themselves to identify new forms of crisis management that no longer required the involvement of increasing numbers of professionals. The Marlborough Family Day Unit, an "institution for change" (Cooklin, Miller, & McHugh, 1983), was founded some 25 years ago, and more than 1,000 children and their families have been treated there since. At the outset, the work of the Marlborough Family Day Unit was very intensive and long: families attended for eight hours per day, five days a week, often over a period of many months if not a whole year. However, subsequently the approach has undergone many changes and transitions, with programmes that now last 12 weeks and a balance between clinic-based and home-based work. Families attend for 3 or 4 whole days one week—and less frequently (1 or 2 whole days) during the following 2 weeks, when families are also seen in their own homes, so as to facilitate the transfer of experiences from the clinic to the home context. This is followed by another intensive 3 or 4 whole days within the space of one week. A similar pattern of attendance prevails for the rest of the multi-family day programme. Nowadays not all families participate for the entire 12 weeks: some may leave early and new families join this "open" group (Asen, Dawson, & McHugh, 2001). The family day unit is a specialist resource, a kind of "pressure cooker", providing intensive whole-day experiences as well as exposure to other families.

During their attendance families have a structured timetable, which requires them to make frequent transitions and changes throughout the day. There are formal groups, involving at various times all families, at times parents and children separately. There is a mixture of action-oriented and reflective work. A major principle of this work is openness and transparency, not only between the families but also between staff and families. The day unit's rooms are well equipped with cameras and one-way screens, and there are many video-feedback sessions when families view their own—and others'—interactions. Families can also take small video cameras home and make a "home movie" about their life or specific issues. These are then edited (by the families) and shown to the whole group of families, who are often more expert at analysing and commenting than extensively (and expensively) trained professionals! In this way families and their individual members become "consultants" to other families. They support each other and reflect on their own process, they observe and comment on unhelpful patterns they see in each other. They form friendships and often create a network of support for isolated families outside the programme. In this way the families are a resource for each other, and this can help to prevent relapse. Experienced families engage new and sceptical families, offering hope.

Transparency is not a one-way process: it also applies to the staff. The "Reflections Meeting", inspired by Tom Andersen's "reflecting team" ideas (Andersen, 1987), takes place at regular—at present fortnightly—intervals. The team of family day unit workers—some three or four staff—convenes a clinical meeting that is videotaped. In this clinical meeting the family workers exchange information and views about each family's dynamics and their work during the previous weeks. The workers are very specific about their observations, and they reflect about each family's interactions and issues. This meeting lasts about 30 minutes, and the videotape recording is given to a systemic consultant who has not been part of the clinical meeting. The consultant meets with the parents (and at times also with older children) to watch the clinical meeting and the staff's views, opinions, and reflections. The remote control for the video-recorder is handed to one of the parents or another adult—a message that it is up to them to let the specific tape segment run for its entirety or to pause so that specific points can be taken up. Most adults opt for stopping and re-starting the tape, as pausing the tape allows family members to respond immediately to the staff's views. It is the systemic consultant's task to stimulate the families' curiosity about one another, as well as encouraging them to provide advice, criticism, and support for one another. The family workers are not in the room for the Reflections Meeting, but some will watch it via a video-link. This is deliberate, as it makes staff temporarily unavailable for being drawn into prolonged discussions with families, feeling that they have to justify what they have said in their staff meeting. It thus allows staff to be in a reflective position, listening to the families' reflections without an opportunity to immediately put the record "straight". This also permits families to reflect on how staff might digest the parents' feedback to what has been said about them. The Reflections Meeting is a popular event, at times more with families than with staff. Families like the idea that not only they themselves but also staff can be observed at work. This adds considerably to the ethos of openness and transparency prevailing in the family day unit. A subsequent Post-reflections Meeting, involving the systemic consultant and staff only, creates yet another layer of context: staff reflect on the families' reflections on the staff's reflections.

The Marlborough Family Day Unit in London has pioneered the establishment of the first permanent multiple family day setting, specifically designed for and solely dedicated to the work with seemingly "hopeless" families (Asen, Dawson, & McHugh, 2001). While the main emphasis is on multiple family work, other forms of treatment—such as single family work and individual interventions—are also used if and when required. This approach is in marked contrast to previous multiple family therapy work, as described above. It has resulted in a significantly improved engagement with seemingly impossible families and helped to neutralize poor relationships with professionals.

A school for pupils—and their parents

The principles and practices of intensive multiple family work have subsequently been adapted to the work with other patient and problem groups. The reason for establishing a "Family School" (Dawson & McHugh, 1986) at the Marlborough Family Service was prompted by needing to make a context to deal with pupils who had been referred as a result of being excluded from their schools because of serious learning "blocks", violence, and disruptive classroom behaviour. The referring teachers seemed to put all the blame for the pupil's problems at the family's door, whereas the family tended to blame the school entirely for the educational failure of the children. The more the family blamed the school, the more the school blamed the family. In this impasse the child is caught in the middle between the warring parties. The families refused to seek psychiatric or psychological help, and the teachers no longer wanted these difficult children in their classes. To overcome this impasse, a "Family School" was created, with the simultaneous attendance of each child's parent(s) being mandatory. This allows parents to witness their children's educational problems, and it permits teachers to witness the family issues that are often transferred into school (Dawson & McHugh, 1994), with the focus not simply on the individual pupil, but on the interactions within the family, between family and school—and within the school system. The multiple family paradigm proves to be a particularly effective way of achieving change. With up to nine families on any day attending with their sons or daughters for three hours four mornings a week, there is a group of families that can reflect on one another and their relationships with the school system. In the Family School's daily meetings all children, parents, and teachers are involved, providing a context for reflection, mutual support, and encouragement for trying out new ways of relating and communicating. With the opportunity for families to challenge and support each other in their struggles for change, the multi-family group is an excellent context for intensification. There is a special atmosphere of immediacy and intensity that is rarely attained during conventional single-family therapy sessions. Moreover, the information relating in a multiple family group to one family frequently has significant meaning for other families in the group. Families often say that they have thought about something that was said several days earlier, and that they decided to try something new as a result of what they had previously seen and heard in the group. Over time, the multiple family group gains its own momentum and becomes a context that drives the participants to expect change in themselves as well as in other group members.

The Marlborough Family School is an intervention from outside the school, and through the attendance of both child and family it can provide an in-depth systemic report as a contribution to the official assessment and placement procedures. Changes made at the Marlborough Family School usually result in the child returning to school full-time, but in a few instances the intervention can also help the local education authority make a decision about more appropriate alternative long-term educational provision for the child (Dawson & McHugh, 2000).

The Family School programme is structured around a core multi-family group. Up to nine children and at least one significant adult per child come together for a maximum of four mornings each week. The morning lasts for about 3 hours. There are two main strands to the functioning of the school: education and therapy. Families can arrive from 9.00 a.m. onwards, and they can have breakfast together and talk informally. The first formal part of a morning session, 9.30–10.10, is a time when the children are taught in the classroom, with all their parents or other family members present. Depending on the presenting difficulty, parents can either sit with their child and help them or talk with the other parents in an informal group, still within the physical space of the classroom. The task of the teacher–therapists during this phase of the morning is to be both teacher and therapist. This is achieved by teaching the children and observing and experiencing the difficulties they present in this domain. In the classroom, children will show their difficulties in their relationship to the curriculum set, their interactions with the teacher, or their interactions with their peers. In the Family School it is possible to undertake "live" observations of difficulties in the intra-family relationships. The task is to convert teacher observations into an issue that is relevant to both child and parent and to use it as a potential vehicle for change. This is very different from the usual position of teachers who, when confronted with problematic behaviour, would expect to have to resolve the situation themselves. In the Family School this would be seen as an opportunity missed, as there would be less potential for new information to be introduced to the child and family system as organized around an educational task.

After the initial "teaching" phase of the morning, all the children and family members come together for a more structured multiple family group meeting (at 10.15 a.m.). This lasts for 40 minutes and happens at the same time every day. Each meeting is chaired by one of the teacher–therapists or by a parent, with two other group members—children or adults—acting a co-chairs and timekeepers. All the families have their own five-minute slot, which is divided into three parts. The family members can use the first two minutes as they wish, but usually to report back to the group on how the last 24 hours have gone in relation to their goals for change. These are clearly defined behavioural targets, for both the school and the home setting, and they are rated on a daily basis. For the next two minutes the rest of the members of the group are invited to make comments. These can be about what has just been said, about changes that someone might have noticed, about an observation of how the child or parent has been trying something different, or about how the family members seem to be getting stuck with each other. The group applauds family members who are meeting their goals. In the remaining one minute the targets are reviewed and specific emerging themes are used to set the next task. The timekeeper only keeps the time and lets everybody know when it is time to move on to the next family. It is the chair's responsibility to elicit and highlight themes as they come up, as well as encouraging the group members to become more expert and vocal in observing their own and others' repeating patterns of behaviour. They attempt to create the conditions in which different families can both challenge and support each other in their struggles for change.

More recently, the Family School has involved the parents in a parallel literacy programme: once a week for one hour they receive help with reading and writing via laptops in another classroom. The parents, initially reserved, quickly become enthusiastic about managing a computer. "Graduate" families—those who have gone successfully through the Family School programme—go on to co-run, with a member of staff, multiple family groups in now 18 mainstream primary and secondary schools in the local area. "Graduate children" mentor or "buddy" other children on these outreach programmes, which are run under the management and supervision of the Marlborough Family School. Pupils leave with 80% success on targets and 95% return to full-time education, with significantly improved attendances and raised academic achievements. Families and teachers consistently report vastly improved relationships between family and school.

Multiple family work for eating-disordered teenagers

A particularly successful application of the multiple family approach can be found in the treatment of teenagers suffering from anorexia nervosa (Dare & Eisler, 2000; Eisler, LeGrange, & Asen, 2003; Scholz & Asen, 2001). When these patients are admitted as inpatients to eating disorder units, their treatment is provided by nursing and medical staff, with their parents tending to feel left out and isolated. In contrast, in a multi-family day programme, parents connect with other parents who have an anorexic child. This helps them to overcome such isolation and allows parents to share their accompanying feelings of guilt and shame. Being in the presence of other families for whole days highlights not only similarities but also differences between them and their anorexic offspring, and it also invites comparisons. Families generally cannot help but become curious about one another. They become very fascinated, for example, by how other parents handle the food refusal of their teenager. Similarly, the young persons cannot help comparing their own parents' responses with those of other eating-disordered teenagers. Furthermore, in a multi-family-day programme the responsibility for the teenagers' weight increase is not left in the hands of expert nursing and medical staff, but the parents are centrally and directly involved in the feeding and eating issues of their children. Here professional staff are in a minority, and this contributes to a "family" rather than a "medical" atmosphere. Working alongside each other allows parents and teenagers to compare notes and to learn from one another. Peer support and peer criticism is more easily heard and taken onboard when coming from fellow sufferers, as teenagers and their parents have all had plenty of direct and painful experiences around eating, dieting, weight loss, life-threatening states, and repeated hospitalizations.

The frequency and duration of multiple family programmes varies from centre to centre. An initial "tasting event" may be a good start, as it enables families who are considering to participate to learn about the approach and to meet other families, including "graduate" (past) service users. This event is followed, some weeks later, by an intensive week of 4 or 5 whole-day (8-hour) attendances, with 6–8 families in one group; 2–3 weeks later the families attend again for 3 whole days, and this is repeated again after another 2–3 weeks. This initial intensive phase consists of up to 10 whole days in the space of about 6 weeks. It requires considerable commitment from the parents, and it is, at one level, quite surprising that almost all parents accept such involvement, given that it may well mean not being able to go to work and having to take annual leave. At another level it is not at all surprising, as these families have already made many sacrifices, usually for years, including taking time off work because of repeated episodes of acute ill health of their child. After this initial "burst"—which is mostly focused around eating and weight gain and is generally very successful—the intervals between the multi-family days become longer, initially 2 days monthly, reduced to 1 day per month and then to one day bi-monthly. The whole programme lasts one year and involves altogether 15–20 whole-day attendances. The treatment approach has now been manualized.

Much of the first phase of the programme is deliberately structured around eating times. Feedback and joint reflection are generated via a whole range of different activities throughout the day, from joint meals and informal encounters to formal large group discussions, creative art work, or outings. Activities include cross-family linkage and "foster" meals, food collages and body image tasks, psychoeducational sessions on "tricks anorexia plays", video reviews and "hot seat" sessions, family life posters and goal trees, clay sculpture work, theatrical dramatizations of family issues and role reversals. Many of these activities are playful, eliciting a whole range of emotions, including humour. Joint laughter can help at times to "zoom out" and experience the problem from a meta-perspective. For example, inverting the roles of anorexic daughter and worried parent in a brief role play often results in the anorexic teenager literally admiring their parent's acting and mimicking abilities when re-staging the drama of refusing to eat the lovingly prepared meal, which is represented by a paper food collage. The anorexic, in the role of her own mother, attempts to persuade and coax her "daughter": and all this in front of other families who recognize—and can laugh about—these all too familiar scenarios. The role of the therapist in multiple family work is that of making contexts that permit such encounters, initially staging and then managing such events. Once an activity has evolved, the therapist can afford to step back and becomes a kind of catalyst, enabling families to connect with one another and encouraging mutual curiosity and feedback. This day programme requires families and their individual members to constantly change context and to adapt to new demands. This feels intensive to the families—and such intensity simply cannot be created in individual family sessions. The sheer energy released provides a "buzz" for adolescents and parents alike, and it creates hope.

Reflections and further perspectives

The metaphor of the "Greek Chorus", introduced by Papp (1980) to describe the activities of her clinical team to reflect on their patients' issues, can be usefully borrowed for understanding the roles of the different families and their members during multiple family group work. In this setting the protagonists—be that an individual or a family—tell their story or enact their issues in front of a group of people who are then asked to comment. In Aeschylus' famous Greek tragedies it was through the chorus that the Gods spoke, and the chorus was literally seen as the preserver of the world order. It amplified and thereby intensified the action on the stage, reflecting on what went on from different perspectives and inviting the spectators to join in these reflections. Adopting new perspectives, as well as seeing things in perspective, are major aims and outcomes in multiple family work. Unlike in the Greek tragedies, the participants in today's multiple family group work are hardly Gods nor major moral forces. Instead, they lend their ordinary voices to the action(s) in front of them, and this makes them both human and pragmatic. The concept of the "outsider witness group" (White, 1997) provides an alternative frame within which to view both the processes and the therapeutic potential of multiple family work: the individuals' and families' stories about life, relationships, and identity become enriched by the group's re-telling of these stories. The outsider witness group—the other families—adds to the person's and family's narrative resources by sharing experiences from listening to the experiences of persons and their lives, triggered by the story told by the family in focus. Other group members can resonate with what is being told and articulate this. Nuances are introduced bit by bit, helping to generate multiple experiences and ideas, with a multiverse for new curious inquiry unfolding.

New developments

Over the past two years a group of clinicians and researchers, mostly drawn from the Anna Freud Centre and The Marlborough Family Service (Peter Fonagy, Mary Target, Eia Asen, N. Dawson, R. Malik, D. Bevington), has been developing a model of service delivery that includes multiple family work as one of its major components. The work concerns a home-based outreach service for acutely mentally ill teenagers and young persons (age 14–21) presenting serious risk of hospital admission because of psychosis, depression, and acute suicidality, acute eating disorder, borderline personality disorder, and severe obsessive–compulsive disorder. The interventions are carried out by mental health professionals who have received special training in a range of interventions. Both ex-users of services and carers are involved significantly in the work. A day setting—the Education Centre—allows the adolescent to have an educational (school, higher education) focus, as well as providing a setting where other service users and families can exchange ideas and learn from one another. The interventions are mainly delivered, in any one case, by two specially trained mental health workers, recruited primarily from nursing, occupational therapy, social work, and psychology backgrounds. These mental health professionals are formally trained (3 months full-time, and then a programme of in-service training) to deliver the various different therapeutic modalities for this specific group of patients and their families. The interventions are all manualized, with clear outcome measurements built in, and they are carried out primarily in the family home or in other relevant community settings, with attendance at an education centre for educational and multi-family work as required.

Future perspectives

Multiple family therapy can be a powerful mode of treatment that assists other treatment approaches, such as the medical, behavioural, and psychotherapeutic regimes developed for patients with schizophrenia. With other client groups, it may play the major part of the overall intervention, as in the case of multiple family work with multi-problem families (Asen, 2002). Day programmes provide intensive "*in vivo*" experiences that are more likely to bring about changes in "stuck" and chronic families than does more traditional single-family therapy. However, even with intensive multi-family day programmes, other interventions have to be carried out simultaneously, such as individual, couple, and single family work. Formal evaluation of multiple family therapy is still somewhat scarce, though a number of studies and audit projects have shown that this form of treatment is very acceptable to families and their individual members (Lim, 2000; Singh, 2000; Summer, 1998). A few prospective outcome studies are on the way to evaluate the long-term effects of multiple family work. Multiple family therapy is now also used in the treatment and management of substance and alcohol misuse (Kaufman & Kaufman, 1979), chronic medical illness (Gonsalez, Steinglass, & Reiss, 1989), Huntingdon's disease (Murburg, Price, & Jalali, 1988), child abuse (Asen, George, Piper, & Stevens, 1989), bulimia nervosa (Wooley & Lewis, 1987), and other presentations. The approach is becoming increasingly popular, in part because of its cost-effectiveness, and also as a result of the more recent social and political emphasis on involving service users more actively in their treatments.

Commentary

Robert A. King

In relation to the renewal of the institutional ties between London (Anna Freud Centre and University College) and New Haven (Yale Child Study Center and Western New England Institute for Psychoanalysis) commemorated in this volume, I am reminded of George Bernard Shaw's famous quip that England and America were two countries divided by a common language. Despite shared clinical concerns, as mental health clinicians, we often find ourselves divided from colleagues by various theoretical or technical formulations. So, it is a special pleasure to be able to discuss Eia Asen's thought-provoking and paradigm-stretching chapter.

Historically, systems-based models have often had "anti-psychiatric" roots, with the mission of de-emphasizing the notion of a "disorder" or "symptoms" residing in an individual designated "patient" and focusing instead on the dysfunctional interactions of the family, community, or care system as a whole. The notion of "therapy" was eschewed as stigmatizing and re-enforcing the passive aspects of "patienthood" (with its insidious implication of the therapist's superior knowledge and privileged position), at the expense of fostering the patient's—and family's—autonomous strengths and skills. (In some cases, an additional facet of this "anti-psychiatric" bias was to reject the notion of intrinsic biological or temperamental factors at work in individuals.) Although one goal of this approach was to de-stigmatize individuals' difficulties, early versions of family systems approaches sometimes shifted the "hot potato" of pathology or blame to the family or society instead.

Over the years, multisystemic interventions have evolved on a more pragmatic and less ideological basis. As Eia Asen describes, important early applications focused on reducing schizophrenic relapses by reducing Expressed Emotion in families. Other applications of multi-family groups have been to provide education about and to help families cope with chronic medical conditions (such as asthma, cystic fibrosis, epilepsy, infertility, and cancer). Beyond education, multi-family groups were soon found to have many benefits, to which Eia Asen has alluded. These include: combating isolation; providing mutual support, encouragement and feedback; building a collaborative alliance with the larger group; emphasizing strengths rather than pathology; providing multiple perspectives on the diverse ways issues and roles are negotiated within different families; and establishing a safe arena for trial identifications and reality testing—all in a setting where issues of authority, perceived criticism, and resistance are diffused by virtue of multiple peers and "safety in numbers".

As a result, it became clear that such models were useful in enhancing family communication and problem-solving skills and empowering families to meet their own needs, including more effectively using community services and resources. Multi-family models have now also been applied to families impacted by a broad array of difficulties: substance or alcohol abuse, bereavement (including by suicide), and children or adolescents with eating, mood, conduct, or anxiety disorders. In addition, multi-family approaches have been used to help to empower families coping with displacement, adversity, or marginalization (e.g., Kosovar refugees, native Americans, and inner-city African–American families).

What is refreshing about Eia Asen's chapter is its integrative approach, which admits the possibility of constitutional neurobiological factors, temperament, and various forms of dysregulation in individuals being among the multiple domains and context to be addressed by any intervention. Like Bion's work with groups, this approach also emphasizes the multi-family group becoming a work group, empowered to observe, comment on, discuss, and foster the participants' own problem-solving abilities.

Here at the Child Study Center, the development of Family Support Services (FSS) and Intensive In-home Child and Adolescent Psychiatric Services (IICAPS) models has prompted much innovative thinking about how to address the overlapping systems affecting children's functioning (Woolston, Adnopoz, & Berkowitz, in press). A key feature of these multi-modal interventions is the emphasis on promoting systems changes in the relation of the child to the parent and of the family to the school, community, and service agencies, with the goal of developing stable connections with supportive services. Like the programmes described by Asen, the FSS and IICAPS models are present-focused, action-oriented, and strength-based. An intrinsic part of the model is an iterative, "no-fault", empirically based evaluation process that continuously reviews the multiple ecodomains (child, family, school, physical environment, and extended support systems) with an eye to identifying the mechanisms by which the child's and family's strengths or weaknesses help to maintain or alleviate current problems. This entails evaluating the quality of fit between the child, the child's internal resources, the family, the school, and the extended community and service system. (The eco-domain diagrams explicitly charted at the regular treatment team meetings are often baroquely complex, as in the recent case of one troubled adolescent and her family who were involved with over 20 service providers!).

The guiding principle for FSS and IICAPS interventions is to not simply change specific behaviours—important though this may be—but to try to identify what interventions will have progressively catalytic effects, such as fostering a shift in approach to a whole domain of rules (e.g., parental leadership style).

Another area of work here at the Child Study Center that resonates with Eia Asen's presentation has been our involvement in helping to develop patient advocacy groups on a local and national level. The Tourette's Syndrome Association has been an exemplary model of such an advocacy group, bringing together affected families, clinicians, educators, and researchers through a panoply of programmes, including support groups, conferences, school presentations, media development, research initiatives, and the like. The most powerful component, however, has been the mutual support, guidance, and encouragement families have provided each other over the years and, at its best, the fostering of a sense of partnership between patients, families, and clinicians.

Although these US programmes share some of the systems emphasis of the setting in which Eia Asen works, they lack the bravura technical virtuosity Asen describes and demonstrates. This emphasizes what Asen describes as the difficult art of being a "context chameleon", simultaneously involved in "context reading, context making, and context managing". And here I must admit to simultaneous anxiety and envy. Michael Balint (1955) spoke of two contrasting personality types: the *ocnophilic* and the *philobatic*. The ocnophile fears wide-open spaces and prefers to cling to secure attachment objects; in contrast, the philobat loves risks and is eager to explore the unknown world. I suspect that clinicians also fall into these two types: those who prefer to stick close to an established technical style of work, with a well-defined therapeutic setting and "frame", versus those at ease with great fluidity of role; considerable flexibility regarding time, place, and style; and an emphasis on high transparency, self-disclosure, and mutuality. Like many in the audience, I find myself a bit vertiginous, wanting to ask Eia Asen, "But how do you do it!?" "How do you keep so many contextual and affect-charged balls in the air at a time, without getting overwhelmed or losing your orientation?" Our professional training socializes us into a theoretical and observational focus, for better or worse, a notion of what to attend to, what to give interventional priority to, how to proceed. Donald Schön's (1987) work on training the reflective practitioner emphasizes how this can be a progressive, rather than a closed process. Perhaps with sufficient immersion, experience, and training in the multi-family, multisystemic, multimodal approach Eia Asen describes (which fosters the growth of the professionals as well as the families), even the ocnophiles among us might be able to achieve a sense of competency.

Phillip Rieff (1959) suggests that Freud found himself temperamentally lacking in the necessary charisma to be a good hypnotist (the prevailing prerequisite for treating hysteria at the time). To compensate for this lack, Freud developed first the "pressure" technique of free association and then its subsequent elaboration into psychoanalysis, transforming charisma, in Rieff's words, into a (mere) "technical function" of the therapist. So perhaps there is hope for the rest of us.

In the end, of course, what matters most is not our aesthetic or stylistic preferences regarding method, but what is effective for the patient (or whatever alternative term we develop for the objects of our interventional concern). The steps Eia Asen describes towards the manualization of his group's approach are important prerequisites to empirically testing its effectiveness. As with Peter Fonagy and Mary Target's development of a manualized approach to psychodynamic child psychotherapy, the more flexible and conceptually complex a therapy is, the greater the challenge and importance of being able to ensure fidelity and reproducibility in its delivery in order to test its effectiveness.

CHAPTER TWELVE

Towards a typology of late adolescent suicide

Robert A. King, Alan Apter, & Ada Zohar

Throughout the industrialized world, adolescent suicide is a leading cause of death in an otherwise vigorous age group. Many of the psychiatric risk factors for youth suicide have been delineated by careful psychological post-mortem studies. For example, in most studies, an Axis I diagnosis, such as a depressive, disruptive, or anxiety disorder or substance abuse, is present in over 90% of young suicides (Gould, Shaffer, & Greenberg, 2003). In addition, impulsive, aggressive, avoidant, inhibited, or perfectionistic traits are also risk factors found in youth suicides, as are poor affect regulation and impaired problem-solving skills (Brent, 1997; Brent, Johnson, et al., 1994; Shaffer, 1974; Shafii, Carrigan, Whittinghill, & Derrick, 1985).

In most cases of youthful suicidal behaviour, these background risk factors interact with acute stressors or life events, such as a disciplinary crisis, perceived humiliation or failure, or threatened loss of an important relationship, to produce a state of acute emotional distress (Beautrais, Joyce, & Mulder, 1997; Brent, 1997). (These stressors themselves are often the result of the vulnerable adolescent's impulsivity or propensity to form intense, insecure, or ambivalent relationships). Suicidal behaviour in adolescents thus usually occurs in the context of an intolerable feeling state, such as rage, grief, painfully intense isolation, self-loathing, or anxious dread, from which the destruction of the self appears to the desperate adolescent as the only means of escape

(Baumeister, 1990; Hawton, Cole, O'Grady, & Osborn, 1982; Hendin, 1991; Shneidman, 1989).

Despite these insights, our ignorance remains encyclopaedic concerning many aspects of adolescent suicide. Diagnostic risk factors are non-specific, in that fewer than 10% of individuals with a major depressive disorder commit suicide. Furthermore, we know little about how risk or protective factors change or interact over time or how gene–environment interactions change over the lifespan.

Most research studies of adolescent suicide emphasize variable-oriented, rather than person-oriented, data analytic approaches. This approach tends to consider variables as independent entities that take on a life of their own, rather than as inhering in individuals; as a result, this approach obscures individual typologies and the interplay of risk and protective factors in individuals over time (King, Ruchkin, Schwab-Stone, 2003). As Cairns and colleagues put it: "Behavioral variables rarely function as independent entities that are separable from the web of influences in which they occur" (Cairns, Cairns, Rodkin, & Xie, 1998, p. 15). With a few notable exceptions (e.g., Fergusson, Woodward, & Horwood, 2000; Lewinsohn, Rohde, Seeley, & Baldwin, 2001; Patton et al., 1997), most studies of adolescent suicidality are cross-sectional and hence give us little information on why—and how—different vulnerabilities come to prominence in different developmental epochs.

A developmental psychodynamic perspective focuses on the origins of vulnerability to suicide and depression in the capacity for self-care and comfort, the ability to develop and make use of protective affiliations, the regulation of self-esteem, and the developmental challenges of adolescence, as well as the more traditional emphasis on the vicissitudes of aggression and impulse control (King, 2003). This perspective also tries to understand how these factors play out over in individuals to increase (or decrease) risk over time.

In this chapter we report on an attempt to use a psychodynamic perspective to predict suicide over the course of late adolescence, using the unique set of prospective and longitudinal data available on individual male adolescents entering universal military service in the Israeli Defence Force.

The Israeli Defence Force context

The age- and sex-specific 1999 suicide rate in Israel for males, age 15–24 years, was 11.4 per 100,000, intermediate between that in the United Kingdom (10.7 per 1,000,000) and in the United States (17.2 per 100,000) (WHOSIS, 2005). Near-universal compulsory military service in Israel provides a unique epidemiological window on the longitudinal risk and protective factors for various forms of psychopathology, including suicide, in successive national cohorts of adolescents. Virtually all Jewish and Druze males undergo intensive pre-induction screening at age 16–17, in preparation for three years of compulsory service between the ages of 18 and 21. This pre-induction screening includes psychometric testing, physical exam, and an interview by a trained psychological technician, with referral for second-stage evaluation by a mental health clinician if indicated. Based on many years' experience, the IDF has developed ratings based on these assessments that have proven reliable and valid for predicting successful service in various military assignments (Gal, 1986). Strikingly, however, these ratings have proven to be of little use in predicting suicide.

An initial study of 43 consecutive suicides of adolescent male recruits done in collaboration with the IDF Mental Health Branch (Apter et al., 1993) found that in general these young men were above average in intelligence (26% with IQs > 135), physical fitness, and pre-induction ratings of suitability for military service. A disproportionately high number came from Ashkenazi (European) background, front-line combat units, or families with a parental divorce or death. As ascertained by an extensive post-mortem investigation, 83% warranted an Axis I diagnosis (with about half having major depression, largely recent and undiagnosed); reflecting Israeli society at the time of the study, none had a history of substance abuse.

Although service in front-line combat units is often demanding and physically and mentally arduous, none of the suicides studied occurred in the context of actual hostilities. Front-line units are highly selective in terms of physical fitness, intelligence, and leadership potential. Despite their rigors, combat unit assignments in the IDF carry high prestige (especially elite units such as pilots and commandos) and were, at the time of the study, highly sought after, both because of their perceived prestige and because of the advantages they confer in post-army life (similar to attendance at an Ivy League college in the United States or Oxbridge in the United Kingdom).

Taken as a group, there appeared to be three principal patterns of suicide.

1. *Impulsive/aggressive suicides.* These were young men who appeared to fit the pattern of what van Praag (1996) has described as "serotonin-related anxiety/aggression stressor-precipitated depression."

2. *Narcissistic, low self-disclosure suicides.* These were young men with very high self-expectations and aspirations for their military service, who were very intolerant of perceived self-failures. At the same time, they were often self-contained emotionally and did not disclose their disappointments or other painful feelings to others.
3. *Suicides involving hopelessness secondary to masked psychiatric disorder.* As seen in retrospect, this group of young men, who overlapped to some extent with Group 2, became depressed and discouraged, often after a physical injury prevented them from functioning in an assignment they wanted.

A heuristic experiment in prediction

As a heuristic exercise to understand better the obstacles to effective suicide prediction (and prevention) in this population, we decided to test our ability to predict outcome (suicide vs. non-suicide) based on the extensive pre-induction psychometrics and standardized interview narratives and ratings available on all recruits.

Method

A colleague selected a sample of 28 cases together with the pre-induction data on each recruit. The sample consisted of 10 recruits who ultimately committed suicide during their army service and 18 non-suicides. To reduce the assessor variability in the pre-induction data, for each suicide case, two non-suicides were selected (to the extent available) who had been interviewed by the same pre-induction psychological technician during the same week as the future suicide.

Blind to outcome, two experienced clinicians (RK and AZ) rated each case on the presence or absence of a series of variables and arrived at a consensus prediction of outcome (suicide during service vs. no suicide). The characteristics on which each subject was rated included such items as parental divorce or death, excessive expectations of service, estrangement from family, mood lability, denial of difficulties, a psychiatric diagnosis given at pre-induction screening, and the presence of conduct disorder.

Results

When the blind was broken, it turned out that the clinicians had correctly identified only 3 of the 10 suicides—a success rate no better than chance. This failure is all the more notable in this "enriched" research sample in which there were 10 suicides among the 28 subjects; in contrast, in the general Israeli male adolescent population, the suicide rate is on the order of about 1 per 10,000, posing an even more daunting task of finding the needle in the haystack. [As with all rare conditions, suicide is statistically difficult to predict in practice because one must correctly identify the one vulnerable individual out of 10,000. This, in turn, leads to the classic trade-off between specificity and sensitivity. If one casts a wide net to avoid the serious consequences of missing the rare true future suicide cases (minimizing "false negatives"), one will incorrectly identify as being at risk an extremely large number of non-suicides ("false positives"), requiring extensive and burdensome second-stage assessment; conversely, minimizing the number of false positives can only be accomplished at the risk of missing true positives.]

Furthermore, after breaking the blind, the only characteristics that significantly distinguished recruits who suicided from those who did not (after correcting for multiple comparisons) were parental divorce or death and excessive expectations of military service.

Predictive successes and failures

In order to understand why our attempts at prediction failed, even in an unrealistically lenient trial, we took a more detailed look at each recruit's pre-induction data, his subsequent experience during military service, and his outcome (including, in the case of the suicides, the findings of the detailed psychological post-mortem conducted on all military suicides).

We present condensed vignettes of several of these cases to illustrate the gap between what might be expected at the time of their induction and how subsequent events actually unfolded during their active duty.

"Avi": a high-functioning kibbutz youth

Pre-induction interview. Avi was described by the interviewer as a serious, hard-working young man. Following his parents' divorce, he went to live on his own on an ideologically committed kibbutz, where, through hard work, he rose to various top youth leadership positions. He described himself as diligent, punctual, and exercising vigorously daily. Despite his family situation, he described himself as never having had to face difficult situations. Although popular with many friends, the interviewer noted he was, "surprisingly, less sociable than expected".

Clinicians' prediction: suicide. Impressed by Avi's seeming overemphasis on high achievement as a means for dealing with loss, his uncertain capacity for intimacy, and his intolerance for failure or sad affect, the research clinicians predicted that Avi would be one of the suicides—or, less likely, a future chief of staff. (Considered un-ironically, this uncertainty underlines the Janus-like nature of traits such as high ambition, which may confer both high achievement and vulnerability).

Outcome: suicide (true positive). Avi injured himself exercising before induction, and consequently, despite his efforts to conceal his problem, he was disqualified from service in an elite combat unit. (In retrospect, his voluntary intensive physical training before induction reflected a probable excess of zeal.) Nonetheless, in basic training he convinced the medical officers to upgrade his physical fitness rating, and he was assigned to the elite unit he coveted. However, because of his injury, he was unable to keep up with the physical rigors of this assignment, and three months after induction he was medically dropped from his combat unit assignment and assigned instead to Intelligence. Even though Intelligence is a high-prestige assignment, Avi was bitterly disappointed not to be in an elite combat unit, and he felt humiliated about going home on leave without the insignia of an elite unit; he complained to friends that "life was not worth living" after losing his dream.

During the month following his transfer, he had some minor disciplinary problems (passive ones, such as lateness or non-completion of assignments), but he appeared cheerful when visiting friends on leave. During the day preceding his suicide he seemed depressed, apathetic, and he refused to go to classes or to engage socially with the soldiers with whom he roomed. Soon after returning to quarters in the evening, he shot himself. There was no identifiable immediate precipitating event to the suicide.

Save for his last day, there were no signs of depression noted by others. In the combat unit he had been very successful socially, was prominent in the unit, and exerted leadership. In retrospect his minor difficulties (lateness, work incompleteness) in his new unit appear to have been signs of distress.

"Ehud": a troubled youth

Pre-induction interview. Ehud's parents divorced when he was young, and he lived with many different relatives while growing up. He was alienated from his better-off peers and hung out with a delinquent crowd, playing truant and occasionally drinking. He was often in trouble with authorities for frequent fist-fights and shoplifting.

During his pre-induction interview, he complained of depression and insomnia. He wanted to serve in an elite combat unit but was rated unfit.

Clinicians' prediction: suicide. The research clinicians predicted a suicidal outcome and saw Ehud as vulnerable due to the confluence of family disruption and estrangement, aggression, conduct problems, social alienation, substance use, and probable depression, as well as unrealistic aspirations regarding service

Outcome: suicide (true positive). On induction, Ehud insisted on joining a special infantry unit, demanding re-classification and claiming he had exaggerated his troubles at the time of his pre-induction assessment and had matured in the interim.

Ehud was assigned to a combat unit, but he soon complained that training was "too hard". He was tearful when denied a weekend leave. After his next leave, one month after induction, he was reluctant to return to base, wanted to be reassigned to a non-combat unit, and shot himself on the way back to base.

During the post-mortem investigation Ehud was described by his peers as "closed, isolative, and introverted". He had been enthusiastic at first about the prospect of serving in a combat unit but was then disappointed and overwhelmed. In retrospect, he had insisted on covering up major vulnerabilities in order to gain a front-line assignment.

"Tsvi": a high-functioning youth

Pre-induction interview. Tsvi was described by the interviewer as level-headed, energetic, conscientious, very sociable, independent-minded, and highly motivated, with good relationships at home and broad interests. He stated that he was willing to serve in a combat unit, but he preferred journalism or an engineering unit.

Clinicians' prediction: non-suicide. Based on the apparent absence of risk factors and his apparent good relationships and coping skills, the research clinicians predicted that Tsvi would be a non-suicide.

Outcome: suicide (false negative). Tsvi was assigned to a combat unit and was disappointed. He asked his parents to give false testimony to the authorities to the effect that mother was being beaten and that his sister was suicidal, in order to justify his transfer to another unit.

When he was issued his weapon, he initially fearfully refused it.

He saw an army psychiatrist, who discussed with him the possibility of transfer to a non-combat unit, but Tsvi was ambivalent about the transfer and agreed to continue trying in his combat unit assignment.

Subsequently, Tsvi lied about a family emergency to get leave, and once home, asked his mother to break his leg, so that he would not have to return. He shot himself the morning he was scheduled to return to base.

Comment. In retrospect, Tsvi had much unrevealed psychopathology. Although he was clearly very anxious at the perceived stress of serving in a combat unit, his attempted confabulations appears to have been more than mere manipulation and bordered on the bizarre. To what extent any dynamic or projective significance can be read into them (concerning suicidality or physical violence and injury) is unclear. Although his initial balking at being issued a weapon may have had to do with fear of the legal responsibility (for example, losing a weapon often results in time in the brig), it may also have been a telltale indicator of his internal struggle with aggressive and suicidal impulses.

"Shmuel": a troubled youth

Pre-induction interview. Shmuel had multiple moves and changes of school growing up; he was a poor student who was often truant and ultimately expelled. Subsequently he was unable to hold down a job and was estranged from his parents, living instead with roommates in a flat to which the police were often called for breach of the peace.

Shmuel was very insistent on having an elite combat unit assignment, but he was rated very low on suitability for service.

Clinicians' prediction: suicide. Based on his estrangement from parents, his impulsive life style, and his excessive expectations of service, the research clinicians predicted that Shmuel would be one of the recruits who committed suicide.

Outcome: non-suicide (false positive). Diagnosed with personality disorder, Shmuel was soon assigned to a rear echelon job as a truck driver. Despite the relatively undemanding nature of his assignment, Shmuel was in the brig (military prison) four times, for a total of 179 days, for disobedience and being absent without leave for a total of one month. He received a dishonourable discharge after 2.5 years.

Comment: Despite his multiple risk factors, Shmuel's easy disregard of army discipline and rules and the consequences of their infraction permitted him to evade the psychological pressures of military life. The ease with which he went AWOL or was insubordinate to orders, as well as the apparent equanimity with which he tolerated disciplinary confinement, served as what Shneidman (1989) would term alternate routes for egression, which obviated the pressures towards suicide experienced by his more conscientious peers.

Discussion

Reasons for failure of prediction

There are several possible reasons for our lack of success in predicting suicide in this study, over and above the inherent difficulties in predicting rare events (even in "enriched" samples such as ours).

1. First and foremost is our lack of a full understanding of how the salient psychopathological variables interact over time with life events to produce what may be fleeting or more persistent suicidal ideation and motivation.
2. Even the detailed pre-induction psychological evaluations used by the IDF for unit assignment may not provide the relevant psychopathological data needed for suicide prediction. Certainly, lack of candour appears to have been a factor in the case of several recruits who minimized their past histories of psychological distress (due in part to a wish for assignment to a unit with perceived prestige); even as they became more distressed, they were unable to use peers, parents, or the trained mental health officers available in virtually all IDF units as alternatives to suicide.

3. Finally, it is impossible to predict from data obtained at the pre-induction assessment (at age 16–17) what will be the vicissitudes of intervening events over the subsequent three years of military service (from age 18 to 21). For example, it seems impossible to have predicted that Avi would have been disqualified for combat unit service because of a subsequent physical injury. It was possible, however, to predict, as we did, that he was likely to have a very adverse reaction to not meeting his extremely high self-expectations. In this sense, suicide prediction will always be a probabilistic matter, involving the stochastic interaction between risk and protective factors on the one hand and current life events on the other.

In our post hoc look at the various psychosocial risk factors rated, two factors—excessive expectations of service and parental loss through divorce, marital separation, or death—distinguished the suicides from the non-suicide cases. As described below, these two variables may parallel two important sets of traits conferring vulnerability to depression—what Blatt (2004) has referred to as self-critical (introjective) versus dependent (anaclitic) forms of depression.

Parental divorce or death

Although studies in the United States find an association between non-intact families and youth suicide, this association decreases markedly once parental psychopathology is controlled for (Brent, Perper, 1994; Gould, Fisher, Parides, Flory, & Shaffer, 1996). Although unstudied, it is possible that in Israel, where divorce was relatively rare at the time of the study, marital separation or divorce may have been a more significant marker than in the United States for family adversity or parental psychopathology (with an attendant more disturbed parent–child relationship and/or greater genetically transmissible vulnerability in the offspring).

Unrealistic expectations of service—self-critical versus dependent depressive traits

As for excessive expectations of service, Blatt (1995, 2004) and others (King, 2003) have discussed two subtypes of vulnerability to depression—dependent (or anaclitic) versus self-critical (or introjective)—with respect to suicide.

Over the past two decades, Blatt and colleagues have delineated two subtypes of vulnerability to depression. The first group of individuals is characterized by what have been termed dependent (or anaclitic) traits. These individuals are characterized by insecure/ambivalent attachments, an overvaluation of dependent relationships, a preoccupation with dependency and the threat of abandonment, and helplessness in the face of perceived loss. As described by Hammen and others (Brown, Hammen, Craske, & Wickens, 1995; Hammen, 2000; Hammen, Ellicott, Gitlin, & Jamison, 1989), depressions in such individuals are often triggered by perceived interpersonal loss or rejection.

The second group of individuals is characterized by self-critical (or introjective) traits, such as compulsive self-reliance, dismissiveness of the importance of intimate relationships, and an anxious preoccupation with self-worth and autonomy. In these individuals depression is often triggered by a perceived failure in achievement, leading to feelings of humiliation, unworthiness, guilt, or loss of control.

Some evidence suggests that the suicide attempts of individuals with dependent vulnerabilities tend to be impulsive, manipulative, and non-lethal, whereas those of self-critical individuals are more planned and serious (Blatt, 1995; Faazia, 2001).

Many suicides among members of elite units, such as Avi, seemed to fit the mould of self-critical (introjective) depression (see also Apter et al., 1993; King, 2003). These were perfectionistic youth who set unrealistically high goals for themselves and for whom a perceived failure to achieve these can lead to a serious or lethal suicide attempt.

Other suicides in which excessive expectations of service played a role were *not* particularly high-functioning or perfectionistic recruits. For some, such as Ehud, the prospect of service in a prestigious unit may have carried the hope of undoing earlier humiliations or adversities, in keeping with the cultural values prevailing in Israel at the time of the study; for these youth, efforts to be assigned to a combat unit entailed covering up important emotional difficulties and vulnerabilities. In those cases (e.g., Ehud, Tsvi) where they did end up assigned to a combat unit, they found themselves in "over their heads" in a stressful setting that exceeded what they perceived to be their ability to cope. In this desperate situation, either their habitual lack of self-disclosure or unrealistic self-expectations may have interfered with their seeking out the mental health officers attached to every unit or accepting the possibility of reassignment to a rear-echelon unit, even when offered (e.g., Tsvi). Combined with poor problem-solving abilities and/or impulsivity, this desperation may have resulted in lethal suicidal behaviour.

Ubiquity of firearms as a risk factor

The ubiquity of firearms in the military may have served as an "amplifier" for suicidal impulses that might, in another setting, have been transient and un-acted-on or have resulted in a less lethal method of attempted suicide.

As summarized by Brent (2001), community case control studies find that the presence of a firearm in the home conveys an increased risk for suicide, especially adolescent suicide. This increased risk is particularly great for suicide in those adolescents *without* apparent psychopathology. Thus, the presence of any gun in the home increased the risk of suicide in adolescents with psychiatric disorder by 3.4-fold. However, the presence of a loaded gun in the home increased the risk of suicide for adolescents without apparent psychopathology by over 32-fold. One possible interpretation of this is that for adolescents with a psychiatric disorder, whose suicidal ideation may more persistent, gun availability amplified the risk of a lethal suicide attempt only moderately; for less impaired adolescents, who may have experienced only transient—but intense—suicidal impulses, the ready presence of a gun made possible an impulsive lethal act that might not have committed in the absence of a gun.

For these young recruits on active duty, gun possession was virtually universal, regardless of unit assignment, both off and on base. As a result, even a passing suicidal impulse, if acted on, was likely to be lethal—attempted suicide with a firearm is usually lethal (resulting in death in over three-quarters of attempts), in comparison with ingestions or cutting, which are far less likely to result in death and permit the possibility of seeking rescue even after the act (Centers for Disease Control, 1995).

Conclusion

The study of these tragically truncated lives promises to give us greater insight into the dynamic interplay of forces over the lifespan that convey changing levels of suicidal risk as the developing individual encounters various challenges and musters or fails to muster the internal and interpersonal resources to meet them. If such studies suggest better means of prediction that prevent even one unnecessary premature death, we can draw comfort from the sages of the Talmud, who wrote: "He who saves a life, saves a world."

Commentary

Duncan J. McLean

Much of the published literature on suicide is devoted to risk factors in relation to completed suicide. This is only of modest usefulness to a clinician when faced with the task of assessing and managing the large number of people who threaten or have attempted suicide. It is of some help to know these risk factors as warning signs for those most in danger, so that we know that elderly, single, physically ill, unemployed males who abuse drugs and alcohol are at the highest risk. However, the vast majority of those who threaten or have attempted suicide will have only one or two risk factors, and in addition this, as Robert King and his colleagues point out in this chapter, completed suicide in itself is a relatively rare event for the individual clinician. Thus predicting who is likely to commit suicide successfully is very difficult.

This is not to say that attempted suicide is not a risk factor in itself. It has been estimated that the mortality of people who attempt suicide is 1% per year in excess of a normal population, so that over a 10-year period 10% of the cohort of attempted suicide would have died in excess of a controlled population.

These figures highlight the importance of managing attempted suicide as effectively as possible, but this needs to be done by attending to factors other than thinking about who is going to be the individual most at risk. In a large London teaching hospital, roughly 1,000 patients attend the casualty department each year following an attempt to kill themselves. About half of these patients are seen for a psychosocial assessment by a team of five mental health workers dedicated to this task. On average, each mental health worker will, in the course of a year, assess one patient who will go on to complete suicide in the following 12 months. Each mental health worker will have assessed about 100 patients, and though risk factors will help them to know who is most at risk, they will be far from being able to predict the rare event of a completed suicide.

When one looks at youth suicide, predictability becomes even more difficult. Even though there is somewhat of a surfeit of young men who kill themselves, nevertheless the suicide rate generally increases relative to age, so that youth suicide remains an even rarer event than the generality of suicide.

Risk factors are only a part of the concern of the clinician dealing with potential suicide, and much broader issues need to be taken into account to guide the clinician in management. In this respect considering psychodynamic issues can come much closer to some of the concerns of a clinician when dealing with the individual patient. In considering psychodynamic factors, Robert King has a very broad conceptualization of multiple factors that can come into play on how a suicide can actually occur. There are so many factors that may play a part that it is difficult to have a coherent idea as to how to establish a hierarchy of their importance. It may well be that this is not possible. The developmental factors that King highlights are ones such as the capacity for self-care and self-comfort, as well as the ability to develop and make positive protective affiliations—that is, the capacity to make relationships that an individual can use to help regulate the way they feel. Other factors he highlights in early development are the way self-esteem evolves and also the way all the above developmental issues are interwoven with and influenced by temperamental factors, as well as the impact of the early environment.

Within adolescent development itself, there are also the specific challenges of that period, such as the integration of sexual drive and the establishment of identity and autonomy that allows separation from the primary family. These developmental factors are impinged upon by the interaction of individuals with their environment and the situation in which they may find themselves with their families; in their peer relationships; and also the wider social and cultural environment.

Added to all the above developmental factors—in terms of a particular episode of self-harm—is the mental state that the individual may be in at the time. For example, depressive affect may be of particular importance. Lastly, accidental factors, such as the means available for self-harm, may be quite critical in terms of outcome. In some of the cases related in the chapter these means are somewhat surprising to English ears because of the method of killing themselves, which is by gunshot. As guns are not readily available in the United Kingdom, this is an extremely rare method of suicide. It is a mistake, however, to think that because one means is not available, another could not be used as readily. In England, when the domestic gas supply was changed from coal gas, which is highly poisonous, to natural gas, which is not, there was a considerable drop in the number of suicides.

King points to an aspect of the dynamics of suicide that I would agree, from a clinical point of view, is of considerable importance—that is, that suicide or attempted suicide can represent an escape from an unbearable affect. However, he also points out that though this may be a central dynamic, there may be considerable difficulty in exploring this in the clinical situation, as very frequently individuals will, at least in the first instance, often give very little information as to what affect is being avoided. Some research attempts to get at the motive for suicide have often not taken us much further. King discusses Hawton's card sort procedure (Hawton et al., 1982), though the results from this—that motivations range from people wanting to die and get the relief from a terrible state of mind—appear to beg the question of what underlies this. There is a fundamental difficulty that most people who have attempted suicide can often give a very poor account of their motives, and there is a question as to the reason for this. Could it be due to the cognitively disorganizing affect of the precipitant, so that the overwhelming affect disables the individual from giving a coherent narrative? On the other hand, could the individual have some longstanding inability, in a developmental sense, about putting feelings into words, and is this developmental deficit linked to the question of poor affect control?

Another perspective is that a defence is operating, so that the person attempting suicide is avoiding looking at what has caused this because it is emotionally painful, and the fact that they acted rather than reflecting on their situation is an indication of this.

The question of whether an individual cannot or will not think about the issues that led to a suicide attempt is central to the clinical situation. It will influence the clinician's technique in trying to establish a narrative about what happened. Establishing a narrative is in itself very important, as only by this means can the issues leading to the suicide attempt be addressed, and the potentially overwhelming affects contained.

In the past psychodynamic theorists have often stressed the importance of unconscious factors leading to suicide attempts. In the literature the dynamic formulation of the underlying motives is rather repetitively stressed as being "turning aggression against the self".

However, there are questions as to how valid this is as a central dynamic, as well as at some level stating the obvious and not being much use to the clinician.

In his chapter King suggests a typology of the motivation leading to suicide that would appear potentially useful, particularly in thinking about how suicidal patients are best managed. He suggests that there are broadly two sorts of people with characteristic personalities that are vulnerable to both depression and suicide. On the one hand are individuals who are rather over-dependent on others, and the second type of those that are highly self critical.

These two types appear to be related to many psychodynamic constructs. The self-critical person who has a severe superego may also be relatively autonomous, independent, and avoidant of seeking help from others. This could be linked to a dismissive type of attachment.

The dependent person has characteristics of a disorganized attachment and angry, over-involved relationships with others. The dependent type would appear to be both less dangerous in terms of suicide and easier to treat, since there is a more readily available relationship that can be used within a therapeutic situation. This particular type also seems to be more congruent with the idea of turning anger and aggression against the self, and certainly recognizing anger within a dependent relationship would be important in these individuals.

Recognition of the self-critical type would also raise the question of adopting a different approach. It is likely that these individuals will be difficult to engage in treatment, since their autonomous, independent style does not lend itself to making a therapeutic relationship. In addition to this, the focus of concern for such individuals is not usually around interpersonal relationships, but much more about self-evaluation. In line with this, anger may not be such a problematic affect—shame may be much more important.

King's typology raises interesting research questions as to how suicidal patients are best treated. Is constructing a coherent narrative about the precipitants of the suicide event potentially a protective factor? Should the two different types be approached in different ways and be given a different type of treatment as a consequence of their differing pathologies?

Though King's chapter is about suicide in adolescence, much of what he writes about is as applicable to suicide at all ages. One might wonder whether the developmental phase of adolescence itself has any importance in relation to suicide at this time in life. Completed suicide in females is lowest in adolescence and rises with age. Since females have to face some developmental tasks that are very similar to those of boys in adolescence, it does tend to undermine the idea that such developmental issues are of critical importance. However, completed suicide in young males does not follow the female patterns: there are increased numbers at this age, which drops in mid-life before rising, as with women, at the end of the life cycle. It is not easy to know why young men are more prone to killing themselves. One possibility is that impulsiveness and aggression is much more readily available in young men, and this lends itself to the deadliness of their self-harm.

In relation to the above, there have been social changes in the United Kingdom that have seen females becoming much more aggressive—joining gangs, being involved in delinquent behaviour, and so on. It will be interesting to see whether such social trends will also be reflected in the statistics for completed suicide in the future.

One of the developmental issues that King discusses is the individuation process that takes place as adolescents move away from their primary family. During this period it is evident that peer relationships are very important. Those who have poor peer relationship at this stage in life are more vulnerable, as they are unable to use others to regulate their feelings and as a source of solace. This might give an indication to the way the self-critical type in particular might best be treated. Could it be that if they were put into a peer group, they would form age-appropriate peer relationships that would mitigate their autonomous and self-critical way of functioning? It seems possible that they would engage with this process more readily perhaps than in individual therapy with an adult.

I would like to end with a clinical vignette on a case that runs somewhat counter to King's typology.

> A mature woman came for psychotherapy treatment following the birth of her first child, a son. She was worried about being a good-enough mother, being concerned that she was too disturbed. At the age of 15 she had jumped out of an upper-story window in a suicide attempt and had only accidentally survived this. She could well have been one of those rare cases of female adolescent completed suicide.
>
> During her therapy she proved to be a well-adjusted adult with a secure type of attachment. She was neither overly dependent nor particularly self critical. Her suicide attempt at 15 was about a year after the death of her father, who had, before he had died, suffered from a degenerative brain condition. His behaviour before

> his death had been distressingly bizarre and frightening. Her suicide attempt could therefore be seen as a consequence of trauma and loss within an adolescent context.

King's model helpfully discriminates between two types of psychopathology that may need to be addressed in relation to the risk of suicide. However, perhaps the clinician is ultimately only able to treat different kinds of psychopathology and not really the risk of suicide as such.

REFERENCES

Aber, L., Slade, A., Berger, B., Bresgi, I., & Kaplan, M. (1985). *The Parent Development Interview*. Unpublished protocol, The City University of New York.

Abramson, L. Y., Metalsky, G. I., & Alloy, L. B. (1989). Hopelessness depression: A theory-based subtype of depression. *Psychological Review, 96*: 358–372.

Abramson, L. Y., Seligman, M. E. P., & Teasdale, J. (1978). Learned helplessness in humans: Critique and reformulation. *Journal of Abnormal Psychology, 87*: 49–74.

Addis, M. E., & Krasnow, A. D. (2000). A national survey of practicing psychologists' attitudes toward psychotherapy treatment manuals. *Journal of Consulting and Clinical Psychology, 68*: 331–339.

Addis, M., Wade, W., & Hatgis, W. (1999). Barriers to dissemination of evidence based practices: Addressing practitioners' concerns about manual based psychotherapies. *Clinical Psychology: Science and Practice, 6*: 430–441.

Adey, W., Bors, E., & Porter, R. (1968). EEG sleep patterns after high cervical lesions in man. *Archives of Neurology, 24*: 377–83.

Adler, A. (1944). Disintegration and restoration of optic recognition in visual agnosia: Analysis of a case. *Archives of Neurology and Psychiatry, 51*: 243–259.

Adler, A. (1950). Course and outcome of visual agnosia. *Journal of Nervous & Mental Diseases, 111*: 41–51.

Ainsworth, M. D., & Bell, S. M. (1970). Attachment, exploration, and separation: Illustrated by the behavior of one-year-olds in a strange situation. *Child Development, 41* (1): 49–67.

Ainsworth, M. D, Blehar, M. C., Waters, E., & Wall, S. (1978). *Patterns of Attachment: A Psychological Study of the Strange Situation.* Hillsdale, NJ: Erlbaum.

Allen, J. (2003). Mentalizing. *Bulletin of the Menninger Clinic, 67* (2): 91–112.

Ambelas, A. (1990). Life events and the onset of mania. *British Journal of Psychiatry, 157*: 450–451.

Amico, J. A., Mantella, R. C., & Vollmer, R. R. (2002). "Plasma Corticosterone Response of Oxytocin Deficient Mice Exposed to Stress." 2002 Abstract Viewer/Itinerary Planner. Society for Neuroscience. Online. Program No. 176.7.

Ammerman, R. T., Hersen, M., & Last, C. G. (Eds.) (1999). *Handbook of Prescriptive Treatments for Children and Adolescents* (2nd edition). Needham Heights, MA: Allyn & Bacon.

Andersen, J., & Adams, C. (1996). Family interventions in schizophrenia: An effective but underused treatment. *British Medical Journal, 313*: 505.

Andersen, T. (1987). The reflecting team. *Family Process, 26*: 415–428.

Anderson, C. M. (1983). A psychoeducational program for families of patients with schizophrenia. In: W.-R. McFarlane (Ed.), *Family Therapy in Schizophrenia.* New York: Guildford Press.

Ankuta, G. Y., & Abeles, N. (1993). Client satisfaction, clinical significance, and meaningful change in psychotherapy. *Professional Psychology: Research and Practice, 24*: 70–74.

Anokhin, P. K. (1964). Systemogenesis as a general regulator of brain development. *Progress in Brain Research, 9*: 54–105.

Apter, A., Bleich, A., King, R. A., Kron, S., Fluch, A., Kotler, M., & Cohen, D. J. (1993). Death without warning? A clinical postmortem study of suicide in 43 Israeli adolescent males. *Archives of General Psychiatry, 50*: 138–142.

Apter, A., Gothelf. D., Orbach, I., Weizman, R., Ratzoni, G., Har-Even, D., & Tyano, S. (1995). Correlation of suicidal and violent behavior in different diagnostic categories in hospitalized adolescent patients. *Journal of the American Academy of Child & Adolescent Psychiatry, 34* (7): 912–918.

Arnold, L. E. (2002). Treatment alternatives for attention deficit hyperactivity disorder. In: P. S. Jensen & J. R. Cooper (Eds.), *Attention Deficit Hyperactivity Disorder: State of the Science, Best Practices* (pp. 13-1–13-29). Kingston, NJ: Civic Research Institute.

Asen, E. (2002). Multiple family therapy: An overview. *Journal of Family Therapy, 24*: 3–16.

Asen, E. (2004). Collaborating in promiscuous swamps—the systemic practitioner as context chameleon? *Journal of Family Therapy, 26*: 280–285.

Asen, E., Dawson, N., & McHugh, B. (2001). *Multiple Family Therapy: The*

Marlborough Model and Its Wider Applications. London/New York: Karnac.

Asen, K. E., George, E., Piper, R., & Stevens, A. (1989). A systems approach to child abuse: Management and treatment issues. *Child Abuse & Neglect, 13*: 45–57.

Asen, K. E., Stein, R., Stevens, A., McHugh, B., Greenwood, J., & Cooklin, A. (1982). A day unit for families. *Journal of Family Therapy, 4*: 345–358.

Aserinsky, E., & Kleitman, N. (1953). Regularly occurring periods of eye motility and concurrent phenomena during sleep. *Science, 118*: 273.

Aserinsky, E., & Kleitman, N. (1955). Two types of ocular motility during sleep. *Journal of Applied Physiology, 8*: 1.

Bakermans-Kranenburg, M. J., van IJzendoorn, M. H., & Juffer, F. (2003). Less is more: Meta-analyses of sensitivity and attachment interventions in early childhood. *Psychological Bulletin, 129* (2): 195–215.

Baldwin, D. A., & Moses, L. J. (1996). The ontogeny of social information gathering. *Child Development, 67*: 1915—1939.

Balint, M. (1955). Friendly expanses—horrid empty spaces. *International Journal of Psychoanalysis, 36*: 225–241.

Barbe, R., Bridge, J., Birmaher, B., Kolko, D., & Brent, D. (2001). "Outcome of a Psychotherapy Treatment in a Population of Suicidal Depressed Adolescents." Paper presented at the Congress on Suicide and Suicide Prevention in Youth, Geneva, Switzerland (November).

Baron, R. M., & Kenny, D. A. (1986). The moderator-mediator variable distinction in social psychological research: Conceptual, strategic, and statistical considerations. *Journal of Personality and Social Psychology, 51*: 1173–1182.

Baron-Cohen, S. (1994). How to build a baby that can read minds: Cognitive mechanisms in mindreading. *Cahiers de Psychologie Cognitive, 13* (5): 513–552.

Baron-Cohen, S. (1995). *Mindblindness: An Essay on Autism and Theory of Mind*. Cambridge, MA: MIT Press.

Baron-Cohen, S., Tager-Flusberg, H., & Cohen, D. (Eds.) (2000). *Understanding Other Minds: Perspectives from Developmental Neuroscience* (2nd edition). Oxford: Oxford University Press.

Barrett, K., & Campos, J. (1987). Perspectives on emotional development: II. A functionalist approach to emotions. In: J. Osofsky (Ed.), *Handbook of Infant Development* (2nd edition, pp. 555–578). New York: Wiley.

Bartels, A., & Zeki, S. (2004). The neural correlates of maternal and romantic love. *NeuroImage, 21* (3): 1155–1166.

Baskin, T. W., Tierney, S. C., Minami, T., & Wampold, B. E. (2003). Establishing specificity in psychotherapy: A meta-analysis of structural equivalence of placebo controls. *Journal of Consulting and Clinical Psychology, 71*: 973–979.

Basso, A., Bisiach, E., & Luzzatti, C. (1980). Loss of mental imagery: A case study. *Neuropsychologia, 18*: 435–442.

Bateman, A. W., & Fonagy, P. (2004a). Mentalization-based treatment of BPD. *Journal of Personal Disorders, 18* (1): 36–51.

Bateman, A. W., & Fonagy, P. (2004b). *Psychotherapy for Borderline Personality Disorders: Mentalization Based Treatment*. Oxford: Oxford University Press.

Bates, E. (1979). On the evolution and development of symbols. In: E. Bates (Ed.), *The Emergence of Symbols: Cognition and Communication in Infancy* (pp. 1–32). New York: Academic Press.

Baumeister, R. F. (1990). Suicide as escape from self. *Psychological Review, 97*: 90–113.

Beautrais, A. L., Joyce, P. R., & Mulder, R. T. (1997). Precipitating factors and life events in serious suicide attempts among youths aged 13 through 24 years. *Journal of the American Academy of Child & Adolescent Psychiatry, 36* (11): 1543–1551.

Beck, A. T., Rush, A. J., Shaw, B. F., & Emery, G. (1979). *Cognitive Therapy of Depression*. New York: Guilford Press.

Beebe, B., Jaffe, J., Feldstein, S., Mays, K., & Alson, D. (1985). Interpersonal timing: The application of an adult dialogue model to mother–infant vocal and kinesic interactions. In: T. Field & N. Fox (Eds.), *Social Perception in Infants* (pp. 217- 247). Norwood, NJ: Ablex.

Bein, E., Andersen, T., Strupp, H. H., et al. (2000). The effects of training in time-limited dynamic psychotherapy: Changes in therapeutic outcome. *Psychotherapy Research, 10*: 119–132.

Benoit, D., Zeanah, D. H., Parker, K. C. H., Nicholson, E., & Coolbear, J. (1997). Working models of the child interview: Infant clinical status related to maternal perceptions. *Infant Mental Health Journal, 18* (1): 107–121.

Benson, D. F., & Greenberg, J. (1969). Visual form agnosia: A specific defeat in visual discrimination. *Archives of Neurology,* 20: 82–89.

Berg, B. L. (2001). *Qualitative Research Methods for the Social Sciences* (4th edition). Needham Heights, MA: Allyn & Bacon.

Bergin, A. E., & S. L. Garfield, S. L. (Eds.) (1971). *Handbook of Psychotherapy and Behavior Change: An Empirical Analysis*. New York: Wiley.

Bickman, L. (1996). A continuum of care: More is not always better. *American Psychologist, 51*: 689–701.

Bigelow, A. E. (2001). Discovering self through other: Infants' preference for social contingency. *Bulletin of the Menninger Clinic, 65*: 335–346.

Birmaher, B., & Brent, D. (1998). Practice parameters for the assessment and treatment of children and adolescents with depressive disorders. *Journal of the American Academy of Child and Adolescent Psychiatry, 37* (Suppl. 10): 63S–83S. (Special Issue: Practice Parameters.)

Birmaher, B., Brent, D. A., Kolko, D., Baugher, M., Bridge, J., Iyengar, S., & Ulloa, R. E. (2000). Clinical outcome after short-term psychotherapy for adolescents with major depressive disorder. *Archives of General Psychiatry, 57*: 29–36.

Bischof, M., & Bassetti, C. (2004). Total dream loss: A distinct neuropsychological dysfunction after bilateral PCA stroke. *Annals of Neurology, 56*: 583–586.

Blakemore, S.-J., & Decety, J. (2001). From the perception of action to the understanding of intention. *Nature Reviews Neuroscience, 2*: 561–567.

Blatt, S. J. (1995). The destructiveness of perfectionism: Implications for the treatment of depression. *American Psychologist, 50*: 1003–1020.

Blatt, S. J. (2004). *Experiences of Depression: Theoretical, Clinical, and Research Perspectives.* Washington, DC: American Psychological Association.

Boccia, M. L., & Pedersen, C. A. (2001). Brief vs. long maternal separations in infancy: Contrasting relationships with adult maternal behavior and lactation levels of aggression and anxiety. *Psychoneuroendocrinology, 26* (7): 657–672.

Boller, F., Wright, D., Cavalieri, R., & Mitsumoto, H. (1975). Paroxysmal "nightmares": Sequel of a stroke responsive to diphenylhydantoin. *Neurology, 25*: 1026–1028.

Bolton, D. (2002). Knowledge in the human sciences. In: S. Priebe & M. Slade (Eds.), *Evidence in Mental Health Care* (pp. 3–10). Hove/New York: Brunner-Routledge.

Bornstein, M. H. (1995). Parenting infants. In: M. Bornstein (Ed.), *Handbook of Parenting, Vol. 1* (pp. 3–39). Hillsdale, NJ: Lawrence Erlbaum.

Botez, M. I., Gravel, J., Attig, E., & Vézina, J.-L. (1985). Reversible chronic cerebellar ataxia after phenytoin intoxication: Possible role of cerebellum in cognitive thought. *Neurology, 35*: 1152.

Bouchard, T. J., & McGue, M. (2003). Genetic and environmental influences on human psychological differences. *Journal of Neurobiology, 54*: 4–45.

Bowlby, J. (1969). *Attachment and Loss, Vol. 1: Attachment* (2nd edition). London: Hogarth Press, 1982; reprinted New York: Basic Books, 2000.

Bowlby, J. (1980). *Attachment and Loss, Vol. 2: Separation.* London: Hogarth Press .

Bowlby, J. (1980). *Attachment and Loss, Vol. 3: Loss: Sadness and Depression.* London: Hogarth Press .

Boyle, J., & Nielsen, J. (1954). Visual agnosia and loss of recall. *Bulletin of the Los Angeles Neurological Society, 19*: 39–42.

Brain, R. (1950). The cerebral basis of consciousness. *Brain, 73*: 465–479.

Brain, R. (1954). Loss of visualization. *Proceedings of the Royal Society of Medicine, 47*: 288–290.

Brandt, K. A., Andrews, C. B., & Kvale. J. (1998). Mother–infant interaction and breastfeeding outcomes 6 weeks after birth. *Journal of Obstetric, Gynecologic and Neonatal Nursing, 27*: 169–174.

Braten, S. (1988). Dialogic mind: The infant and the adult in protoconversation. In: M. Carvallo (Ed.), *Nature, Cognition, and System, Vol. 1* (pp. 187–205). Dordrecht: Kluwer Academic Publishers.

Braten, S. (1992). The virtual other in infants' minds and social feelings. In: H. Wold (Ed.), *The Dialogical Alternative* (pp. 77–97). Oslo: Scandinavian University Press.

Braten, S. (Ed.) (1998). *Intersubjective Communication and Emotion in Early Ontogeny*. Cambridge : Cambridge University Press.

Braun, A., et al. (1997). Regional cerebral blood flow throughout the sleep–wake cycle. *Brain, 120*: 1173.

Braun, A., et al. (1998). Dissociated pattern of activity in visual cortices and their projections during human rapid eye movement sleep. *Science, 279*: 91.

Brazelton, T. B., Koslowski, B., & Main, M. (1974). The origins of reciprocity: The early mother–infant interaction. In: M. Lewis & L. Rosenblum (Eds.), *The Effect of the Infant on Its Caregiver* (pp. 49–76). New York: Wiley.

Brazelton, T. B., & Tronick, E. (1980). Preverbal communication between mothers and infants. In: D. R. Olson (Ed.), *The Social Foundations of Language and Thought* (pp. 299–315). New York: Norton.

Brent, D. A. (1997). The aftercare of adolescents with deliberate self-harm. *Journal of Child Psychology and Psychiatry, 38*: 277–286.

Brent, D. A. (2001). Firearms and suicide. *Annals of the New York Academy of Sciences, 932*: 225–239; discussion, 239–240.

Brent, D. A., Holder, D., Kolko, D., Birmaher, B., Baugher, M., Roth, C., & Johnson, B. (1997). A clinical psychotherapy trial for adolescent depression comparing cognitive, family, and supportive treatments. *Archives of General Psychiatry, 54:* 877–885.

Brent, D. A., Johnson, B. A., Perper, J., Connolly, J., Bridge, J., Bartle, S., & Rather, C. (1994). Personality disorder, personality traits, impulsive violence, and completed suicide in adolescents. *Journal of the American Academy of Child & Adolescent Psychiatry, 33* (8): 1080–1086.

Brent, D. A., Kolko, D., Birmaher, B., Baugher, M., Bridge, J., Roth, C., & Holder, D. (1998). Predictors of treatment efficacy in a clinical trial of three psychosocial treatments for adolescent depression. *Journal of the American Academy of Child & Adolescent Psychiatry, 37*: 906–914.

Brent, D. A., Perper, J. A., Moritz, G., et al. (1994). Familial risk factors for adolescent suicide: A case-control study. *Acta Psychiatrica Scandinavica, 89*: 52–58.

Bretherton, I. (1987). New perspectives on attachment relations: Security, communication, and internal working models. In: J. D. Osofsky (Ed.), *Handbook of Infant Development* (pp. 1061–1100). New York: Wiley.

Bretherton, I., & Munholland, K. A. (1999). Internal working models in attachment relations—a construct revisited. In: J. Cassidy & P. R. Shaver (Eds.), *Handbook of Attachment: Theory, Research, and Clinical Implications* (pp. 89–111). New York: Guildford Press.

Bretherton, I., Ridgeway, D., & Cassidy, J. (1990). Assessing internal working models of the attachment relationship: An Attachment Story Completion Task for 3-year olds. In: M. T. Greenberg, D. Cicchetti, & E. M. Cummings (Eds.), *Attachment in the Preschool Years* (pp. 273–310). Chicago, IL: University of Chicago Press.

Bridges, R. S., Numan, M., Ronsheim, P. M., Mann, P. E., & Lupini, C. E. (1990). Central prolactin infusions stimulate maternal behavior in steroid-treated, nulliparous female rats. *Proceedings of the National Academy of Sciences USA, 87*: 8003–8007.

Brodzinsky, D. M. (1987). Adjustment to adoption: A psychological perspective. *Clinical Psychology Review, 7*: 25–47.

Brooks-Gunn, J., Klebanov, P. K., Liaw, F., & Spiker, D. (1993). Enhancing the development of low-birthweight, premature infants: Changes in cognition and behavior over the first three years. *Child Development, 64* (3): 736–753.

Brown, G. P., Hammen, C. L., Craske, M. G., & Wickens, T. D. (1995). Dimensions of dysfunctional attitudes as vulnerabilities to depressive symptoms. *Journal of Abnormal Psychology, 104*: 431–435.

Brown, G. W., Bifulco, A., & Harris, T. O. (1987). Life events, vulnerability and onset of depression: Some refinements. *British Journal of Psychiatry, 150*: 30–42.

Brown, J. (1972). *Aphasia, Apraxia, Agnosia: Clinical and Theoretical Aspects.* Springfield, IL: Charles C Thomas.

Brown, L. P. (1990). Neighborhood-oriented policing. *American Journal of Police, 9* (3).

Bruner, J. (1990). *Acts of Meaning.* Cambridge, MA: Harvard University Press.

Bruner, J., Olver, P., & Greenfield, P. M. (1966). *Studies on Cognitive Growth.* New York: Wiley.

Bureau of Justice Assistance (1994). *Understanding Community Policing: A Framework for Action.* Washington, DC.

Burges Watson, I., Hoffman, L., & Wilson, G. (1988). The neuropsychiatry of post-traumatic stress disorder. *British Journal of Psychiatry, 152*: 164–173.

Burt, V. K., & Stein, K. (2002). Epidemiology of depression throughout the female life-cycle. *Journal of Clinical Psychiatry, 63* (Suppl. 7): 9–15.

Buzsáki, G., & Draguhn, A. (2004). Neuronal oscillations in cortical networks. *Science, 304*: 1926–1929.

Cahill, L. T., Kaminer, R. K., & Johnson, P. G. (1999). Developmental, cognitive, and behavioral sequelae of child abuse. *Child and Adolescent Psychiatric Clinics of North America, 8* (4): 827–843.

Cairns, R. B., Cairns, B. D., Rodkin, P., & Xie, H. (1998). New directions in developmental research: Models and methods. In: R. Jessor (Ed.), *New Perspectives on Adolescent Risk Behavior* (pp. 13–40). Cambridge: Cambridge University Press.

Caldji, C., Francis, D., Sharma, S., Plotsky, P. M., & Meaney, M. J. (2000). The effects of early rearing environment on the development of GABAA and central benzodiazepine receptor levels and novelty-induced fearfulness in the rat. *Neuropsychopharmacology, 22* (3): 219–229.

Caldji, C., Tannenbaum, B., Sharma, S., Francis, D., Plotsky, P. M., & Meaney, M. J. (1998). Maternal care during infancy regulates the development of neural systems mediating the expression of fearfulness in the rat. *Proceedings of the National Academy of Sciences USA, 95* (9): 5335–5340.

Camille, N., Coricelli, G., Sallet, J., Pradat-Diehl, P., Duhamel, J., & Sirigu, A. (2004). The involvement of the orbitofrontal cortex in the experience of regret. *Science, 304*: 1167–1170.
Campos, J. J., & Sternberg, C. R. (1981). Perception, appraisal, and emotions: The onset of social referencing. In: M. E. Lamb & L. R. Sherrod (Eds.), *Infant Social Cognition*. Hillsdale, NJ: Lawrence Erlbaum.
Camras, L. A. (1992). Expressive development and basic emotions. *Cognition and Emotion, 6*: 269–283.
Camras, L. A. (2000). Surprise! Facial expressions can be coordinative motor structures. In: M. D. Lewis & I. Granic (Eds.), *Emotion, Development, and Self-Organization: Dynamic Systems Approaches to Emotion-al Development* (pp. 100–124). Cambridge: Cambridge University Press.
Carlson, E. A. (1998). A prospective longitudinal study of attachment disorganization/disorientation. *Child Development, 69* (4): 1107–1128.
Carlson, V., Cicchetti, D., Barnett, D., et al. (1989). Disorganized/disoriented attachment relationships in maltreated infants. *Developmental Psychology, 25*: 525–531.
Caron, A. J., Caron, R. F., & MacLean, D. J. (1988). Infant discrimination of naturalistic emotional expressions: The role of face and voice. *Child Development, 59*: 604–616.
Caron, R. F., Caron, A. J., & Myers, R. S. (1985). Do infants see facial expressions in static faces? *Child Development, 56*: 1552–1560.
Carr, L., Iacoboni, M., Dubeau, M. C., Mazziotta, J. C., & Lenzi, G. L. (2003). Neural mechanisms of empathy in humans: A relay from neural systems for imitation to limbic areas. *Proceedings of the National Academy of Sciences USA, 100* (9): 5497–5502.
Carter, S. C. (1998). Neuroendocrine perspectives on social attachment and love. *Psychoneuroendocrinology, 23*: 779–818.
Casey, R. J., & Berman, J. S. (1985). The outcome of psychotherapy with children. *Psychological Bulletin, 98:* 388–400.
Caspi, A., McClay, J., Moffitt, T. E., Mill, J., Martin, J., Craig, I. W., et al. (2002). Role of genotype in the cycle of violence in maltreated children. *Science, 297*: 851–854.
Caspi, A., Sugden, K., Moffitt, T. E., Taylor, A., Craig, I. W., Harrington, H., et al. (2003). Influence of life stress on depression: Moderation by a polymorphism in the 5-HTT gene. *Science, 301*: 386–389.
Cassidy, J., & Shaver, P. R. (Eds.) (1999). *Handbook of Attachment*. New York: Guilford Press.
Cassidy, J., Woodhouse, S., Cooper, G., Hoffman, K., Powell, B., & Rodenberg, M. (2005). Examination of the precursors of infant attachment security: Implications for early intervention and intervention research. In: L. Berlin, Y. Ziv, L. Amaya-Jackson, & M. Greenberg (Eds.), *Enhancing Early Attachments: Theory, Research, Intervention, and Policy*. New York: Guilford Press.
Cathala, H., Laffont, F., Siksou, M., Esnault, S., Gilbert, A., Minz, M., Moret-Chalmin, C., Burzaré, M., & Waisbord, P. (1983). Sommeil et

rêve chez des patients atteints de lesions parietals et frontales. *Revue Neruologique, 139*: 497–508.

Cavallero, C., et al. (1992). Slow wave sleep dreaming. *Sleep, 15*: 562.

Centers for Disease Control. (1995). Fatal and nonfatal suicide attempts among adolescents—Oregon, 1988–1993. *Morbidity and Mortality Weekly Report (MMWR), 44* (16): 312–315, 321–323.

Champagne, F., Chretien, P., Stevenson, C. W., Zhang, T. Y., Gratton, A., & Meaney, M. J. (2004). Variations in nucleus accumbens dopamine associated with individual differences in maternal behavior in the rat. *Journal of Neuroscience, 24* (17): 4113–4123.

Champagne, F., Diorio, J., Sharma, S., & Meaney M. J. (2001). Naturally occurring variations in maternal behavior in the rat are associated with differences in estrogen-inducible central oxytocin receptors. *Proceedings of the National Academy of Sciences USA, 98* (22): 12736–12741.

Champagne, F., & Meaney, M. J. (2001). Like mother, like daughter: Evidence for non-genomic transmission of parental behavior and stress responsivity. *Progress in Brain Research, 133*: 287–302.

Champagne, F., Weaver, I. C. G., Diorio, J., Sharma, S., & Meaney, M. J. (2003). Natural variations in maternal care are associated with estrogen receptor alpha expression and estrogen sensitivity in the medial preoptic area. *Endocrinology, 144* (11): 4720–4724.

Charcot, J.-M. (1883). Un cas de suppression brusque et isolée de la vision mentale des signes et des objets, (formes et couleurs) [On a case of sudden isolated suppression of the mental vision of signs and objects (forms and colours)]. *Progrès Médical, 11*: 568–571.

Charmandari, E., Kino, T., Souvatzoglou, E., & Chrousos, G. P. (2003). Pediatric stress: Hormonal mediators and human development. *Hormone Research, 59* (4): 161–179.

Chase, T., Moretti, L., & Prensky, A. (1968). Clinical and electroencephalographic manifestations of vascular lesions of the pons. *Neurology, 18*: 357–368.

Chiodera, P., & Coiro, V. (1987). Oxytocin reduces metyrapone-induced ACTH secretion in human subjects. *Brain Research, 420* (1): 178–181.

Chisholm, K., Bigelow, A. E., Gillis, R., & Myatt, T. (2001). "Continuity of Maternal Sensitivity throughout Infancy: Impact on Infants' Joint Attention, Maturity of Play, and Attachment." Poster presented at the Society for Research in Child Development Conference (SRCD), Minneapolis, Minnesota.

Christophersen, E. R., & Mortweet, S. L. (2001). *Treatments That Work with Children: Empirically Supported Strategies for Managing Childhood Problems*. Washington, DC: American Psychological Association.

Churchland, P. S., Ramachandran, V. S., & Sejnowski, T. J. (1994). A critique of pure vision. In: C. Koch & J. L. Davis (Eds.), *Large-Scale Neuronal Theories of the Brain: Computational Neuroscience* (pp. 23–60). Cambridge, MA: MIT Press.

Clark, A. (1999). An embodied cognitive science? *Trends in Cognitive Science, 3*: 345–351.

Clarke, G. N., Hawkins, W., Murphy, M., Sheeber, L. B., Lewinsohn, P. M., & Seeley, J. R. (1995). Targeted prevention of unipolar depressive disorder in an at-risk sample of high school adolescents: A randomized trial of a group of cognitive intervention. *Journal of the American Academy of Child and Adolescent Psychiatry, 34:* 312–321.

Clarke, G., Hops, H., Lewinsohn, P. M., Andrews, J., Seeley, J. R., & Williams, J. (1992). Cognitive-behavioral group treatment of adolescent depression: Prediction of outcome. *Behavior Therapy, 23:* 341–354.

Clarke, G. N., Hornbrook, M., Lynch, F., Polen, M., Gale, J., Beardslee, W., O'Connor, E., & Seeley, J. (2001). A randomized trial of a group cognitive intervention for preventing depression in adolescent offspring of depressed parents. *Archives of General Psychiatry, 58:* 1127–1134.

Clarke, G. N., Hornbrook, M., Lynch, F., Polen, M., Gale, J., O'Connor, E., Seeley, J. R., & Debar, L. (2002). Group cognitive-behavioral treatment for depressed adolescent offspring of depressed parents in a health maintenance organization. *Journal of the American Academy of Child and Adolescent Psychiatry, 41:* 305–313.

Clarke, G. N., Lewinsohn, P. M., Rohde, P., Hops, H., & Seeley, J. R. (1999). Cognitive-behavioral group treatment of adolescent depression: Efficacy of acute group treatment and booster sessions. *Journal of the American Academy of Child and Adolescent Psychiatry, 38:* 272–279.

Clarke, L. P. (1915). The nature and pathogenesis of epilepsy. *New York Medical Journal, 101*: 522, 567–573, 623–628.

Clarkin, J. F., Kernberg, O. F., & Yeomans, F. (1999). *Transference-Focused Psychotherapy for Borderline Personality Disorder Patients.* New York: Guilford Press.

Clement, P. W. (1999). *Outcomes and Incomes: How to Evaluate, Improve, and Market Your Practice by Measuring Outcomes in Psychotherapy.* New York: Guilford Press.

Clutton-Brock, T. H. (1991). *The Evolution of Parental Care.* Princeton, NJ: Princeton University Press.

Cohen, D. J. (2001). Into life: Autism, Tourette's syndrome and the community of clinical research. *Israeli Journal of Psychiatry and Related Sciiences, 38*: 226–234.

Comings, D. E., & Blum, K. (2000). Reward deficiency syndrome: Genetic aspects of behavioral disorders. *Progress in Brain Research, 126*: 325–341.

Compton, S. N., March, J. S., Brent, D. A., Albano, A. M., Weersing, V. R., & Curry, J. (2004). Cognitive-behavioral psychotherapy for anxiety and depressive disorders in children and adolescents: An evidence-based medicine review. *Journal of the American Academy of Child and Adolescent Psychiatry, 43:* 930–959.

Consumers Union (1995). Mental health: Does therapy help? *Consumer Reports, 60* (November): 734–739.

Cooklin, A. (1982). Change in here-and-now systems vs. systems over time. In: A. Bentovim, G. Gorell-Barnes, & A. Cooklin (Eds.), *Fam-*

ily Therapy: Complementary Frameworks of Theory and Practice. London: Academic Press.
Cooklin, A., Miller, A., & McHugh, B. (1983). An institution for change: Developing a family day unit. *Family Process, 22*: 453–468.
Cooper, R. P., & Aslin, R. N. (1990). Preference for infant-directed speech in the first month after birth. *Child Development, 61*: 1584–1595.
Corsini, C. A., & Viazzo, P. (1997). *The Decline of Infant and Child Mortality: The European Experience, 1750–1990.* The Hague: Kluwer Law International.
Cotgrove, A., Cottrell, D. J., Goodyer, I. M., Whittington, C. J., Kendall, T., Fonagy, P., & Boddington, C. (2004). *Sampling Methods in Trials of SSRIs for the Treatment of Depression in Children and Young People.* Unpublished manuscript.
Crittenden, P. M. (2002). Special article: Attachment, information processing, and psychiatric disorder. *World Psychiatry, 1* (2): 72–75.
Crittenden, P. M. (2004). *Patterns of Attachment in Adulthood: A Dynamic-Maturational Approach to Analyzing "The Adult Attachment Interview".* Unpublished manuscript, Family Relations Institute, Miami, FL.
Csibra, G., & Gergely, G. (2006). Social learning and social cogniton: The case for pedagogy. In: M. H. Johnson & Y. Munakata (Eds.), *Progress of Change in Brain and Cognitive Development. Attention and Performance XXI* (pp. 249–274). Oxford: Oxford University Press.
Cummings, J. L., & Greenberg R. (1977). Sleep patterns in the "locked in" syndrome. *Electroencephalography and Clinical Neurophysiology, 43*: 270–271.
Damasio, A. R. (1994). *Descartes' Error: Emotion, Reason, and the Human Brain.* New York: Putnam.
Dare, C., & Eisler, I. (2000). A multi-family group day treatment programme for adolescent eating disorder. *European Eating Disorders Review, 8*: 4–18.
Darwin, C. (1872). *The Expression of the Emotions in Man and Animals.* Chicago, IL: University of Chicago Press, 1965.
Dawson, N., & McHugh, B. (1986). Families as partners. *Pastoral Care in Education, 4* (2): 102–109.
Dawson, N., & McHugh, B. (1994). Parents and children: Participants in change. In: E. Dowling & E. Osborne (Ed.), *The Family and the School: A Joint Systems Approach to Problems with Children.* London: Routledge.
Dawson, N., & McHugh, B. (2000). Family relationships, learning and teachers: Keeping the connections. In: R. Best & C. Watkins (Eds.), *Tomorrow's Schools.* London: Routledge.
De Bellis, M. D., Baum, A., Birmaher, B., Keshavan, M. S., Eccard, C. H., Boring, A. M., et al. (1999). Developmental traumatology, Part I: Biological stress systems. *Biological Psychiatry, 45*: 1259–1270.
Dement, W., & Kleitman, N. (1957a). Cyclic variations in EEG during sleep and their relation to eye movements, body mobility and dreaming. *Electroencephalography and Clinical Neurophysiology, 9*: 673.

Dement, W., & Kleitman, N. (1957b). The relation of eye movements during sleep to dream activity: An objective method for the study of dreaming. *Journal of Experimental Psychology, 53*: 89.

Denenberg, V. H., Hoplight, B. J., & Mobraaten, L. E. (1998). The uterine environment enhances cognitive competence. *Neuroreport, 9*: 1667–1671.

Denenberg, V. H., Rosenberg, K. M., Paschke, R., & Zarrow, M. X. (1969). Mice reared with rat aunts: Effects on plasma corticosterone and open-field activity. *Nature, 221*: 73–74.

Dennett, D. C. (1991). *Consciousness Explained*. Boston, MA: Little, Brown.

Denzin, N. H., & Lincoln, Y. S. (Eds.) (2000). *Handbook of Qualitative Research* (2nd edition). Thousand Oaks, CA: Sage.

DeRubeis, R. J., Evans, M. D., Hollon, S. D., Garvey, M. J., Grove, W. M., & Tuason, V. B. (1990). How does cognitive therapy work? Cognitive change and symptom change in cognitive therapy and pharmacotherapy for depression. *Journal of Consulting and Clinical Psychology, 58*: 862–869.

De Sanctis, S. (1896). *Il sogni é il sonno*. Rome: Alighieri.

Dettling, A. C., Feldon, J., & Pryce, C. R. (2002). Repeated parental deprivation in the infant common marmoset (*Callithrix jacchus*, primates) and analysis of its effects on early development. *Biological Psychiatry, 52* (11): 1037–1046.

Dozier, M., Stovall, K. C., & Albus, K. E. (1999). Attachment and psychopathology in adulthood. In: J. Cassidy & P. R. Shaver (Eds.), *Handbook of Attachment* (pp. 497–519). New York: Guilford Press.

Dubowitz, H. (1999). *Neglected Children: Research, Practice, and Policy*. Thousand Oaks, CA: Sage.

Dunn, J. B. (1977). Patterns of early interaction: Continuities and consequences. In: H. R. Schaffer (Ed.), *Studies in Mother–Infant Interaction* (pp 438–456). London: Academic Press.

Eckenrode, J., Ganzel, B., Henderson, C. R. Jr., Smith, E., Olds, D. L., Powers, J., et al. (2000). Preventing child abuse and neglect with a program of nurse home visitation: The limiting effects of domestic violence. *Journal of the American Medical Association, 284* (11): 1385–1391.

Efron, R. (1968). *What Is Perception? Boston Studies in the Philosophy of Science*. New York: Humanities Press.

Egeland, B., & Sroufe, L. A. (1981). Developmental sequelae of maltreatment in infancy. *New Directions for Child Development, 11*: 77–92.

Egyed, K., Király, I., & Gergely, G. (2004). "Object-Centered versus Agent-Centered Interpretations of Referential Attitude Expressions in 14-Month-Olds." Poster presented at the 14th Biennial International Conference on Infant Studies, Chicago (May).

Eisler, I., LeGrange, D., & Asen, E. (2003). Family treatments. In: J. Treasure, U. Schmidt, & E. van Furth (Eds.), *Handbook of Eating Disorders: Theory, Treatment and Research*. Chichester: Wiley.

Ekman, P. (1992). Facial expressions of emotion: New findings, new questions. *Psychological Science, 3* (1): 34–38.

Ekman, P., Friesen, W. V., & Ellsworth, P. (1972). *Emotion in the Human Face.* New York: Pergamon Press.

Elman, J. L., Bates, E. A., Johnson, M. K., Karmiloff-Smith, A., Parisi, D., & Plunkett, K. (1996). *Rethinking Innateness: A Connectionist Perspective on Development.* Cambridge, MA: MIT Press.

Emde, R. E., Wolf, D. P., & Oppenheim, D. (2003). *Revealing the Inner Worlds of Young Children: The MacArthur Story Stem Battery and Parent–Child Narratives.* New York: Oxford University Press.

Engel, A. K., Fries, P., & Singer, W. (2001). Dynamic predictions: Oscillations and synchrony in top-down processing. *Nature Reviews Neuroscience, 2*: 704–716.

Entwisle, D. R., & Doering, S. G. (1981). *The First Birth: A Family Turning Point.* Baltimore, MD: Johns Hopkins University Press.

Epstein, A. (1964). Recurrent dreams: Their relationship to temporal lobe seizures. *Archives of General Psychiatry, 10*: 49–54.

Epstein, A. (1967). Body image alterations during seizures and dreams of epileptics. *Archives of Neurology, 16*: 613–619.

Epstein, A. W. (1979). Effect of certain cerebral hemispheric diseases on dreaming. *Biological Psychiatry, 14*: 77–93.

Epstein, A., & Ervin, F. (1956). Psychodynamic significance of seizure content in psycho-motor epilepsy. *Psychosomatic Medicine, 18*: 43–55.

Epstein, A., & Freeman, N. (1981). The uncinate focus and dreaming. *Epilepsia, 22*: 603–605.

Epstein, A., & Hill, W. (1966). Ictal phenomena during REM sleep of a temporal lobe epileptic. *Archives of Neurology, 15*: 367–375.

Epstein, E., & Simmons, N. (1983). Aphasia with reported loss of dreaming. *American Journal of Psychiatry, 140*: 109.

Ettlinger, G., Warrington, E., & Zangwill, O. (1957). A further study of visual-spatial agnosia. *Brain, 80*: 335–361.

Even, C., Siobud-Dorocant, E., & Dardennes, R. M. (2000). Critical approach to antidepressant trials: Blindness protection is necessary, feasible and measurable. *British Journal of Psychiatry, 177*: 47–51.

Evidence-Based Mental Health (1998). [Journal devoted to evidence-based treatments and linking research to practice.] Vol. 1, No. 1.

Eysenck, H. J. (1952). The effects of psychotherapy: An evaluation. *Journal of Consulting Psychology, 16*: 319–324..

Faazia, N. (2001). *Dependency, Self-Criticism and Suicidal Behavior.* Unpublished Master's thesis, University of Windsor, Windsor, Ontario.

Fantz, R. (1963). Pattern vision in newborn infants. *Science, 140*: 296–297.

Farah, M., Levine, D., & Calviano, D. (1988). A case study of mental imagery deficit. *Brain and Cognition, 8*: 147–164.

Farr, R. M. (1984). Interviewing: The social psychology of the interview. In: C. L. Cooper & P. Makin (Eds.), *Psychology for Managers.* London: Macmillan.

Farrell, B. (1969). *Pat & Roald.* London: Hutchinson.

Farroni, T., Csibra, G., Simion, F., & Johnson, M. H. (2002). Eye contact detection in humans from birth. *Proceedings of the National Academy of Sciences USA, 99* (14): 9602–9605.

Farroni, T., Massaccesi, S., Pividori, D., Simion, F., & Johnson, M. H. (2004). Gaze following in newborns. *Infancy, 5*: 39–60.

Fechner, G. (1889). *Elemente der Psychophysik.* Leipzig: Breitkopf & Härtel.

Feldman, M. H. (1971). Physiological observations in a chronic case of "locked-in" syndrome. *Neurology, 21*: 459–478.

Feldman, R. (2003). "From Biological Rhythms to Interaction Rhythms: Physiological Precursors of Mother–Infant Synchrony." Paper presented at the biennial meeting of the Society for Research in Child Development, Tampa, FL (April 24–27).

Feldman, R. (2004). Mother–infant skin-to-skin contact and the development of emotion regulation. In: S. P. Shohov (Ed.), *Advances in Psychology Research Vol. 27* (pp. 113–131). Hauppauge, NY: Nova Science.

Feldman, R., & Eidelman, A. I. (2003). Direct and indirect effects of maternal milk on the neurobehavioral and cognitive development of premature infants. *Developmental Psychobiology, 43*: 109–119.

Feldman, R., Eidelman, A. I., Sirota, L., & Weller, A. (2002). Comparison of skin-to-skin (kangaroo) and traditional care: Parenting outcomes and preterm infant development. *Pediatrics, 110*: 16–26.

Feldman, R., Greenbaum, C. W., & Yirmiya, N. (1999). Mother–infant affect synchrony as an antecedent to the emergence of self-control. *Developmental Psychobiology, 35*: 223–231.

Feldman, R., & Keren, M. (2004). Expanding the scope of infant mental health assessment: A community-based approach. In: R. Delcarmen-Wiggins & A. S. Carter (Eds.), *Handbook of Infant Mental Health Assessment* (pp. 443–465). New York: Oxford Press.

Feldman, R., Weller, A., Leckman, J. F., Kvint, J., & Eidelman, A. I. (1999). The nature of the mother's tie to her infant: The formation of parent–infant bonding in healthy and at-risk dyads. *Journal of Child Psychology and Psychiatry, 40*: 929–939.

Feldman, R., Weller, A., Sirota, L., & Eidelman, A. I. (2002). Skin-to-skin contact (Kangaroo Care) promotes self-regulation in premature infants: Sleep–wake cyclicity, arousal modulation, and sustained exploration. *Developmental Psychology, 38*: 194–207.

Feldman, R., Weller, A., Sirota, L., & Eidelman, A. I. (2003). Testing a family intervention hypothesis: The contribution of mother–infant skin-to-skin contact (Kangaroo Care) to family interaction, proximity, and touch. *Journal of Family Psychology, 17* (1): 94–107.

Ferber, S. G., & Feldman, R. (2005). Delivery pain and the development of mother–infant interaction. *Infancy, 8* (1): 43–62.

Ferguson, J. N., Aldag, J. M., Insel, T. R., & Young, L. J. (2001). Oxytocin in the medial amygdala is essential for social recognition in the mouse. *Journal of Neuroscience, 21* (20): 8278–8285.

Ferguson, J. N., Young, L. J., & Insel, T. R. (2002). The neuroendocrine basis of social recognition. *Frontiers in Neuroendocrinology, 23* (2): 200–224.

Fergusson, D. M., Woodward, L. J., & Horwood, L. J. (2000). Risk factors and life processes associated with the onset of suicidal behavior during adolescence and early adulthood. *Psychological Medicine, 30*: 23–39.

Fernald, A. (1985). Four-month-old infants prefer to listen to motherese. *Infant Behavior and Development, 8*: 181–195.

Fernald, A. (1992). Human maternal vocalizations to infants as biological signals: An evolutionary perspective. In: J. H. Barkow, J. Tooby, & L. C. Cosmides (Eds.), *The Adapted Mind: Evolutionary Psychology and the Generation of Culture* (pp. 391–428). Oxford: Oxford University Press.

Ferrari, P. F., Gallese, V., Rizzolatti, G., & Fogassi, L. (2003). Mirror neurons responding to the observation of ingestive and communicative mouth actions in the monkey ventral premotor cortex. *European Journal of Neuroscience, 17* (8): 1703–1714.

Field, T. (1992). Infants of depressed mothers. *Developmental Psychopathology, 4*: 49–66.

Field, T., Woodson, R., Cohen, D., Garcia, R., & Greenberg, R. (1983). Discrimination and imitation of facial expressions by term and preterm neonates. *Infant Behavior and Development, 6*: 485–490.

Flavell, J. H. (2004). Theory-of-mind development: Retrospect and prospect. *Merrill-Palmer Quarterly, 50* (3): 274–290.

Flavell, J. H., Botkin, P. T., Fry, C. L., Jr., Wright, J. W., & Jarvis, P. E. (1968). *The Development of Role-Taking and Communication Skills in Children*. New York: Wiley.

Fleming, A. S., O'Day, D. H., & Kraemer, G. W. (1999). Neurobiology of mother–infant interactions: Experience and central nervous system plasticity across development and generations. *Neuroscience and Biobehavioral Reviews, 23* (5): 673–685.

Fleming, A. S., Steiner, M., & Corter, C. (1997). Cortisol, hedonics, and maternal responsiveness in human mothers. *Hormones and Behavior, 32* (2): 85–98.

Fleming, A. S., Vaccarino, F., & Luebke, C. (1980). Amygdaloid inhibition of maternal behavior in the nulliparous female rat. *Physiology & Behavior, 25*: 731–743.

Floccia, C., Christophe, A., & Bertoncini, J. (1997). High-amplitude sucking and newborns: The quest for underlying mechanisms. *Journal of Experimental Child Psychology, 64*: 175–189.

Fogel, A., Nwokah, E., Dedo, J. Y., Messinger, D., Dickson, K. L., Matusov, E., & Holt, S. A. (1992). Social process theory of emotion: A dynamic systems approach. *Social Development, 2*: 122–142.

Fónagy, I. (2000). *Languages within Language: An Evolutive Aproach*. Amsterdam: John Benjamins.

Fónagy, I., & Fonagy, P. (1995). Communications with pretend actions in language, literature, and psychoanalysis. *Psychoanalysis and Contemporary Thought, 18*: 363–418.

Fonagy, P. (2001). Introduction to attachment theory. In: *Attachment Theory and Psychoanalysis* (pp. 5–18). New York: Other Press.

Fonagy, P., Gergely, G., Jurist, E., & Target, M. (2002). *Affect Regulation, Mentalization, and the Development of the Self*. New York: Other Press.

Fonagy, P., & Moran, G. S. (1990). Studies on the efficacy of child psychoanalysis. *Journal of Consulting and Clinical Psychology, 58*: 684–695.

Fonagy, P., Steele, H., & Steele, M. (1991). Maternal representations of attachment during pregnancy predict the organization of infant–mother attachment at one year of age. *Child Development, 62*: 891–905.

Fonagy, P., Steele, H., Steele, M., Leigh, T., Kennedy, R., Mattoon, G., & Target, M. (1995). Attachment, the reflective self, and borderline states: The predictive specificity of the Adult Attachment Interview and pathological emotional development. In: S. Goldberg, R. Muir, & J. Kerr (Eds.), *Attachment Theory: Social, Developmental, and Clinical Perspectives* (pp. 233–278). New York: Analytic Press.

Fonagy, P., & Target, M. (1995). Playing with reality: I. Theory of mind and the normal development of psychic reality. *International Journal of Psychoanalysis, 77*: 217–233.

Fonagy, P., & Target, M. (1997). Attachment and reflective function: Their role in self-organization. *Development and Psychopathology, 9*: 679–700.

Fonagy, P., & Target, M. (in press). The rooting of the mind in the body: New links between attachment theory and psychoanalytic thought. *Journal of the American Psychoanalytic Association.*

Fonagy, P., Target, M., Cottrell, D., Phillips, J., & Kurtz, Z. (2002). *What Works for Whom? A Critical Review of Treatments for Children and Adolescents*. New York: Guilford Press.

Fonagy, P., Target, M., & Gergely, G. (2000). Attachment and borderline personality disorder: A theory and some evidence. *Psychiatric Clinics of North America, 23* (1): 103–123.

Foulkes, D. (1962). Dream reports from different stages of sleep. *Journal of Abnormal and Social Psychology, 65*: 14.

Foulkes, D., & Vogel, G. (1965). Mental activity at sleep onset. *Journal of Abnormal and Social Psychology, 70*: 231.

Foulkes, D., Spear, P., & Symonds, J. (1966). Individual differences in mental activity at sleep onset. *Journal of Abnormal and Social Psychology, 71*: 280.

Fox, R., & McDaniel, C. (1982). The perception of biological motion by human infants. *Science, 218*: 486–487.

Fraiberg, S. (1980). *Clinical Studies in Infant Mental Health*. New York: Basic Books.

Fraiberg, S., Adelson, E., & Shapiro, V. (1975). Ghosts in the nursery: A psychoanalytic approach to the problems of impaired infant–mother relationships. *Journal of the American Academy of Child and Adolescent Psychiatry, 14*: 387–421.

Francis, D. D., Caldji, C., Champagne, F., Plotsky, P. M., & Meaney, M. J. (1999). The role of corticotropin-releasing factor–norepinephrine systems in mediating the effects of early experience on the development of behavioral and endocrine responses to stress. *Biological Psychiatry, 46* (9): 1153–1166.

Francis, D. D., Champagne, F. C., & Meaney, M. J. (2000). Variations in maternal behavior are associated with differences in oxytocin receptor levels in the rat. *Journal of Neuroendocrinology, 12*: 1145–1148.

Francis, D. D., Diorio, J., Liu, D, & Meaney M. J. (1999). Non-genomic transmission across generations of maternal behavior and stress responses in the rat. *Science, 286*: 1155–1158.

Francis, D. D., Diorio, J., Plotsky, P. M., & Meaney, M. J.(2002). Environmental enrichment reverses the effects of maternal separation on stress reactivity. *Journal of Neuroscience, 22* (18): 7840–7843.

Francis, D. D., & Meaney, M. J. (1999). Maternal care and the development of stress responses. *Current Opinion in Neurobiology, 9* (1): 128–134.

Francis, D. D., Szegda, K., Campbell, G., Martin, W. D., & Insel, T. R. (2003). Epigenetic sources of behavioral differences in mice. *Nature Neuroscience, 6* (5): 445–446.

Francis, D. D., Young, L. J., Meaney, M. J., & Insel, T. R. (2002). Naturally occurring differences in maternal care are associated with the expression of oxytocin and vasopressin (V1a) receptors: Gender differences. *Journal of Neuroendocrinology, 14* (5): 349–353.

Franck, G., Salmon, E., Poirrier, R., Sadzot, B., Franco, G., & Maquet, P. (1987). Evaluation of human cerebral glucose uptake during wakefulness, slow wave sleep and paradoxical sleep. *Sleep, 16*: 46.

Frank, J. (1946). Clinical survey and results of 200 cases of prefrontal leucotomy. *Journal of Mental Science, 92*: 497.

Frank, J. (1950). Some aspects of lobotomy (prefrontal leucotomy) under psychoanalytic scrutiny. *Psychiatry, 13*: 35.

Franzini, C. (1992). Brain metabolism and blood flow during sleep. *Journal of Sleep Research, 1*: 3–16.

Freemantle, N., Anderson, I. M., & Young, P. (2000). Predictive value of pharmacological activity for the relative efficacy of antidepressant drugs: Metaregression analysis. *British Journal of Psychiatry, 177*: 292–302.

Freud, A. (1936). *The Ego and the Mechanisms of Defence*. London: Hogarth Press; New York: International Universities Press, 1966..

Freud, A. (1965). *Normality and Pathology in Childhood: Assessments of Development*. New York: International Universities Press.

Freud, A. (1968). Indications and contraindications for child analysis. *The Writings of Anna Freud, Vol. 7* (pp. 110–123). New York: International Universities Press.

Freud, A., & Burlingham, D. T. (1943). *War and Children*. New York: Medical War Books.

Freud, S. (1900a). *The Interpretation of Dreams. S.E.*, 4/5.

Freud, S. (1920g). *Beyond the Pleasure Principle. S.E.*, 18.

Freud, S. (1926d [1925]). *Inhibitions, Symptoms and Anxiety. S.E.*, 20: 77–174.

Freud, S. (1937c). Analysis terminable and interminable. *S.E.*, 23: 209–253.
Freud, S. (1940a [1938]). *An Outline of Psychoanalysis. S.E.*, 23.
Freud, S. (1950 [1895]). Project for a scientific psychology. *S.E.*, 1.
Frith, C. D., & Frith, U. (1999). Interacting minds: A biological basis. *Science, 286* (5445): 1692–1695.
Futó, J., Bátki, A., Koós, O., Fonagy, P., & Gergely, G. (2004). "Early Social-Interactive Determinants of Later Representational and Affect-Regulative Competence in Pretend Play." Poster presented at the 14th Biennial International Conference on Infant Studies, Chicago (May).
Gaffan, E. A., Tsaousis, I., & Kemp-Wheeler, S. M. (1995). Researcher allegiance and meta-analysis: The case of cognitive therapy for depression. *Journal of Consulting and Clinical Psychology, 63*: 966–980.
Gal, R. (1986). *A Portrait of the Israeli Soldier.* New York: Greenwood Press.
Gallassi, R., Morreale, A., Montagna, P., Gambetti, P., & Lugaresi, E. (1992). Fatal familial insomnia: Neuropsychological study of a disease with thalamic degeneration. *Cortex, 28*: 175–187.
Gallese, V., & Goldman, A. (1998). Mirror neurons and the simulation theory of mind reading. *Trends in Cognitive Sciences, 12*: 493–501.
Gallese, V., Keysers, C., & Rizzolatti, G. (2004). A unifying view of the basis of social cognition. *Trends in Cognitive Sciences, 8*: 396–403.
Gardner, H. (1985). Psychology: The wedding of methods to substance. *The Mind's New Science: A History of the Cognitive Revolution* (chap. 5). New York: Basic Books
Garfield, S. L., & Bergin, A. E. (Eds.) (1978). *Handbook of Psychotherapy and Behavior Change* (2nd edition). New York: Wiley.
Gauthier, I., Tarr, M., Anderson, A., Skudlarski, P., & Gore, J. (1999). Activation of the middle fusiform face area increases with expertise in recognizing novel objects. *Nature Neuroscience*, 2: 568–573.
George, C., Kaplan, N., & Main, M. (1985). *Adult Attachment Interview* (2nd edition). Unpublished manuscript, University of California at Berkeley.
George, C., Kaplan, N., & Main, M. (1996). *The Adult Attachment Interview.* Unpublished protocol (3rd edition). Department of Psychology, University of California at Berkeley.
George, C., & Solomon, J. (1989). Internal working models of caregiving and security of attachment at age six. *Infant Mental Health Journal, 10* (3): 222–238.
Gergely, G. (2002). The development of understanding self and agency. In: U. Goshwami (Ed.), *Blackwell Handbook of Childhood Cognitive Development* (pp. 26–46). Oxford: Blackwell.
Gergely, G. (2003). The development of teleological versus mentalizing observational learning strategies in infancy. *Bulletin of the Menninger Clinic, 67* (2): 113–131.
Gergely, G. (2004). The role of contingency detection in early affect-regulative interactions and in the development of different types of infant attachment. *Social Development, 13* (3): 468–488.

Gergely, G., Bekkering, H., & Király, I. (2002). Rational imitation in preverbal infants. *Nature, 415*: 755.

Gergely, G., & Csibra, G. (2006). Sylvia's recipe: Human culture, imitation, and pedagogy. In: N. J. Enfield & S. C. Levinson (Eds.), *Roots of Human Sociality: Culture, Cognition, and Human Interaction* (pp. 229–255). London: Berg Press.

Gergely, G., Fonagy, P., & Watson, J. S. (in preparation). *Attachment Security and Early Social Sensitization to Internal versus External Cues of State-expressive Behaviors in the Self and the Other.*

Gergely, G., Nadasdy, Z., Csibra, G., & Biro, S. (1995). Taking the intentional stance at 12 months of age. *Cognition, 56*: 165–193.

Gergely, G., & Watson, J. (1996). The social biofeedback model of parental affect-mirroring. *International Journal of Psychoanalysis, 77*: 1181–1212.

Gergely, G., & Watson, J. S. (1999). Early social-emotional development: Contingency perception and the social biofeedback model. In: P. Rochat (Ed.), *Early Social Cognition* (pp. 101–137). Hillsdale, NJ: Lawrence Erlbaum.

Gianino, A., & Tronick, E. Z. (1988). The mutual regulation model: The infant's self and interactive regulation and coping and defensive capacities. In: T. M. Field, P. M. McCabe, & N. Schneiderman (Eds.), *Stress and Coping across Development* (pp. 47–68). Hillsdale, NJ: Lawrence Erlbaum.

Gibbons, M. C., Crits-Christoph, P., Levinson, J., & Barber (2003). Flexibility in manual-based psychotherapies: Predictors of therapist interventions in interpersonal and cognitive-behavioural therapy. *Psychotherapy Research, 13*: 169–185.

Gloning, K., & Sternbach, I. (1953). Überdas Träumen bei zerebralen Herdläsionen. *Wiener Zeitschrift für Nervenheilkunde, 6*: 302–329.

Goldman, A. I. (1993). The psychology of folk psychology. *Behavioral & Brain Sciences, 16* (1): 15–28.

Goldstein, H. (1977). *Policing a Free Society.* Cambridge, MA: Ballinger.

Goldstein, J., Freud, A., & Solnit, A. (1973). *Beyond the Best Interests of the Child, Vol. 1.* New York: Free Press.

Goldstein, J., Freud, A., & Solnit, A. J. (1979). *Before the Best Interests of the Child, Vol. 2.* New York: Free Press.

Goldstein, J., Freud, A., & Solnit, A. (1983). *In the Best Interests of the Child, Vol. 3.* New York: Free Press.

Gonsalez, S., Steinglass, P., & Reiss, D. (1989). Putting the illness in its place: Discussion groups for families with chronic medical illnesses. *Family Process, 28*: 69–87.

Goodman, S. H., & Gottlieb, I. H. (1999). Risk for psychopathology in the children of depressed mothers: A developmental model for understanding mechanisms of transmission. *Psychological Review, 106*: 458–490.

Goodyer, I. M., & Cooper, P. J. (1993). A community study of depression in adolescent girls: 2. The clinical features of identified disorder. *British Journal of Psychiatry, 163*: 374–380.

Gopnik, A. (1993). How we know our minds: The illusion of 1st-person knowledge of intentionality. *Behavioral and Brain Sciences, 16*: 1–14.

Gordon, R. M. (1995). Simulation without introspection or inference from me to you. In: M. Davies & T. Stone (Eds.), *Mental Simulation: Evaluations and Applications* (pp. 53–67). Oxford: Blackwell.

Gould, M. S., Fisher, P., Parides, M., Flory, M., & Shaffer, D. (1996). Psychosocial risk factors of child and adolescent completed suicide. *Archives of General Psychiatry, 53*: 1155–1162.

Gould, M. S., Shaffer, D., & Greenberg, T. (2003). The epidemiology of youth suicide. In: R. A. King & A. Apter (Eds.), *Suicide in Children & Adolescents* (pp. 1–40). Cambridge: Cambridge University Press.

Grienenberger, J., Kelly, K., & Slade, A. (2005). Maternal reflective functioning, mother–infant affective communication, and infant attachment: Exploring the link between mental states and observed caregiving behavior in the intergenerational transmission of attachment. *Attachment and Human Development, 7* (3): 299–311.

Grelotti, D. J., Klin, A., Volkmar, F. R., Gauthier, I., Skudlarski, P., Cohen, D. J., Gore, J. C., & Schultz, R. T. (2005). FMRI activation of the fusiform gyrus and amygdala to cartoon characters but not faces in a boy with autism. *Neuropsychologia, 43* (3): 373–385.

Grienenberger, J., Popek, P., Stein, S., Solow, J., Morrow, M., Levine, N., Alexandre, D., Ibarra, M., Wilson, A., Thompson, J., & Lehman, J. (2004). *The Wright Institute Reflective Parenting Program Workshop Training Manual.* Unpublished manual, The Wright Institute, Los Angeles, CA.

Grigorenko, E. L., Klin, A., Pauls, D. L., Senft, R., Hooper, C., & Volkmar, F. R. (2002). A descriptive study of hyperlexia in a clinically referred sample of children with developmental delays. *Journal of Autism and Developmental Disorders, 32* (1): 3–12.

Grissom, R. J. (1996). The magical number .7 +/- .2: Meta-meta-analysis of the probability of superior outcome in comparisons involving therapy, placebo, and control. *Journal of Consulting and Clinical Psychology, 64*: 973–982.

Grossman, F. K., Pollack, W. S., & Golding E. (1988). Fathers and children: Predicting the quality and quantity of fathering. *Developmental Psychology, 24* (1): 82–91.

Grünstein, A. (1924). Die Erforschung der Träume al seine Methode der topischen Diagnostik bei Grosshirnerkrankungen. *Zeitschrift für die gesamte Neurologie und Psychatrie, 93*: 416–420.

Guedeney, N., Guedeney, A., Rabouanan, C., Mintz, A. S., Danon, G., Heut, M. M., & Jacquemain, F. (2003). The Zero-to-Three diagnostic classification: A contribution to the validation of this classification from a sample of 85 under-threes. *Infant Mental Health Journal, 24:* 313–336.

Gunderson, J., Carpenter, W., & Strauss, J. (1975). Borderline and schizophrenic patients: A comparative study. *American Journal of Psychiatry, 132*: 1257–1264.

Gunnar, M. R., Brodersen, L., Nachmias M., Buss, K., & Rigatuso, J. (1996). Stress reactivity and attachment security. *Developmental Psychobiology, 29* (3): 191–204.

Gutelius, M. F., Kirsch, A. D., MacDonald, S., Brooks, M. R., & McErlean, T. (1977). Controlled study of child health supervision: Behavioral results. *Pediatrics, 60* (3): 294–304.

Gutelius, M. F., Kirsch, A. D., MacDonald, S., Brooks, M. R., McErlean, T., & Newcomb, C. (1972). Promising results from a cognitive stimulation program in infancy. A preliminary report. *Clinical Pediatrics, 11* (10): 585–593.

Haaga, D. A. F. (2000). Introduction to the special section on stepped-care models in psychotherapy. *Journal of Consulting and Clinical Psychology, 68*: 547–548.

Habib, M., & Sigiru, A. (1987). Pure topographical disorientation: A definition and anatomical basis. *Cortex, 23*: 73–85.

Hagoort, P., Hald, L., Bastiaansen, M., & Petersson, K. M. (2004). Integration of word meaning and world knowledge in language comprehension. *Science, 304*: 438–441.

Haigh, R. (2002). Therapeutic community research: Past, present and future. *Psychiatric Bulletin, 26*: 68–70.

Haith, M. M., Bergman, T., & Moore, M. J. (1979). Eye contact and face scanning in early infancy. *Science, 198* (4319): 853–855.

Hamer, D. H., Hu, S., Magnuson, V. L., Hu, N., & Pattatucci, A. M. L. (1993). A linkage between DNA markers on the X-chromosome and male sexual orientation. *Science, 261*: 321–327.

Hammen, C. (2000). Interpersonal factors in an emerging developmental model of depression. In: S. L. Johnson, A. M. Hayes, T. M. Field, N. Schneiderman, & P. McCabe (Eds.), *Stress, Coping, and Depression* (pp. 71–88). Mahwah, NJ: Lawrence Erlbaum.

Hammen, C., Ellicott, A., Gitlin, M., & Jamison, K. R. (1989). Sociotrophy/autonomy and vulnerability to specific life events in patients with unipolar and bipolar disorder. *Journal of Abnormal Psychology, 98*: 154–160.

Hammen, C., Rudolph, K., Weisz, J., Rao, U., & Burge, D. (1999). The context of depression in clinic-referred youth: Neglected areas in treatment. *Journal of the American Academy of Child and Adolescent Psychiatry, 38*: 64–71.

Hansen, S., Harthon, C., Wallin, E., Lofberg, L., & Svensson, K. (1991). Mesotelencephalic dopamine system and reproductive behavior in the female rat: Effects of ventral tegmental 6-hydroxy-dopamine lesions on maternal and sexual responsiveness. *Behavioral Neuroscience, 105*: 588–598.

Happé, F. G. (2005). The weak central coherence account of autism. In: F. R. Volkmar, R. Paul, A. Klin, & D. J. Cohen (Eds)., *Handbook of Autism and Pervasive Developmental Disorders* (3rd edition, pp. 640–649). New York: Wiley.

Harlow, H. F. (1963). The maternal affectional system of rhesus monkeys.

In: H. L. Rheingold (Ed.), *Maternal Behavior in Mammals* (pp. 254–281). New York: Wiley.

Harris, P. L. (1991). The work of imagination. In: A. Whiten (Ed.), *Natural Theories of Mind: Evolution, Development, and Simulation in Everyday Mindreading* (pp. 283–304). Oxford: Blackwell.

Harris, P. L. (1992). From simulation to folk psychology: The case for development. *Mind & Language, 7* (1–2): 120–144. [Special Issue, Mental simulation: Philosophical and psychological essays.]

Harris, P. L., & Kavanaugh, R. D. (1993). Young children's understanding of pretence. *Monographs of the Society of Research on Child Development. 58* (Serial No. 237): 1.

Harris, T. O., Brown, G. W., & Bifulco, A. T. (1990). Depression and situational helplessness/mastery in a sample selected to study childhood parental loss. *Journal of Affective Disorders, 20* (1): 27–41.

Hartmann, B., Russ, D., Oldfield, M., Falke, R., & Skoff, B. (1980). Dream content: Effects of L-Dopa. *Sleep Research, 9*: 153.

Hasson, U., Nir, Y., Levy, I., Fuhrmann, G., & Malach, R. (2004). Intersubject synchronization of cortical activity during natural vision. *Science, 303* (5664): 1634–1640.

Haviland, J., & Lelwicka, M. (1987). The induced affect response: 10-week old infants' responses to three emotional expressions. *Developmental Psychology, 23*: 97–104.

Hawe, P., Shiell, A., & Riley, T. (2004). Complex interventions: How "out of control" can a randomised controlled trial be? *British Medical Journal, 328*: 1561–1563.

Hawton, K., Cole, D., O'Grady, J., & Osborn, M. (1982). Motivational aspects of deliberate self-poisoning in adolescents. *British Journal of Psychiatry, 141*: 286–291.

Hayes, S. C., Follette, V. M., Dawes, R. M., & Grady, K. E. (1995). *Scientific Standards of Psychological Practice: Issues and Recommendations*. Reno, NV: Context Press.

Hebb, D. O. (1949). *Organization of Behavior*. New York: Wiley.

Heider, F., & Simmel, M. (1944). An experimental study of apparent behavior. *American Journal of Psychology, 57* (2): 243–259.

Heinicke, C. (1995). Determinants of the transition to parenting. In: M. Bornstein (Ed.), *Handbook of Parenting, Vol. 3* (pp. 277–303). Mahwah, NJ: Lawrence Erlbaum.

Heiss, W.-D., Pawlik, G., Herholz, K., Wagner, R., & Weinhard, K. (1985). Regional cerebral glucose metabolism in man during wakefulness, sleep and dreaming. *Brain Research, 327*: 362–366.

Hellman, I. (1962). Hampstead Nursery follow-up studies: I. Sudden separation and its effect followed over twenty years. *Psychoanalytic Study of the Child, 17*: 159–174.

Hellman, I. (1983). Work in the Hampstead war nurseries. *International Journal of Psychoanalysis, 64*: 435–439.

Henderson, K., Steele, M., & Hillman, S. (2001). *Experience of Parenting*

Coding Manual. Unpublished manuscript, The Anna Freud Centre, London.

Hendin, H. (1991). Psychodynamics of suicide, with particular reference to the young. *American Journal of Psychiatry, 148*: 1150–1158.

Henry, W. P., Strupp, H. H., Butler, S. F., et al. (1993). The effects of training in time-limited psychotherapy: Changes in therapists' behaviour. *Journal of Consulting and Clinical Psychology, 61*: 434–440.

Herpertz, S. C., Dietrich, T. M., Wenning, B., Krings, T., Erberich, S. G., Willmes, K., Thron, A., & Sass, H. (2001). Evidence of abnormal amygdala functioning in borderline personality disorder: A functional MRI study. *Biological Psychiatry, 50* (4): 292–298.

Herzberg, A. (1945). *Active Psychotherapy.* New York: Grune & Stratton.

Hill, J., Pickles, A., Byatt, M., & Rollinson, L. (2004). Juvenile versus adult onset depression: Multiple differences imply different pathways. *Psychological Medicine, 34*: 1483–1493.

Hoagwood, K., Hibbs, E., Brent, D., & Jensen, P. J. (1995). Efficacy and effectiveness in studies of child and adolescent psychotherapy. *Journal of Consulting and Clinical Psychology, 63*: 683–687.

Hobson, J. (1988). *The Dreaming Brain.* New York: Basic Books.

Hobson, J., & McCarley, R. (1977). The brain as a dream-state generator. *American Journal of Psychiatry, 134*: 1335.

Hobson, J., Stickgold, R., & Pace-Schott, E. (1998). The neuropsychology of REM sleep dreaming. *NeuroReport, 9*: R1.

Hobson, P. (2002). *The Cradle of Thought: Exploring the Origins of Thinking.* London: Macmillan.

Hobson, R. P. (1993). *Autism and the Development of Mind.* Hove: Lawrence Erlbaum.

Hobson, R. P., Ouston, J., & Lee, A. (1988). What's in a face? The case of autism. *British Journal of Psychology, 79*: 441–453.

Hodges, J., & Steele, M. (2000). Effects of abuse on attachment representations: Narrative assessments of abused children. *Journal of Child Psychotherapy, 26*: 433–455.

Hodges, J., Steele, M., Hillman, S., & Henderson, K. (2002). *Coding Manual for Story Stem Assessment Profile.* Unpublished manuscript, The Anna Freud Centre, London.

Hodges, J., Steele, M., Hillman, S., & Henderson, K. (2003). Mental representations and defences in severely maltreated children: A story stem battery and rating system for clinical assessment and research applications. In: R. Emde, D. Wolf, & D. Oppenheim (Eds.), *Narrative Processes and the Transition from Infancy to Early Childhood.* Chicago, IL: University of Chicago Press.

Hodges, J., Steele, M., Hillman, S., Henderson, K., & Kaniuk, J. (2003). Changes in attachment representations over the first year of adoptive placement: Narratives of maltreated children. *Clinical Child Psychology and Psychiatry, 8* (3): 351–367.

Hollon, S. D., & Beck, A. T. (2004). Cognitive and cognitive behavioral therapies. In: M. J. Lambert (Ed.), *Bergin and Garfield's Handbook of Psychotherapy and Behavior Change* (5th edition, pp. 447–492). New York: Wiley.

Hong, C. C., Gillin, J. C., Dow, B. M., Wu, J., & Buchsbaum, M. S. (1995). Localised and lateralized cerebral glucose metabolism associated with rapid eye movements during REM sleep and wakefulness. A positron emission tomography (PET) study. *Sleep, 18*: 570–580.

Hopfield, J. J., & Tank, D. W. (1985). "Neural" computation of decisions in optimization problems. *Biological Cybernetics, 52*: 141–152.

Horowitz, L. M., Rosenberg, S. E., & Bartholomew, K. (1993). Interpersonal problems, attachment styles and outcome in brief dynamic therapy. *Journal of Consulting and Clinical Psychology, 61*: 549–560.

Horowitz, M. J. (1988). Psychodynamic phenomena and their explanation. In: M. J.Horowitz (Ed.), *Psychodynamics and Cognition* (pp. 3–20). Chicago, IL: University of Chicago Press.

Horowitz, M. J., Fridhandler, B., & Stinson, C. D. (1991). Person schemas and emotion. *Journal of the American Psychoanalytic Association, 39*: 173–208.

Hrdy, S. (1999). *Mother Nature: A History of Mother, Infants and Natural Selection*. New York: Pantheon Books.

Hughes, C. W., Emslie, G. J., Crismon, L., Wagner, K. D., Birmaher, B., Geller, B., Pliszka, S. R., Ryan, N. D., Strober, M., Trivedi, M. H., Toprac, M. G., Sedillo, A., Llana, M. E., Lopez, M., Rush, A. J., & The Texas Consensus Conference Panel on Medication Treatment of Childhood Major Depressive Disorder (1999). The Texas children's medication algorithm project: Report of the Texas consensus conference panel on medication treatment of childhood major depressive disorder. *Journal of the American Academy of Child and Adolescent Psychiatry, 38:* 1442–1454.

Humphrey, M., & Zangwill, O. (1951). Cessation of dreaming after brain injury. *Journal of Neurology, Neurosurgery and Psychiatry, 14*: 322–325.

Huot, R. L., Plotsky, P. M., Lenox, R. H., & McNamara, R. K. (2002). Neonatal maternal separation reduces hippocampal mossy fiber density in adult Long Evans rats. *Brain Research, 950* (1–2): 52–63.

Hurst, N., Valentine, C., & Renfro, L. (1997). Skin-to-skin holding in the neonatal intensive care unit influences maternal milk volume. *Journal of Perinatology, 17*: 213–217.

Iacoboni, M. (2000). Attention and sensorimotor integration: Mapping the embodied mind. In: A. W. Toga & J. C. Mazziotta (Eds.), *Brain Mapping: The Systems* (pp. 463–490). San Diego, CA: Academic Press.

Insel, T. R. (2003). Is social attachment an addictive disorder? *Physiology & Behavior, 79* (3): 351–357.

Insel, T. R., & Harbaugh, C. R. (1989). Lesions of the hypothalamic paraventricular nucleus disrupt the initiation of maternal behavior. *Physiology and Behavior, 45*: 1033–1041.

Insel, T. R., & Young, L. J. (2001). The neurobiology of attachment. *Nature Reviews Neuroscience, 2* (2): 129–136.

Izard, C. E. (1979). *The Maximally Discriminative Facial Movement Coding System (MAX)*. Newark, DE: University of Delaware, Office of Instructional Technology.

Izard, C. E. (1991). *The Psychology of Emotions*. New York: Plenum Press.

Izard, C. E., Dougherty, L. M., & Hembree, E. A. (1983). *A System for Identifying Affect Expressions by Holistic Judgments (AFFEX)*. Newark, DE: University of Delaware, Office of Instructional Technology.

Izard, C. E., & Malatesta, C. Z. (1987). Perspectives on emotional development. I. Differential emotions theory of early emotional development. In: J. D. Osofsky (Ed.), *Handbook of Infant Development* (2nd edition, pp. 494–554). New York: Wiley.

Jackendoff, R. (1987). *Consciousness and the Computational Mind*. Cambridge, MA: MIT Press.

Jacobs, N., Van Gestel, S., Derom, C., Thiery, E., Vernon, P., Derom, R., et al. (2001). Heritability estimates of intelligence in twins: Effect of chorion type. *Behavior Genetics, 31*: 209–217.

Jaffee, S. R., Moffitt, T. E., Caspi, A., Fonbonne, E., Poulton, R., & Martin, J. (2002). Differences in early childhood risk factors for juvenile-onset and adult-onset depression. *Archives of General Psychiatry, 59*: 215–222.

Janz, D. (1974). Epilepsy and the sleep–waking cycle. In: P. Vinken & G. Bruyn (Eds.), *Handbook of Clinical Neurology, Vol. 15*. Amsterdam: Elsevier.

Jayson, D., Wood, A., Kroll, L., Fraser, J., & Harrington, R. (1998). Which depressed patients respond to cognitive-behavioral treatment? *Journal of the American Academy of Child and Adolescent Psychiatry, 37*: 35–39.

Jensen, A. L., & Weisz, J. R. (2002). Assessing match and mismatch between practitioner-generated and standardized interviewer-generated diagnoses for clinic-referred children and adolescents. *Journal of Consulting and Clinical Psychology, 70*: 158–168.

Johansson, G. (1973). Visual perception of biological motion and a model for its analysis. *Perception and Psychophysics, 14*: 201–211.

Johnson, J. G., Cohen, P., Brown, J., Smailes, E. M., & Bernstein, D. P. (1999). Childhood maltreatment increases risk for personality disorders during early adulthood. *Archives of General Psychiatry, 56* (7): 600–606.

Johnson, M. (1987). *The Body in the Mind: The Bodily Basis of Meaning, Imagination, and Reason*. Chicago, IL: University of Chicago Press.

Johnson, S., Slaughter, V., & Carey, S. (1998). Whose gaze will infants follow? The elicitation of gaze-following in 12-month-olds. *Developmental Science, 1*: 233–238.

Jones, B. (1979). Elimination of paradoxical sleep by lesions of the pontine gigantocellular tegmental field in the cat. *Neuroscience. Letters, 13*: 285.

Jouvet, M. (1962). Recherches sur les structures nerveuses et les mécanismes responsables des differentes phases du sommeil physiologique. *Archives Italiennes de Biologie, 153*: 125.

Jus, A., et al. (1973). Studies on dream recall in chronic schizophrenic patients after prefrontal lobotomy. *Biological Psychiatry, 6*: 275.

Kagan, J. (1992). The conceptual analysis of affects. In: T. Shapiro, & R. N. Emde (Eds.), *Affects: Psychoanalytic Perspectives*. Madison, CT: International Universities Press.

Kanner, L. (1943). Autistic disturbances of affective contact. *The Nervous Child, 2*: 217–253.

Kanwisher, N., McDermott, J., & Chun, M. (1997). The fusiform face area: A module in human extrastriate cortex specialized for face perception. *Journal of Neuroscience, 17*: 4302–4311.

Kapur, S. (2003). Psychosis as a state of aberrant salience: A framework linking biology, phenomenology, and pharmacology in schizophrenia. *American Journal of Psychiatry, 160*: 13–23.

Kardiner, A. (1932). The bio-analysis of the epileptic reaction. *Psychoanalytic Quarterly, 1*: 375–483.

Karpf, J. C. (2004). *The Functional Implications of Early Parental Imitation: A Prospective Study of Infants From Two to 18 Months*. Unpublished Ph.D. thesis, University of Reading.

Kaslow, N. J., & Thompson, M. P. (1998). Applying the criteria for empirically supported treatments to studies of psychosocial interventions for child and adolescent depression. *Journal of Clinical Child Psychology, 27*: 146–155.

Kaufman, E., & Kaufman, P. (1979). Multiple family therapy with drug abusers. In: E. Kaufman & P. Kaufman (Eds.), *Family Therapy of Drug and Alcohol Abuse*. New York: Gardner.

Kazdin, A. E. (1978). *History of Behavior Modification: Experimental Foundations of Contemporary Research*. Baltimore, MD: University Park Press.

Kazdin, A. E. (1981). Drawing valid inferences from case studies. *Journal of Consulting and Clinical Psychology, 49*: 183–192.

Kazdin, A. E. (1993). Evaluation in clinical practice: Clinically sensitive and systematic methods of treatment delivery. *Behavior Therapy, 24*: 11–45.

Kazdin, A. E. (1999). The meanings and measurement of clinical significance. *Journal of Consulting and Clinical Psychology, 67*: 332–339.

Kazdin, A. E. (2000a). Developing a research agenda for child and adolescent psychotherapy research. *Archives of General Psychiatry, 57*: 829–835.

Kazdin, A. E. (2000b). *Psychotherapy for Children and Adolescents: Directions for Research and Practice*. New York: Oxford University Press.

Kazdin, A. E. (2001). Almost clinically significant (*p* < .10): Current measures may only approach clinical significance. *Clinical Psychology: Science and Practice, 8*: 455–462.

Kazdin, A. E. (2005). *Parent Management Training: Treatment for Oppositional, Aggressive, and Antisocial Behavior in Children and Adolescents*. New York: Oxford University Press.

Kazdin, A. E. (2006). Mechanisms of change in psychotherapy: Advances, breakthroughs, and cutting-edge research (do not yet exist). In: R. R. Bootzin (Ed.). *Festschrift in Honor of Lee Sechrest*. Washington, DC: American Psychological Association.

Kazdin, A. E., Bass, D., Ayers, W. A., & Rodgers, A. (1990). The empirical and clinical focus of child and adolescent psychotherapy research. *Journal of Consulting and Clinical Psychology, 58*: 729–740.

Kazdin, A. E., & Weisz, J. R. (1998). Identifying and developing empirically supported child and adolescent treatments. *Journal of Consulting and Clinical Psychology, 66:* 19–36.

Kazdin, A. E., & Weisz, J. R. (Eds.) (2003). *Evidence-Based Psychotherapies for Children and Adolescents*. New York: Guilford Press.

Kellaway, P., & Frost, J. (1983). Biorythmic modulation of epileptic events. In: T. Pedley & B. Meldrum (Eds.), *Recent Advances in Epilepsy, Vol. 1* (pp. 139–154). Edinburgh/London: Churchill Livingstone.

Kelling, G. L., & Moore, M. H. (1989). *The Evolving Strategy of Policing.* Washington, DC: U.S. Dept. of Justice, Office of Justice Programs, National Institute of Justice.

Kendall, P. C. (Ed.) (1999). Special section: Clinical significance. *Journal of Consulting and Clinical Psychology, 67*: 283–339.

Kendall, P. C., & Grove, W. M. (1988). Normative comparisons in therapy outcome. *Behavioral Assessment, 10:* 147–158.

Kendall, P. C., & Southam-Gerow, M. A. (1995). Issues in the transportability of treatment: The case of anxiety disorders for youth. *Journal of Consulting and Clinical Psychology, 63:* 702–708.

Kendler, K. S., Kessler, R. C., Neale, M. C., Heath, A. C., & Eaves, L. J. (1993). The prediction of major depression in women: Toward an integrated etiologic model. *American Journal of Psychiatry, 150* (8): 1139–1148.

Keren, M., Feldman, R., Eidelman, A. I., Sirota, L., & Lester, B. (2003). Clinical Interview for high-risk parents of premature infants (CLIP): Relations to mother–infant interaction. *Infant Mental Health Journal, 24*: 93–110.

Keren, M., Feldman, R., & Tyano, S. (2001). Emotional disturbances in infancy: Diagnostic classification and interactive patterns of infants referred to a community-based infant mental health clinic. *Journal of the American Academy of Child and Adolescent Psychiatry, 40*: 27–35.

Kerr, N. H., Foulkes D., & Jurkovic, G. (1978). Reported absence of visual dream imagery in a normally sighted subject with Turner's syndrome. *Journal of Mental Imagery, 2*: 247–264.

King, M. (1998). *Bangin'* [videorecording]. Boston, MA: Boston Productions, Inc.

King, R. A. (2003). Psychodynamic approaches to youth suicide. In: R. A. King & A. Apter (Eds.), *Suicide in Children and Adolescents*. New York: Cambridge University Press.

King, R. A., Ruchkin, V. V., & Schwab-Stone, M. (2003). Suicide and the "continuum of adolescent self destructiveness": Is there a connection? In: R. A. King & A. Apter (Eds.), *Suicide in Children and Adolescents.* New York: Cambridge University Press.

King-Casas, B., Tomlin, D., Anen, C., Carmerea, C., Quartz, S., & Montague, P. R. (2005). Getting to know you: Reputation and trust in a two-person economic exchange. *Science, 38*: 78–82.

Király, I., Csibra, G., & Gergely, G. (2004). "The Role of Communicative-Referential Cues in Observational Learning during the Second Year." Poster presented at the 14th Biennial International Conference on Infant Studies, Chicago (May).

Kitzman, H., Olds, D. L., Sidora, K., Henderson, C. R. Jr., Hanks, C., Cole, R., Luckey, D. W., Bondy, J., Cole, K., & Glazner, J. (2000). Enduring effects of nurse home visitation on maternal life course: A 3-year follow-up of a randomized trial. *Journal of the American Medical Association, 283* (15): 1983–1989.

Klawans, H., Moskowitz, C., Lupton, N., & Scharf, B. (1978). Induction of dreams by levodopa. *Harefuah, 45*: 57.

Klin, A. (2000). Attributing social meaning to ambiguous visual stimuli in higher functioning autism and Asperger syndrome: The Social Attribution Task. *Journal of Child Psychology and Psychiatry, 41*: 831–846.

Klin, A., Chawarska, K., Paul, R., Rubin, E., Morgan, T., Wiesner, L., & Volkmar, F. (2004). Autism in a 15-month-old child. *American Journal of Psychiatry, 161* (11): 1981–1988.

Klin, A., & Jones, W. (2006). Attributing social and physical meaning to ambiguous visual stimuli in higher functioning individuals with autism spectrum disorders. *Brain & Cognition, 61*: 40–53.

Klin, A., & Jones, W. (submitted). Watching a face but not seeing a person: Social engagement in a 15-month-old toddler with autism.

Klin, A., Jones, W., Schultz, R. T., & Volkmar, F. R. (2003). The enactive mind—from actions to cognition: Lessons from autism. *Philosophical Transactions of the Royal Society, Biological Sciences, 358*: 345–360.

Klin, A., Jones, W., Schultz, R., Volkmar, F., & Cohen, D. (2002a). Defining and quantifying the social phenotype in autism. *American Journal of Psychiatry, 159* (6): 895–908.

Klin, A., Jones, W., Schultz, R., Volkmar, F. R., & Cohen, D. (2002b). Visual fixation patterns during viewing of naturalistic social situations as predictors of social competence in individuals with autism. *Archives of General Psychiatry, 59* (9): 809–816.

Klin, A., Schultz, R., & Cohen, D. (2000). Theory of mind in action: Developmental perspectives on social neuroscience. In: S. Baron-Cohen, H. Tager-Flusberg, & D. Cohen (Eds.), *Understanding Other Minds: Perspectives from Developmental Neuroscience* (2nd edition, pp. 357–388). Oxford: Oxford University Press.

Klin, A., Sparrow, S. S., de Bildt, A., Cicchetti, D. V., Cohen, D. J., & Volkmar, F. R. (1999). A normed study of face recognition in autism and related disorders. *Journal of Autism and Developmental Disorders, 29* (6): 497–507.

Kondo, T., Antrobus, J., & Fein, C. (1989). Later REM activation and sleep mentation. *Sleep Research, 18*: 147.

Koob, G. F., & Le Moal, M. (1997). Drug abuse: Hedonic homeostatic dysregulation. *Science, 278* (5335): 52–58.

Koós, O., & Gergely, G. (2001). A contingency-based approach to the etiology of "disorganized" attachment: The "flickering switch" hypothesis. *Bulletin of the Menninger Clinic, 65* (3): 397–410.

Kosslyn, S. (1994). *Image and Brain*. Cambridge, MA: MIT Press.

Kovacs, M. (1992). *Children's Depression Inventory Manual.* North Tonawanda, NY: Multi-Health Systems.

Kovacs, M. (1996). Presentation and course of major depressive disorder during childhood and later years of the life span. *Journal of the American Academy of Child and Adolescent Psychiatry, 35:* 705–715.

Kovacs, M., Obrosky, D. S., Gatsonis, C., & Richards, C. (1997). First-episode major depressive and dysthymic disorder in childhood: Clinical and sociodemographic factors in recovery. *Journal of the American Academy of Child and Adolescent Psychiatry, 36:* 777–784.

Kraemer, H. C., Stice, E., Kazdin, A. E., Offord, D. R., & Kupfer, D. J. (2001). How do risk factors work together? Mediators, moderators, independent, overlapping, and proxy-risk factors. *American Journal of Psychiatry, 158*: 848–856.

Kraemer, H. C., Wilson, G. T., Fairburn, C. G., & Agras, W. S. (2002). Mediators and moderators of treatment effects in randomized clinical trials. *Archives of General Psychiatry, 59*: 877–883.

Kreisler, L., Fain, M., & Soulé, M. (1974). *L'enfant et son corps.* Paris: Presses Universitaires de France.

Kuhl, P. (2004). Early language acquisition: Cracking the speech code. *Nature Reviews Neuroscience, 5* (11): 831–843.

Kuipers, L., Leff, J., & Lam, D. (1992). *Family Work for Schizophrenia: A Practical Guide*. London: Gaskell.

Kwon, S., & Oei, T. P. S. (2003). Cognitive processes in a group cognitive behavior therapy of depression. *Journal of Behavior Therapy and Experimental Psychiatry, 34*: 73–85.

Ladd, C. O., Huot, R. L., Thrivikraman, K. V., Nemeroff, C. B., Meaney, M. J., & Plotsky, P. M. (2000). Long-term behavioral and neuroendocrine adaptations to adverse early experience. In: E. A. Mayer & C. B. Saper (Eds.), *Progress in Brain Research: The Biological Basis for Mind Body Interactions, Vol. 122* (pp. 81–103). Amsterdam: Elsevier.

Lakoff, G., & Johnson, M. (1999). *Philosophy in the Flesh: The Embodied Mind and Its Challenge to Western Thought*. New York: Basic Books.

Lambert, M. J. (2004). *Bergin and Garfield's Handbook of Psychotherapy and Behaviour Change*. New York: Wiley.

Lambert, W., Salzer, M. S., & Bickman, L. (1998). Clinical outcome, consumer satisfaction, and ad hoc ratings of improvement in children's mental health. *Journal of Consulting and Clinical Psychology, 66*: 270–279.

Laor, N., Wolmer, L., & Cohen, D. J. (2001). Mothers' functioning and children's symptoms 5 years after a SCUD missile attack. *American Journal of Psychiatry, 158*: 1020–1026.

Laor, N., Wolmer, L., Kora, M., Yucel, D., Spirinan, S., & Yazgan, Y. (2002). Posttraumatic, dissociative and grief symptoms in Turkish children exposed to the 1999 earthquakes. *Journal of Nervous and Mental Disease, 190*: 824–832.

Laor, N., Wolmer, L., Mayes, L. C., Golomb, A., Silverberg, D. S., Weizman, R., & Cohen, D. J. (1996). Israeli preschoolers under Scud missile attacks: A developmental perspective on risk-modifying factors. *Archives of General Psychiatry, 53*: 416–423.

Lapsley, P. (2004). Commentary: Patients in medical education and research. *British Medical Journal, 329*: 334.

Laqueur, H. P. (1972). Mechanisms of change in multiple family therapy. In: C. J. Sager & H. S. Kaplan (Eds.), *Progress in Group and Family Therapy*. New York: Bruner/Mazel.

Laqueur, H. P. (1973). Multiple family therapy: Questions and answers. In: D. Bloch (Ed.), *Techniques of Family Psychotherapy*. New York: Grune & Stratton.

Laqueur, H. P., La Burt, H. A., & Morong, E. (1964). Multiple family therapy: Further developments. *International Journal of Social Psychiatry, 10*: 69–80.

Lavie, P., & Tzichinsky, O. (1984). Cognitive asymmetries after waking from REM and nonREM sleep: Effects of delayed testing and handedness. *International Journal of Neuroscience, 23*: 311–315.

Leckman, J. F., Carter, C. S., Hennessy, M. B., Hrdy, S. B., Kervene, E. B., Klann-Delius, G., Schradin, C., Todt, D., & von Holst, D. (2006). Biobehavioral processes in attachment and bonding. In: C. S. Carter, L. Ahnert, K. E. Grossman, S. B. Hrdy, M. E. Lamb, S. W. Porges, & N. Sachser (Eds.), *Attachment and Bonding: A New Synthesis* (pp. 301–348). Dahlem Workshop Report 92. Cambridge, MA: MIT Press.

Leckman, J. F., Feldman, R., Swain, J. E., Eicher, V., Thompson, N., & Mayes, L. C. (2004). Primary parental preoccupation: Circuits, genes, and the crucial role of the environment. *Journal of Neural Transmission, 111*: 753–771.

Leckman, J. F., & Herman, A. (2002). Maternal behavior and developmental psychopathology. *Biological Psychiatry, 51* (1): 27–43.

Leckman, J. F., & Mayes, L. C. (1998). Understanding developmental psychopathology: How useful are evolutionary perspectives? *Journal of the American Academy of Child and Adolescent Psychiatry*, 37: 1011–1021.

Leckman, J. F., Mayes, L. C., & Cohen, D. J. (2002). Primary maternal preoccupation—revisited: Circuits, genes, and the crucial role of early life experience. *South African Psychiatry Review, 5* (2): 4–12.

Leckman, J. F., Mayes, L. C., Feldman, R., Evans, D., King, R. A., & Cohen, D. J. (1999). Early parental preoccupations and behaviors and their possible relationship to the symptoms of obsessive-compulsive disorder. *Acta Psychiatrica Scandinavica, 100* (Suppl. 396): 1–26.

LeDoux, J. (2002). *Synaptic Self: How Our Brains Become Who We Are*. New York: Viking/Penguin.

Legros, J. J., Chiodera, P., & Geenen, V. (1988). Inhibitory action of exogenous oxytocin on plasma cortisol in normal human subjects: Evidence of action at the adrenal level. *Neuroendocrinology, 48* (2): 204–206.

Leibenluft, E., Gobbini, M. I., Harrison, T., & Haxby, J. V. (2004). Mothers' neural activation in response to pictures of their children and other children. *Biological Psychiatry, 56* (4): 225–232.

Leichter, E., & Shulman, G. L. (1974). Multiple family group therapy: A multidimensional approach. *Family Process, 13*: 95–110.

Lena, I., Deschaux, O., Muffat, S., Parrot, S., Sauvinet, V., Suaud-Chagny, M.-F., Renaud, B., & Gottesmann, C. (2004). Dreaming and schizophrenia have the same neurochemical background. *Sleep Research, 13* (Suppl. 1): 141.

Leslie, A. M. (1987). Pretense and representation: The origins of "Theory of Mind." *Psychological Review, 94*: 412–426.

Lester, B. M., Hoffman, J., & Brazelton, T. B. (1985). The rhythmic structure of mother–infant interaction in term and preterm infants. *Child Development, 56*: 15–27.

Levine, A., Feldman, R., & Weller, A. (2004). "A Psychoneuroendocrinological Study of Antenatal Depression and Bonding." Paper presented at the 37th annual meeting of the International Society for Developmental Psychobiology, Aix-en-Provence, France (25–28 June).

Levine, S. (1975). Psychosocial factors in growth and development. In: L. Levi (Ed.), *Society, Stress and Disease* (pp. 43–50). London: Oxford University Press.

Levitt, E. E. (1957). The results of psychotherapy with children: An evaluation. *Journal of Consulting Psychology, 21*: 189–196.

Levitt, E. E. (1963). Psychotherapy with children: A further evaluation. *Behaviour Research and Therapy, 60*: 326–329.

Lewinsohn, P. M., & Clarke, G. N. (1999). Psychosocial treatments for adolescent depression. *Clinical Psychology Review, 19*: 329–342.

Lewinsohn, P. M., Clarke, G. N., Hops, H., & Andrews, J. (1990). Cognitive-behavioral treatment for depressed adolescents. *Behavior Therapy, 21*: 385–401.

Lewinsohn, P. M., Clarke, G. N., Rohde, P., Hops, H., & Seeley, J. R. (1996). A course in coping: A cognitive-behavioral approach to the treatment of adolescent depression. In: E. D. Hibbs & P. S. Jensen (Eds.), *Psychosocial Treatments for Child and Adolescent Disorders: Empirically Based Strategies for Clinical Practice* (pp. 109–135). Washington, DC: American Psychological Association.

Lewinsohn, P. M., Gotlib, I. H., & Hautzinger, M. (1998). Behavioral treatment of unipolar depression. In: V. E. Caballo (Ed.), *International Handbook of Cognitive and Behavioural Treatments for Psychological Disorders* (pp. 441–488). Oxford: Pergamon.

Lewinsohn, P. M., Hops, H., Roberts, R. E., Seeley, J. R., & Andrews, J. A. (1993). Adolescent psychopathology, I: Prevalence and incidence of depression and other DSM-III-R disorders in high school students. *Journal of Abnormal Psychology, 102*: 133–144.

Lewinsohn, P. M., Rohde, P., Seeley, J. R., & Baldwin, C. L. (2001). Gender differences in suicide attempts from adolescence to young adulthood. *Journal of the American Academy of Child and Adolescent Psychiatry, 40* (4): 427–434.

Lewis, M., Allessandri, S. M., & Sullivan, M. W. (1990). Violation of expectancy, loss of control and anger expressions in young infants. *Developmental Psychology, 26* (5): 745–751.

Lewis, M., & Brooks, J. (1978). Self-knowledge and emotional development. In: M. Lewis & L. A. Rosenblum (Eds.), *The Development of Affect* (pp. 205–226). New York: Plenum Press.

Lewis, M., & Granic, I. (2000). *Emotion, Development, and Self-Organization: Dynamic Systems Approaches to Emotional Development*. Cambridge: Cambridge University Press.

Lewis, M., & Michalson, L. (1983). *Children's Emotions and Moods: Developmental Theory and Measurement*. New York: Plenum Press.

Li, M., Diorio, J., Day, J. C., Francis, D. D., & Meaney, M. J. (2000). Maternal care, hippocampal synaptogenesis and cognitive development in rats. *Nature Neuroscience, 3*: 799–806.

Li, M., Diorio, J., Tannenbaum, B., Caldji, C., Francis, D., Freedman, A., Sharma, S., Pearson, D., Plotsky, P. M., & Meaney, M. J. (1997). Maternal care, hippocampal glucocorticoid receptors, and hypothalamic-pituitary-adrenal responses to stress. *Science, 277*: 1659–1662.

Li, M., & Fleming, A. S. (2003). The nucleus accumbens shell is critical for normal expression of pup-retrieval in postpartum female rats. *Behavioural Brain Research, 145* (1–2): 99–111.

Lieberman, A., Silverman, R., & Pawl, J. (1999). Infant–parent psychotherapy: Core concepts and current approaches. In: C. H. Zeanah (Ed.), *Handbook of Infant Mental Health* (pp. 472–485). New York: Guilford Press.

Lim, C. (2000). *A Pilot Study of Families: Experiences of a Multi-Family Group Day Treatment Programme*. Unpublished MSc thesis, Institute of Psychiatry, London.

Linehan, M. M. (1993). *Cognitive-Behavioural Treatment of Borderline Personality Disorder*. New York: Guilford Press.

Liu, D., Diorio, J., Day, J. C., Francis, D. D., & Meaney, M. J. (2000). Maternal care, hippocampal synaptogenesis and cognitive development in rats. *Nature Neuroscience, 3* (8): 799–806.

Liu, D., Diorio, J., Tannenbaum, B., Caldji, C., Francis, D., Freedman, A., et al. (1997). Maternal care, hippocampal glucocorticoid receptors, and hypothalamic-pituitary-adrenal responses to stress. *Science, 277* (5332): 1659–1662.

Liu, Y., & Wang, Z. X. (2003). Nucleus accumbens oxytocin and dopamine interact to regulate pair bond formation in female prairie voles. *Neuroscience, 121* (3): 537–544.

Llinás, R., Ribary, U., Contreras, D., & Pedroarena, C. (1998). The neuronal basis for consciousness. *Philosophical Transactions of the Royal Society London, B, Biological Sciences, 353*: 1929–1933.

Loewald, H. (1960). On the therapeutic action of psychoanalysis. *International Journal of Psychoanalysis, 41*: 16–33.

Lonigan, C. J., & Elbert, J. C. (Eds.) (1998). Special issue on empirically supported psychosocial interventions for children. *Journal of Clinical Child Psychology, 27* (2).

Lorberbaum, J. P., Newman, J. D., Horwitz, A. R., Dubno, J. R., Lydiard, R. B., Hamner, M. B., Bohning, D. E., & George, M. S. (2002). A potential role for thalamocingulate circuitry in human maternal behavior. *Biological Psychiatry, 51* (6): 431–445.

Lord, C., & Paul, R. (1997). Language and communication in autism. In: D. Cohen & F. Volkmar (Eds.), *Handbook of Autism and Pervasive Developmental Disorders* (pp. 195–225). New York: Wiley.

Loup, F., Tribollet, E., Dubois-Dauphin, M., & Dreifuss, J. J. (1991). Localization of high-affinity binding sites for oxytocin and vasopressin in the human brain. An autoradiographic study. *Brain Research, 555* (2): 220–232.

Lovic, V., Gonzalez, A., & Fleming, A. S. (2001). Maternally separated rats show deficits in maternal care in adulthood. *Developmental Psychobiology, 39* (1): 19–33.

Luborsky, L., Crits-Christoph, P., Mintz, J., & Auerbach, A. (1988). *Who Will Benefit from Psychotherapy? Predicting Therapeutic Outcomes*. New York: Basic Books.

Luborsky, L., Diguer, L., Seligman, D. A., et al. (1999). The researcher's own therapy allegiances: A "wild card" in comparisons of treatment efficacy. *Clinical Psychology: Science and Practice, 6*: 95–106.

Luborsky, L., Singer, B., & Luborsky, L. (1975). Comparative studies of psychotherapies: Is it true that "everyone has won and all must have prizes"? *Archives of General Psychiatry, 32*: 995–1008.

Lugaresi, E., Medori, R., Montagna, P., Baruzzi, A., Cortelli, P., Lugaresi, A., Tinuper, P., Zucconi, M., & Gambetti, P. (1986). Fatal familial insomnia and dysautonomia with selective degeneration of thalamic nuclei. *New England Journal of Medicine, 315*: 997–1003.

Luria, A. (1973). *The Working Brain*. Harmondsworth: Penguin.

Lyman, R., Kwan, S., & Chao, W. (1983). Left occipito-parietal tumour with observations on alexia and agraphia in Chinese and in English. *Chinese Medical Journal, 54*: 491–516.

Lyons-Ruth, K., & Jacobvitz, D. (1999). Attachment disorganization: Unresolved loss, relational violence, and lapses in behavioral and attentional strategies. In: J. Cassidy & P. Shaver (Eds.), *Handbook of Attachment: Theory, Research, and Clinical Implications* (pp. 520–554). New York: Guilford Press.

Macrae, D., & Trolle, E. (1956). The defect of function in visual agnosia. *Brain, 79*: 94–110.

Madsen, P. C. (1993). Blood flow and oxygen uptake in the human brain during various states of sleep and wakefulness. *Acta Neurologica Scandinavia, 88*: 919.

Madsen, P. C., Holm, S., Vorstup, S., Friberg, L., Lassen. N. A., & Wildschiodtz, L. F. (1991a). Human regional cerebral blood flow during rapid eye movement sleep. *Journal of Cerebral Flow and Metabolism, 11*: 502–507

Madsen, P. C., Schmidt, J. F., Wildschiodtz, L. F., Holm, S., Vorstup, S., & Lassen, N. A. (1991b). Cerebral O_2 metabolism and cerebral blood flow in humans during deep and rapid eye movement sleep. *Journal of Applied Physiology, 70*: 2597–2601.

Madsen, P. C., & Vorstrup, S. (1991). Cerebral blood flow and metabolism during sleep. *Cerebrovascular and Brain Metabolism Reviews, 3*: 281–296.

Mahler, M., Pine, F., & Bergman, A. (1975). *The Psychological Birth of the Human Infant: Symbiosis and Individuation*. New York: Basic Books.

Main, M. (1997). The organized categories of infant, child, and adult attachment: Flexible vs. inflexible attention under attachment-related stress. *Journal of the American Psychoanalytic Association, 48* (4): 1055–1095.

Main, M., & Hesse, E. (1990). Parents' unresolved traumatic experiences are related to infant disorganised attachment status: Is frightened and/or frightening parental behaviour the linking mechanism? In: M. T. Greenberg, D. Cicchetti, & E. M. Cummings (Eds.), *Attachment in the Preschool Years: Theory, Research and Intervention* (pp. 161–182). Chicago, IL: University of Chicago Press.

Main, M., Kaplan, N., & Cassidy, J. (1985). Security in infancy, childhood, and adulthood: A move to the level of representation. In: I. Bretherton & E. Waters (Eds.), *Growing Points of Attachment Theory and Research. Monographs of the Society for Research in Child Development, 50* (1–2, Serial No. 209): 66–104.

Main, M., & Solomon, J. (1990). Procedures for identifying infants as disorganized/disoriented during Ainsworth Strange Situation. In: M. Greenberg, D. Cicchetti, & E. Cummings (Eds.), *Attachment in the Preschool Years: Theory Research and Intervention* (pp. 121–160). Chicago, IL: University of Chicago Press.

Maina, G., Albert, U., Bogetto, F., Vaschetto, P., & Ravizza, L. (1999). Recent life events and obsessive-compulsive disorder (OCD): The role of pregnancy/delivery. *Psychiatry Research, 89* (1): 49–58.

Malatesta, C. Z., & Izard, C. E. (1984). The ontogenesis of human social signals: From biological imperative to symbol utilization. In: N. A. Fox & R. J. Davidson (Eds.), *The Psychobiology of Affective Development* (pp. 161–206). Hillsdale, NJ: Lawrence Erlbaum.

Malatesta, C. Z., Culver, C., Tesman, R. J., & Shepard, B. (1989). The development of emotion expression during the first two years of life. *Monographs of the Society for Research in Child Development, 54* (Serial No. 219).

Mandler, J. (1992). How to build a baby: II. Conceptual primitives. *Psychological Review, 99* (4): 587–604.

Maquet, P., Dive, D., Salmon, E., Sadzot, B., Granco, G., Poirrier, R., & Franck, G. (1990). Cerebral glucose utilization during sleep–wake cycle in man determined by positron emission tomography and [18F]-2-fluoro-2 deoxy-D glucose method. *Brain Research, 513*: 136–143.

Maquet, P., Peters, J.-M., Aerts, J., Delfiore, G., Degueldre, C., Luxen, A., & Franck, G. (1996). Functional neuroanatomy of human rapid-eye-movement sleep and dreaming. *Nature, 383*: 163–166.

Marans, S. (1994). Community violence and children's development: Collaborative interventions. In: C. Chiland & J. G. Young (Eds.), *Children and Violence* (pp. 109–124). Northvale, NJ: Aronson.

Marans, S. (2004). Psychoanalytic responses to violent trauma: The Child Development-Community Policing Partnership. In: B. Skalrew, S. Twemlow, & S. Wilkinson (Eds.), *Analysts in the Trenches: Streets, Schools, War Zones* (pp. 211–236). Hillsdale, NJ: Analytic Press.

Marans, S., & Adelman, A. (1997). Experiencing violence in a developmental context. In: J. D. Osofsky (Ed.), *Children in a Violent Society* (pp. 202–222). New York: Guilford Press.

Marans, S., Berkman, M., & Cohen, D. (1996). Child development and adaptation to catastrophic circumstances. In: R. J. Apfel & B. Simon (Eds.), *Minefields in Their Hearts: The Mental Health of Children in War and Communal Violence* (pp. 104–127). New Haven, CT: Yale University Press.

Marans, S., & Cohen, D. J. (1993). Children and inner-city violence: Strategies for intervention. In: L. A. Leavitt & N. A. Fox (Eds.), *The Psychological Effects of War and Violence on Children* (pp. 281–301). Hillsdale, NJ: Lawrence Erlbaum Associates.

Markand, O., & Dyken, M. (1976). Sleep abnormalities in patients with brain stem lesions. l. *Neurology, 26*: 769–776.

Markman, A. N., & Dietrich, E. (2000). Extending the classical view of representation. *Trends in Cognitive Science, 4*: 470–475.

Marrs, R. W. (1995). A meta-analysis of bibliotherapy studies. *American Journal of Community Psychology, 23*: 843–870.

Masserman, J. H. (1943). *Behavior and Neurosis: An Experimental Psycho-Analytic Approach to Psychobiologic Principles.* Chicago, IL: University of Chicago Press.

Matthiesen, A. S., Ransjo-Arvidson, A. B., Nissen, E., & Uvnas-Moberg, K. (2001). Postpartum maternal oxytocin release by newborns: Effects of infant hand massage and sucking. *Birth, 28*: 13–19.

Maughan, B., & Lindelow, M. (1997). Secular change in psychosocial risks: The case of teenage motherhood. *Psychological Medicine, 27* (5): 1129–1144.

Mayes, L. C. (2003). "Reflections on Future Challenges for Psychoanalysis." Paper presented at the Meeting of the Western New England Psychoanalytic Society, New Haven, CT (October).

Mayes, L., Swain, J., & Leckman, J. (2005). Parental attachment systems: Neural circuits, genes, and experiential contributions to parental engagement. *Clinical Neuroscience Research, 4*: 301–313.

McBeath, M., Shaffer, D., & Kaiser, M. (1995). How baseball outfielders determine where to run to catch fly balls. *Science, 268*: 569–573.

McCarley, R., & Hobson, J. A. (1975). Neuronal excitability modulation over the sleep cycle: A structural and mathematical model. *Science, 189*: 58.

McCarley, R., & Hobson, J. A. (1977). The neurobiological origins of psychoanalytic dream theory. *American Journal of Psychiatry, 134*: 1211.

McCarton, C. M., Brooks-Gunn, J., Wallace, I. F., Bauer, C. R., Bennett, F. C., Bernbaum, J. C., Broyles, R. S., Casey, P. H., McCormick, M. C., Scott, D. T., Tyson, J., Tonascia, J., & Meinert, C. L. (1997). Results at age 8 years of early intervention for low-birth-weight premature infants: The Infant Health and Development Program. *Journal of the American Medical Association, 277* (2): 126–132.

McClelland, J. L., & Rumelhart, D. E. (1986). *Parallel Distributed Processing: Explorations in the Microstructure of Cognition, Vol. 2: Psychological and Biological Models*. Cambridge, MA: MIT Press.

McCloskey, M. S., Phan, K. L., & Coccaro, E. F. (2005). Neuroimaging and personality disorders. *Current Psychiatry Reports, 7* (1): 65–72.

McClure, S. M., Daw, N. D., & Montague, P. R. (2003). A computational substrate for incentive salience. *Trends in Neuroscience, 26* (8): 423–428.

McDonough, S. C. (2000). Interaction guidance: An approach for difficult-to-engage families. In: C. H. Zeanah (Ed.), *Handbook of Infant Mental Health* (2nd edition, pp. 485–493). New York: Guildford Press.

McFarlane, W. R. (1982). Multiple family in the psychiatric hospital. In: H. Harbin (Ed.), *The Psychiatric Hospital and the Family*. New York: Spectrum.

McFarlane, W. R. (Ed.) (1993). Multiple family groups and the treatment of schizophrenia. In: *Family Therapy in Schizophrenia*. New York: Guilford Press.

Mead, G. H. (1934). *Mind, Self, and Society*. Chicago, IL: University of Chicago Press.

Meaney, M. J. (2001). Maternal care, gene expression, and the transmission of individual differences in stress reactivity across generations. *Annual Review of Neuroscience, 24* (1): 1161–1192.

Meaney, M. J., Brake, W., & Gratton, A. (2002). Environmental regulation of the development of mesolimbic dopamine systems: A neurobiological mechanism for vulnerability to drug abuse? *Psychoneuroendocrinology, 27* (1–2): 127–138.

Meltzoff, A. N. (1995). Understanding the intention of others: Re-enactment of intended acts by 18-month-old children. *Developmental Psychology, 31*: 838–850.

Meltzoff, A. N. (2002). Imitation as a mechanism of social cognition: Origins of empathy, theory of mind, and the representation of action. In: U. Goshwami (Ed.), *Blackwell Handbook of Childhood Cognitive Development* (pp. 6–25). Oxford: Blackwell.

Meltzoff, A. N., & Gopnik, A. (1993). The role of imitation in understanding persons and developing a theory of mind. In: S. Baron-Cohen, H.

Tager-Flusberg, & D. J. Cohen (Eds.), *Understanding Other Minds: Perspectives from Autism* (pp. 335–365). Oxford: Oxford University Press.
Meltzoff, A. N., & Moore, M. K. (1977). Imitation of facial and manual gestures by human neonates. *Science, 198*: 75–78.
Meltzoff, A. N., & Moore, M. K. (1989). Imitation in newborn infants: Exploring the range of gestures imitated and the underlying mechanisms. *Developmental Psychology, 25*: 954–962.
Meltzoff, A. N., & Moore, M. K. (1997). Explaining facial imitation: Theoretical model. *Early Development and Parenting, 6*: 179–192.
Meltzoff, A. N., & Moore, M. K. (1998). Infant intersubjectivity: Broadening the dialogue to include imitation, identity and intention. In: S. Braten (Ed.), *Intersubjective Communication and Emotion in Early Ontogeny* (pp. 47–62). Cambridge: Cambridge University Press.
Michel, F., & Sieroff, E. (1981). Une approache anatomo-clinique des deficits de l'imagerie oreirique, est-elle possible? In: *Sleep: Proceedings of an International Colloquium*. Milan: Carlo Erba Formitala.
Mill, J. S. (1843). *A System of Logic*. London: John W. Parker.
Miller, L., Kramer, R., Warner, V., Wickramaratne, P., & Weissman, M. (1997). Intergenerational transmission of parental bonding among women. *Journal of the American Academy of Child & Adolescent Psychiatry, 36* (8): 1134–1139.
Mills, M., & Melhuish, E. (1974). Recognition of mother's voice in early infancy. *Nature, 252*: 123–124.
Moncrieff, J. (2002). The antidepressant debate. *British Journal of Psychiatry, 180*: 193–194.
Montague, P. R., Hyman, S. E., & Cohen, J. D. (2004). Computational roles for dopamine in behavioural control. *Nature, 431* (7010): 760–767.
Moran, G. (1984). Psychoanalytic treatment of diabetic children. *Psychoanalytic Study of the Child, 39*: 407–447.
Moran, G., & Fonagy, P. (1987). Psychoanalysis and diabetic control. *British Journal of Medical Psychology, 60*: 357–372.
Morris, M., Bowers, D., Chatterjee, A., & Heilman, K. (1992). Amnesia following a discreet basal forebrain lesion. *Brain, 115*: 1827–1847.
Morton, J., & Johnson, M. H. (1991). CONSPEC and CONLEARN: A two-process theory of infant face recognition. *Psychological Review, 98*: 164–181.
Moss, C. S. (1972). *Recovery with Aphasia: The Aftermath of My Stroke*. Urbana, IL: Illinois University Press.
Movellan, J. R., & Watson, J. S. (2002). *The Development of Gaze Following as a Bayesian Systems Identification Problem*. San Diego, CA: UCSD, Machine Perception Laboratory Technical Reports 2002.01.
Müller, F. (1892). Ein Beitrag zur Kenntniss de Seelenblindheit. *Archiv für Psychiatrie und Nervenkrankenheiten, 24*: 856–917.
Murburg, M., Price, L., & Jalali, B. (1988). Huntington's disease: Therapy strategies. *Family Systems Medicine, 6*: 290–303.
Murphy, R. A. (2002). Mental health, juvenile justice, and law enforcement

responses to youth psychopathology. In: D. Marsh & M. Fristad (Eds.), *Handbook of Serious Emotional Disturbance in Children and Adolescents*. New York: Wiley.

Murri, L., Massetani, R., Siciliano, G., & Arena, R. (1985). Dream recall after sleep interruption in brain-injured patients. *Sleep, 8*: 356–362.

Nagel, T (1974). What is it like to be a bat? *Philosophical Review, 83*: 435–450.

NAMHC (1999). *Bridging Science and Service*. National Advisory Mental Health Council. NIH Publication No. 99-4353. Washington, DC: NIH.

NAMHC (2001). *Blueprint for Change: Research on Child and Adolescent Mental Health*. National Advisory Mental Health Council. Workgroup on Child and Adolescent Mental Health Intervention Development and Deployment. Washington, DC: NIH.

Nathan, P. E., & Gorman, J. M. (Eds.) (2002). *Treatments That Work* (2nd edition). New York: Oxford University Press.

Nausieda, P., et al. (1982). Sleep disruption in the course of chronic levodopa therapy: An early feature of the levodopa psychosis. *Clinical Neuropharmacology, 5*: 183.

Naville, F., & Brantmay, H. (1935). Contribution à étude des équivalents épileptiques chez les enfants [Contribution to the study of epilepsy in infancy]. *Archives Suisses de Neurologie et de Psychiatry, 35*: 92–122.

Neal, P. (1988). *As I Am*. London: Century.

Nelson, C. A. (1987). The recognition of facial expression in the first two years of life: Mechanisms of development. *Child Development, 58*: 889–909.

Nemeroff, C. B., Heim, C. M., Thase, M. E., Klein, D. N., Rush, A. J., Schatzberg, A. F., Ninan, P. T., McCullough, J. P. Jr., Weiss, P. M., Dunner, D. L., Rothbaum, B. O., Kornstein, S., Keitner, G., & Keller, M. B. (2003). Differential responses to psychotherapy versus pharmacotherapy in patients with chronic forms of major depression and childhood trauma. *Proceedings of the National Academy of Sciences USA, 100* (24): 14293–14296.

Neumann, I. D., Torner, L., & Wigger, A. (2000). Brain oxytocin: Differential inhibition of neuroendocrine stress responses and anxiety-related behaviour in virgin, pregnant and lactating rats. *Neuroscience, 95* (2): 567–575.

Newell, A. (1991). *Unified Theories of Cognition*. Cambridge, MA: Harvard University Press.

NICE (2005). *Guideline for the Treatment of Depression in Children and Young People*. London: National Institute of Clinical Excellence.

NICHD Early Child Care Research Network (1999). Child care and mother–child interaction in the first 3 years of life. *Developmental Psychology, 35* (6): 1399–1413.

Nielson, J. (1955). Occipital lobes, dreams and psychosis. *Journal of Nervous and Mental Disease, 121*: 50–52.

Nissen, E., Lilja, G., Widstrom, A. J., & Uvnas-Moberg, K. (1995). Elevation of oxytocin levels early post partum in woman. *Acta Obstetricia et Gynecologica Scandinavica, 74*: 530–533.

Nitschke, J. B., Nelson, E. E., Rusch, B. D., Fox, A. S., Oakes, T. R., & Davidson, R. J. (2004). Orbitofrontal cortex tracks positive mood in mothers viewing pictures of their newborn infants. *NeuroImage, 21* (2): 583–592.

Norton, K. (1992). A culture of enquiry—its preservation or loss. *Therapeutic Communities, 13* (1): 3–25.

Numan, M. (1994). Maternal behavior. In: E. Knobil & J. F. Neill (Eds.), *The Physiology of Reproduction* (pp. 221–301). New York: Raven Press.

Numan, M., Rosenblatt, J. S., & Kiminsaruk, B. R. (1997). Medial preoptic area and onset of maternal behavior in the rat. *Journal of Comparative and Physiological Psychology, 91*: 146–164.

Numan, M., & Sheehan, T. P. (1997). Neuroanatomical circuitry for mammalian maternal behavior. *Annals of the New York Academy of Science, 807*: 101–125.

Olds, D. L., Eckenrode, J., Henderson, C. R. Jr., Kitzman, H., Powers, J., Cole, R., Sidora, K., Morris, P., Pettitt, L. M., & Luckey, D. (1997). Long-term effects of home visitation on maternal life course and child abuse and neglect: Fifteen-year follow-up of a randomized trial. *Journal of the American Medical Association, 278* (8): 637–643.

Olds, D., Henderson, C. R. Jr., Cole, R., Eckenrode, J., Kitzman, H., Luckey, D., Pettitt, L., Sidora, K., Morris, P., & Powers, J. (1998). Long-term effects of nurse home visitation on children's criminal and antisocial behavior: 15-year follow-up of a randomized controlled trial. *Journal of the American Medical Association, 280* (14): 1238–1244.

Olds, D. L., Henderson, C. R. Jr., Kitzman, H. J., Eckenrode, J. J., Cole, R. E., & Tatelbaum, R. C. (1999). Prenatal and infancy home visitation by nurses: Recent findings. *Future Child, 9* (1): 44–65, 190–191.

Olds, D. L., Robinson, J., O'Brien, R., Luckey, D. W., Pettitt, L. M., Henderson, C. R. Jr, Ng, R. K., Sheff, K. L., Korfmacher, J., Hiatt, S., & Talmi, A. (2002). Home visiting by paraprofessionals and by nurses: A randomized, controlled trial. *Pediatrics, 110* (3): 486–496.

Oppenheim, D., Emde, R. N., & Warren, S. (1997). Children's narrative representations of mothers: Their development and associations with child and mother adaptation. *Child Development, 68*: 127–138.

Oppenheim, D., Goldsmith, D., & Koren-Karie, N. (2004). Maternal insightfulness and preschoolers' emotion and behaviour problems: Reciprocal influences in a therapeutic preschool program. *Infant Mental Health Journal, 25*: 352–367.

Oram, M. W., & Perrett, D. I. (1994). Response of anterior superior temporal polysensory (STPa) neurons to "biological motion" stimuli. *Journal of Cognitive Neuroscience, 6* (2): 99–116.

Osorio, I., & Daroff, R. (1980). Absence of REM and altered NREM sleep in patients with spinocerebellar degeneration and slow saccades. *Annals of Neurology, 7*: 277–280.

Oster, H., Hegley, D., & Nagel, L. (1992). Adult judgments and fine-grained analysis of infant facial expressions: Testing the validity of a priori coding formulas. *Developmental Psychology, 28:* 1115–1131.

Ostow, M. (1954). Psychodynamic disturbances in patients with temporal lobe disorder. *Journal of the Mount Sinai Hospital, 20*: 293–308.

Panksepp, J. (1985). Mood changes. In: P. Vinken, C. Bruyn, & H. Klawans (Eds.), *Handbook of Clinical Neurology, Vol. 45*. Amsterdam: Elsevier.

Panksepp, J. (1998). *Affective Neuroscience*. Oxford: Oxford University Press.

Papp, P. (1980). The Greek Chorus and other techniques of paradoxical therapy. *Family Process, 19*: 45–57.

Partridge, M. (1950). *Pre-frontal Leucotomy: A Survey of 300 Cases Personally Followed for 1½–3 Years*. Oxford: Blackwell.

Patterson, G. R. (1982). *Coercive Family Process*. Eugene, OR: Castalia.

Patterson, G. R., Reid, J. B., & Dishion, T. J. (1992). *Antisocial Boys*. Eugene, OR: Castalia.

Patton, G. C., Harris, R., Carlin, J. B., Hibbert, M. E., Coffey, C., Schwartz, M., & Bowes, G. (1997). Adolescent suicidal behaviours: A population-based study of risk. *Psychological Medicine, 27*: 715–724.

Pearce, W. B., & Cronen, V. E. (1980). *Communication, Action and Meaning*. New York: Praeger.

Pedersen, C. A. (1997). Oxytocin control of maternal behavior: Regulation by sex steroids and offspring stimuli. *Annals of the New York Academy of Sciences, 807*: 126–145.

Pedersen, C. A., & Boccia, M. L. (2002). Oxytocin links mothering received, mothering bestowed and adult stress responses. *Stress, 5* (4): 259–267.

Pedersen, C. A., Caldwell, J. D., Walker, C., Ayers, G., & Mason, G. A. (1994). Oxytocin activates the postpartum onset of rat maternal behavior in the ventral tegmental and medial preoptic areas. *Behavioral Neuroscience, 108*: 1163–1171.

Pedersen, C. A., & Prange, A. J. (1979). Induction of maternal behavior in virgin rats after intracerebroventricular administration of oxytocin. *Proceedings of the National Academy of Sciences USA, 76*: 6661–6665.

Pekarik, G., & Wolff, C. B. (1996). Relationship of satisfaction to symptom change, follow-up adjustment, and clinical significance. *Professional Psychology: Research and Practice, 27*: 202–208.

Peña-Casanova, J., Roig-Rovira, T., Bermudez, A., & Tolosa-Sarro, E. (1985). Optic aphasia, optic apraxia, and loss of dreaming. *Brain and Language, 26*: 63–71.

Penfield, W. (1938). The cerebral cortex in man. I: The cerebral cortex and consciousness. *Archives of Neurology and Psychiatry, 40*: 417.

Penfield, W., & Erickson, T. (1941). *Epilepsy and Cerebral Localization*. Springfield, IL: Charles C Thomas.

Penfield, W., & Rasmussen, T. (1955). *The Cerebral Cortex of Man*. New York: Macmillan.

Perry, B. D. (1994). Neurobiological sequelae of childhood trauma: PTSD in children. In: M. M. Murburg (Ed.), *Catecholamine Function in Post-*

traumatic Stress Disorder: Emerging Concepts (pp. 233–255). Washington, DC: American Psychiatric Press.

Peterfreund, E. (1971). *Information, Systems, and Psychoanalysis: An Evolutioniary Biological Approach to Psychoanalytic Theory*. New York: International Universities Press.

Peterfreund, E. (1975). The need for a new general theoretical frame of reference for psychoanalysis. *Psychoanalytical Quarterly, 44*: 534–549.

Peterfreund, E. (1980). On information and systems models for psychoanalysis. *International Review of Psycho-Analysis, 7*: 327–345.

Piaget, J. (1970). *Genetic Epistemology*. New York: Norton.

Piaget, J. (1973). The affective unconscious and the cognitive unconscious. *Journal of the American Psychoanalytic Association, 21*: 249–261.

Piehler, R. (1950). Über das Traumleben leukotomierter (Vorläufige Mitteilung). *Nervenärzt, 21*: 517–21.

Plotsky, P. M., & Meaney, M. J. (1993). Early, postnatal experience alters hypothalamic corticotropin-releasing factor (CRF) mRNA, median eminence CRF content and stress-induced release in adult rats. *Brain Research. Molecular Brain Research, 18* (3): 195–200.

Pompeiano, O. (1979). Cholinergic activation of reticular and vestibular mechanisms controlling posture and eye movements. In: J. A. Hobson & N. Brazier (Eds.), *The Reticular Formation Revisited*. New York: Raven Press.

Premack, D., & Woodruff, G. (1978). Does the chimpanzee have a theory of mind? *Behavioral and Brain Sciences, 1* (4): 515–526.

Prizant, B., & Duchan, J. (1981). The functions of immediate echolalia in autistic children. *Journal of Speech and Hearing Disorders, 46* (3): 241–249.

Pruessner, J. C., Champagne, F., Meaney, M. J., & Dagher, A. (2004). Dopamine release in response to a psychological stress in humans and its relationship to early life maternal care: A positron emission tomography study using [11C]raclopride. *Journal of Neuroscience, 24* (11): 2825–2831.

Pryce, C. R., Bettschen, D., & Feldon, J. (2001). Comparison of the effects of early handling and deprivation on maternal care in the rat. *Developmental Psychobiology, 38* (4): 239–251.

Putnam, H. (1973). Reductionism and the nature of psychology. *Cognition, 2* (1): 131–146.

Pylyshyn, Z. W., & Demopoulos, W. (Eds.) (1986). *Meaning and Cognitive Structure: Issues in the Computational Theory of Mind*. Westport, CT: Ablex.

Pynoos, R. S., & Nader, K. (1989). Children's memory and proximity to violence. *Journal of the American Academy of Child & Adolescent Psychiatry, 28*: 236–241.

Pynoos, R. S., Steinberg, A. M., & Wraith, R. (1995). A developmental model of childhood traumatic stress. In: D. Cicchetti & D. J. Cohen (Eds.), *Developmental Psychopathology, Vol. 2: Risk, Disorder, and Adaptation* (pp. 72–95). New York: Wiley.

Quinton, D., Rushton, A., Dance, C., & Mayes, D. (1998). *Joining New Families: A Study of Adoption and Fostering in Middle Childhood*. Chichester: Wiley.

Ranote, S., Elliott, R., Abel, K. M., Mitchell, R., Deakin, J. F. W., & Appleby, L. (2004). The neural basis of maternal responsiveness to infants: An fMRI study. *Neuroreport, 15* (11): 1825–1829.

Regolin, L., Tommasi, L., & Vallortigara, G. (2000). Visual perception of biological motion in newly hatched chicks as revealed by an imprinting procedure. *Animal Cognition, 3* (1): 53–60.

Reinecke, M. A., Ryan, N. E., & DuBois, L. (1998). Cognitive-behavioral therapy of depression and depressive symptoms during adolescence: A review and meta-analysis. *Journal of the American Academy of Child and Adolescent Psychiatry, 37*: 26–34.

Rice, G., Anderson, C., Risch, N., & Ebers, G. (1999). Male homosexuality: Absence of linkage to microsatellite markers at Xq28. *Science, 284*: 665–667.

Rieff, P. (1959). *Freud: The Mind of the Moralist*. New York: Viking.

Ritchie, D. (1959). *Stroke: A Diary of Recovery*. London: Faber & Faber.

Rizzolatti, G., & Craighero, L. (2004). The mirror-neuron system. *Annual Review of Neuroscience, 27*: 169–192.

Robertson, J., & Robertson, J. (1969). *John, Seventeen Months, in Residential Nursery for Nine Days*. New York: Distributed by New York University Film Library.

Rodin, E., Mulder, D., Faucett, R., & Bickford, R., (1955). Psychologic factors in convulsive disorders of focal origin. *Archives of Neurology, 74*: 365–374.

Rogers, S. (1999). An examination of the imitation deficits in autism. In: J. Nadel & G. Butterworth (Eds.), *Imitation in Infancy: Cambridge Studies in Cognitive Perceptual Development* (pp. 254–283). New York: Cambridge University Press.

Rogosch, F. A., Cicchetti, D., Shields, A., et al. (1995). Parenting dysfunction in child maltreatment. In: M. Bornstein (Ed.), *Handbook of Parenting, Vol. 4* (pp. 127–159). Mahwah, NJ: Lawrence Erlbaum.

Rohde, P., Clarke, G. N., Lewinsohn, P. M., Seeley, J. R., & Kaufman, N. K. (2001). Impact of comorbidity on a cognitive-behavioral group treatment for adolescent depression. *Journal of the American Academy of Child and Adolescent Psychiatry, 40*: 795–802.

Rohde, P., Lewinsohn, P. M., & Seeley, J. R. (1994). Are adolescents changed by an episode of major depression? *Journal of the American Academy of Child and Adolescent Psychiatry, 33* (9): 1289–1298.

Rosenblatt, A., & Thickstun, J. T. (1977). *Modern Psychoanalytic Concepts in a General Psychology, Part 1: General Concepts and Principles. Part 2: Motivation*. New York: International Universities Press.

Rosenblatt, A., & Thickstun, J. (1994). Intuition and consciousness. *Psychoanalytic Quarterly, 63*: 696–714.

Rosenblatt, J. S. (1994). Psychobiology of maternal behavior: Contribution to the clinical understanding of maternal behavior among humans. *Acta Paediatrica* (Suppl. 397): 3–8.

Roth, A., & Fonagy, P. (2005). *What Works for Whom: Implications and Limitations of the Research Literature* (2nd edition). New York: Guilford Press.

Rubino, G., Barker, C., Roth, T., et al. (2000). Therapist empathy and depth of interpretation in response to potential alliance ruptures: The role of therapist and patient attachment styles. *Psychotherapy Research, 10*: 408–420.

Rumbaugh, D. M., & Washburn, D. A. (2003). *Intelligence of Apes and Other Rational Beings*. New Haven, CT: Yale University Press.

Rumelhart, D. E., & McClelland, J. L. (1986). *Parallel Distributed Processing: Explorations in the Microstructure of Cognition, Vol. 1: Foundations*. Cambridge, MA: MIT Press.

Rycroft, P. (2004). When theory abandons us—wading through the "swampy lowlands" of practice. *Journal of Family Therapy, 26*: 245–259.

Sacks, O. (1985). *The Man Who Mistook His Wife for a Hat*. London: Duckworth.

Sacks, O. (1990). *Awakenings*. New York: HarperCollins.

Sacks, O. (1991). Neurological dreams. *MD Medical Newsmagazine, 35* (2, February), pp. 29–32.

Sacks, O. (1995). *An Anthropologist on Mars*. London: Picador.

Sacks, O., & Wasserman, R. (1987). The case of the colorblind painter. *New York Review of Books, 34* (18): 25–34.

Sanchez, M. M., Ladd, C. O., & Plotsky, P. M. (2001). Early adverse experience as a developmental risk factor for later psychopathology: Evidence from rodent and primate models. *Developmental Psychopathology, 13* (3): 419–449.

Scharf, B., Moskovitz, C., Lupton, C., & Klawans, H. (1978). Dream phenomena induced by chronic levodopa therapy. *Journal of Neural Transmission, 43*: 143.

Schindler, R. (1953). Das Traumleben der Leukotomierten. *Wiener Zeitschrift für die Nervenheilkunde, 6*: 330.

Scholz, M., & Asen, E. (2001). Multiple family therapy with eating disordered adolescents: Concepts and preliminary results. *European Eating Disorders Review, 9*: 33–42.

Schön, D. A. (1987). *Training the Reflective Practitioner: Toward a New Design for Teaching and Learning in the Professions*. San Francisco, CA: Jossey-Bass.

Schore, A. J. (2001). The effects of secure attachment relationship on right brain development, affect regulation, and infant mental health. *Infant Mental Health Journal, 22* (1): 7–66.

Schultz, R. T. (2005). Neuroimaging studies in autism spectrum disorders. In: F. R. Volkmar, R. Paul, A. Klin, & D. J. Cohen (Eds.), *Handbook of Autism and Pervasive Developmental Disorders* (3rd edition). New York: Wiley.

Schultz, R. T., Gauthier, I., Klin, A., Fulbright, R., Anderson, A., Volkmar, F.

R., Skudlarski, P., Lacadie, C., Cohen, D. J., & Gore, J. C. (2000). Abnormal ventral temporal cortical activity among individuals with autism and Asperger syndrome during face discrimination. *Archives of General Psychiatry, 57*: 331–340.

Schultz, W. (1998). Predictive reward signal of dopamine neurons. *Journal of Neurophysiology, 80* (1): 1–27.

Searle, J. (1980). *Speech Act Theory and Pragmatics*. Boston, MA: Reidel.

Searle, J. R. (2004). *Mind: A Brief Introduction (Fundamentals of Philosophy)*. New York: Oxford University Press.

Sechrest, L., Stewart, M., Stickle, T. R., & Sidani, S. (1996). *Effective and Persuasive Case Studies*. Cambridge, MA: Human Services Research Institute.

Seidenberg, M. S., & McClelland, J. L. (1989). A distributed, developmental model of word recognition and naming. *Psychological Review, 96*: 523–568.

Shaffer, D. (1974). Suicide in childhood and early adolescence. *Journal of Child Psychology and Psychiatry, 15*: 275–291.

Shafii, M., Carrigan, S., Whittinghill, J. R., & Derrick, A. (1985). Psychological autopsy of completed suicide in children and adolescents. *American Journal of Psychiatry, 142*: 1061–1064.

Sheehan, T. P., Cirrito, J., Numan, M. J., & Numan, M. (2000). Using c-Fos immunocyto-chemistry to identify forebrain regions that may inhibit maternal behavior in rats. *Behavioral Neuroscience, 114*: 337–352.

Sheehan, T., Paul, M., Amaral, E., Numan, M. J., & Numan, M. (2001). Evidence that the medial amygdala projects to the anterior/ventromedial hypothalamic nuclei to inhibit maternal behavior in rats. *Neuroscience, 106* (2): 341–356.

Shernoff, E. S., Kratochwill, T. R., & Stoiber, K. C. (2003). Training in evidence-based interventions (EBIs): What are school psychology programs teaching? *Journal of School Psychology, 41*: 467–483.

Shirk, S. R., & Karver, M. (2003). Prediction of treatment outcome from relationship variables in child and adolescent therapy: A meta-analytic review. *Journal of Consulting and Clinical Psychology, 71*: 452–464.

Shneidman, E. S. (1989). Overview: A multidimensional approach to suicide. In: D. Jacobs & H. N. Brown (Eds.), *Suicide: Understanding and Responding* (pp. 1–30). Madison, CT: International Universities Press.

Silbersweig, D. A., Stern, E., Frith, C., Cahill, C., Holmes, A., Grootoonk, S., Seaward, J., McKenna, P., Chua, S. E., Schnorr, L., Jones, T., & Frackowiak, R. S. J. (1995). A functional neuroanatomy of hallucinations in schizophrenia. *Nature, 378*: 176–179.

Singer, B., & Ryff, C. D. (1999). Hierarchies of life histories and associated health risks. *Annals of the New York Academy of Sciences, 896*: 96–115.

Singer, T., Seymour, B., O'Doherty, J., Kaube, H., Dolan, R. J., & Frith, C. D. (2004). Empathy for pain involves the affective but not the sensory components of pain. *Science, 303*: 1157–1161.

Singh, R. (2000). *A Retrospective Clinical Audit of the Families Who Attended*

the Family Day Unit between 1997–1999. Unpublished manuscript, Marlborough Family Service, BKCW Trust, London.
Singleton, J. (1991). *Boyz n the Hood*. [Videorecording.] Culver City, CA: Columbia Pictures.
Slade, A. (2002). Keeping the baby in mind: A critical factor in perinatal mental health. *Zero to Three* (June/July): 10–16. [Special Issue, Perinatal Mental Health, ed. A. Slade, L. Mayes, & N. Epperson.]
Slade, A. (2005). Parental reflective functioning: An introduction. *Attachment and Human Development, 7*: 269–281.
Slade, A. (in press). Reflective parenting programs: Theory and development. *Psychoanalytic Inquiry*.
Slade, A., Aber, J. L., Cohen, L. J., Fiorello, J., Meyer, J., DeSear, P., & Walter, S. (1993). *Parent Development Interview Coding System*. Unpublished manuscript, City University of New York.
Slade, A., Aber. J. L., Fiorello, J., DeSear, P., Meyer, J., Cohen, L. J., & Wallon, S. (1994). *Parent Development Interview Coding System*. New York: City University of New York.
Slade, A., Belsky, J., Aber, J. L., & Phelps, J. (1999). Maternal representations of their relationship with their toddlers: Links to adult attachment and observed mothering. *Developmental Psychology, 35*: 611–619.
Slade, A., Grienenberger, J., Bernbach, E., Levy, D., & Locker, A. (2005). Maternal reflective functioning and attachment: Considering the transmission gap. *Attachment and Human Development, 7*: 283–292.
Slade, A., Sadler, L., de Dios-Kenn, C., Webb, D., Ezepchick, J., & Mayes, L. (2005). Minding the baby: A reflective parenting program. *Psychoanalytic Study of the Child, 60*: 74–100.
Slade, A., Sadler, L. S., & Mayes, L. (2005). Minding the baby: Enhancing reflective functioning in a nursing/mental health home visiting program. In: L. Berlin, Y. Ziv, L. Amaya-Jackson, & M. Greenberg (Eds.), *Enhancing Early Attachments: Theory, Research, Intervention, and Policy* (pp. 152–177). New York: Guilford Press.
Smith, M. L., & Glass, G. V. (1977). Meta-analysis of psychotherapy outcome studies. *American Psychologist, 32*: 752–760.
Smith, M. L., Glass, G. V., & Miller, T. I. (1980). *The Benefits of Psychotherapy*. Baltimore, MD: Johns Hopkins University Press.
Smyth, J. M. (1998). Written emotional expression: Effect sizes, outcome types, and moderating variables. *Journal of Consulting and Clinical Psychology, 66*: 174–184.
Snyder, H. (1958). Epileptic equivalents in children. *Pediatrics, 18*: 308–318.
Sobell, L. C., Sobell, M. B., & Agrawal, S. (2002). Self-change and dual recoveries among individuals with alcohol and tobacco problems: Current knowledge and future directions alcoholism. *Alcoholism: Clinical and Experimental Research, 26*: 1936–1938.
Sofroniew, M. V., & Weindl, A. (1981). Central nervous system distribution of vasporessin, oxytocin, and neurophysin. In: J. L. Martinex, R. A.

Jensen, R. B. Messing, H. Rigter, & J. L. McGraugh (Eds.), *Endogenous Peptides and Learning and Memory Processes*. New York: Academic Press.
Solms, M. (1977). What is consciousness? *Journal of the American Psychoanalytic Association, 45*: 681–778.
Solms, M. (1995). New findings on the neurological organization of dreaming: Implications for psychoanalysis. *Psychoanalytic Quarterly, 64*: 43–67.
Solms, M. (1997). *The Neuropsychology of Dreams: A Clinico-Anatomical Study*. Mahwah, NJ: Lawrence Erlbaum.
Solms, M. (1998). Psychoanalytische Beobachtungen an vier Patienten mit ventromesialen Frontalhirnlasionen. *Psyche. 52*: 919–962.
Solms, M. (2000). Dreaming and REM sleep are controlled by different brain mechanisms. *Behavioral and Brain Sciences, 23*: 843–850.
Solnit, A. J., Adnopoz, J., Saxe, L., Gardner, J., & Fallon, T. (1997). Evaluating systems of care for children: Utility of the clinical case conference. *American Journal of Orthopsychiatry, 67*: 554–567.
Solomon, J., & George, C. (1999). The measurement of attachment security in infancy and childhood. In: J. Cassidy & P. R. Shaver (Eds.), *Handbook of Attachment*. New York: Guilford Press.
Solomon, J., & George, C. (2002). The place of disorganisation in attachment theory: Linking classical observations with contemporary findings. In: J. Solomon & C. George (Eds.), *Attachment Disorganization*. New York: Guilford Press.
Southwick, S. M., Krystal, J. H., Morgan, C., Johnson, D., Nagy, L. M., Nicolaou, A., Heninger, G. R., & Charney, D. S. (1993). Abnormal noradrenergic function in posttraumatic stress disorder. *Archives of General Psychiatry*, 50: 266–274.
Sperber, D. (1996). *Explaining Culture: A Naturalistic Approach*. Oxford: Blackwell.
Sperber, D. (2006). Why a deep understanding of cultural evolution is incompatible with shallow psychology. In: N. J. Enfield & S. C. Levinson (Eds.), *Roots of Human Sociality: Culture, Cognition, and Human Interaction*. London: Berg Press.
Sperber, D., & Wilson, D. (1986). *Relevance: Communication and Cognition*. Oxford: Blackwell.
Spitz, R. (1946). Anaclitic depression: An inquiry into the genesis of psychiatric conditions in early childhood. *Psychoanalytic Study of the Child, 1*: 47–53.
Sroufe, L. A. (1979). Socioemotional development. In: J. D. Osofsky (Ed.), *Handbook of Infant Development* (pp. 462–516). New York: Wiley.
Sroufe, L. A. (1983). Infant–caregiver attachment and patterns of adaptation in preschool: The roots of maladaptation and competence. In: M. Perlmutter (Ed.), *Minnisota Symposium in Child Psychology* (pp. 41–83). Hillsdale, NJ: Lawrence Erlbaum.
Sroufe, L. A. (1995). *Emotional Development: The Organization of Emotional Life in the Early Years*. Cambridge: Cambridge University Press.

Sroufe, L. A. (1997). Psychopathology as an outcome of development. *Developmental Psychopathology, 9* (2): 251–268.

Sroufe. L. A., Carlson, E. A., Levy, A. K., & Egeland, B. (1999). Implications of attachment theory for developmental psychopathology. *Developmental Psychopathology, 11* (1): 1–13.

Sroufe, L. A., Carlson, E., & Shulman, S. (1993). Individuals in relationships: Development from infancy through adolescence. In: D. C. Funder, R. Parke, C. Tomlinson-Keesey, & K. Widaman (Eds.), *Studying Lives through Time: Approaches to Personality and Development* (pp. 315–342). Washington, DC: American Psychological Association.

Stack, E. C., & Numan, M. (2000). The temporal course of expression of c-Fos and Fos B within the medial preoptic area and other brain regions of postpartum female rats during prolonged mother–young interactions. *Behavioral Neuroscience, 114* (3): 609–622.

Stams, J., Juffer, F., & van IJzendoorn, M. (2002). Maternal sensitivity, infant attachment, and temperament in early childhood predict adjustment in middle childhood: The case of adopted children and their biologically unrelated parents. *Developmental Psychology, 38* (5): 806–821.

Stanley, C., Murray, L., & Stein, A. (2004). The effect of postnatal depression on mother–infant interaction, infant response to the Still-face perturbation, and performance on an Instrumental Learning task. *Development & Psychopathology, 16* (1): 1–18.

Steele, M., Hodges, J., Kaniuk, J., Hillman, S., & Henderson K. (2003). Attachment representations in newly adopted maltreated children and their adoptive parents: Implications for placement and support. *Journal of Child Psychotherapy, 29*: 187–205.

Steele, H., Steele, M., & Fonagy, P. (1996). Associations among attachment classifications of mothers, fathers, and their infants: Evidence for a relationship-specific perspective. *Child Development, 67*: 541–555.

Steele, M., Steele, H., Woolgar, M., Yabsley, S., Johnson, D., Fonagy, P., & Croft,, C. (2003). An attachment perspective on children's emotion narratives: Links across generations. In: R. Emde, D. Wolf, & D. Oppenheim (Eds.), *Narrative Processes and the Transition from Infancy to Early Childhood*. Chicago, IL: University of Chicago Press.

Stern, D. N. (1974). Mother and infant at play: The dyadic interaction involving facial, vocal, and gaze behaviors. In: M. Lewis & L. A. Roseblum (Eds.), *The Effect of the Infant on Its Caregiver*: New York: Wiley-Interscience.

Stern, D. N. (1985). *The Interpersonal Word of the Infant*. New York: Basic Books.

Stern, D. N. (1995). Self/other differentiation in the domain of intimate socio-affective interaction: Some considerations. In: P. Rochat (Ed.), *The Self in Infancy: Theory and Research* (pp. 419–429). Amsterdam: Elsevier.

Stern, D. N. (1997a). *The Motherhood Constellation: A Unified View of Parent–Infant Psychopathology.* New York: Basic Books.

Stern, J. M. (1997b). Offspring-induced nurturance: Animal–human parallels. *Developmental Psychobiology, 31* (1): 19–37.

Stirman, S. W., DeRubeis, R. J., Crits-Christoph, P., & Brody, P. E. (2003). Are samples in randomized controlled trials for psychotherapy representative of community outpatients? A new methodology and initial findings. *Journal of Consulting and Clinical Psychology, 71*: 963–972.

Strathearn, L., Gray, P. H., O'Callaghan, M., & Wood, D. O. (2001). Childhood neglect and cognitive development in extremely low birth weight infants: A prospective study. *Pediatrics, 108* (1): 142–151.

Strathearn, L., & McClure, S. M. (2002). A functional MRI study of maternal responses of infant facial cues. Annual Scientific Meeting of the Society for Neuroscience, Program No. 517.5. *2002 Abstract Viewer/Itinerary Planner*. Washington, DC: Society for Neuroscience (online).

Strathearn, L., O'Callaghan, M. J., Najman, J. M., Williams, G., Bor, W., & Anderson, M. (2002). A 14-year longitudinal study of child neglect: Cognitive development and head growth. *Abstracts of the 14th International Congress on Child Abuse and Neglect*. Durban, South Africa.

Stricker, G. (1992). The relationship of research to clinical practice. *American Psychologist, 47*: 543–549.

Summer, J. (1998). *Multiple Family Therapy: Its Use in the Assessment and Treatment of Child Abuse. A Pilot Study.* Unpublished MSc thesis, Birkbeck College and Institute of Family Therapy, London.

Suomi, S. J. (1995). Influence of Bowlby's Attachment Theory on research on non-human primate biobehavioral development. In: S. Goldberg, R. Muir, & J. Kerr (Eds.), *Attachment Theory: Social, Developmental, and Clinical Perspectives* (pp. 185–201). Hillsdale, NJ: Analytic Press.

Suomi, S. J. (1997). Early determinants of behaviour: Evidence from primate studies. *British Medical Bulletin, 53* (1): 170–184.

Suomi, S. J., Delizio, R., & Harlow, H. F. (1976). Social rehabilitation of separation-induced depressive disorders in monkeys. *American Journal of Psychiatry, 133* (11): 1279–1285.

Suomi, S. J., & Ripp, C. (1983). A history of motherless mothering at the University of Wisconsin Primate Laboratory. In: M. Reite & N. Caine (Eds.), *Child Abuse: The Non-Human Data* (pp. 49–78). New York: Liss.

Sur, M., & Leamey, C. A. (2001). Development and plasticity of cortical areas and networks. *Nature Reviews Neuroscience, 2*: 251–262.

Swain, J. E., Leckman, J. F., Mayes, L. C., Feldman, R., Constable, R. T., & Schultz, R. T. (2004). *Brain Circuitry and Psychopathology of Human Parent–Infant Attachment in the Postpartum.* Abstract P-020–369, International Association for Child and Adolescent Psychiatry and Allied Professions 16th World Congress, Berlin, Germany (22–26 August). Darmstadt: Steinkopff Verlag.

TADS Team (2004). Fluoxetine, cognitive-behavioral therapy, and their combination for adolescents with depression: Treatment for Adolescents with Depression Study (TADS) randomized controlled trial. *Journal of the American Medical Association, 292:* 807–820.

Tang, Y. P., Shimizu, E., Dube, G. R., Rampon, C., Kerchner, G. A., Zhuo,

M., et al. (1999). Genetic enhancement of learning and memory in mice. *Nature, 401*: 63–69.

Task Force on Promotion and Dissemination of Psychological Procedures (1995). Training in and dissemination of empirically-validated psychological treatments: Report and recommendations. *Clinical Psychologist, 48*: 3–24.

Teasdale, J. D., Moore, R. G., Hayhurst, H., Pope, M., Williams, S., & Segal, Z. V. (2002). Metacognitive awareness and prevention of relapse in depression: Empirical evidence. *Journal of Consulting and Clinical Psychology, 70* (2): 275–287.

Terr, L. (1991). Childhood trauma: An outline and overview. *American Journal of Psychiatry, 148*: 10–20.

Thelen, E., & Smith, L. (1994). *A Dynamic Systems Approach to the Development of Cognition and Action*. Cambridge, MA: MIT Press.

Thelen, E., Schoener, G., Scheier, C., & Smith, L. B. (2001). The dynamics of embodiment: A field theory of infant perseverative reaching. *Behavioral and Brain Sciences, 24* (1): 1–86.

Thomas, J. M., & Guskin, K. A. (2001). Disruptive behavior in young children: What does it mean? *Journal of the American Academy of Child & Adolescent Psychiatry, 40*: 44–51.

Thomas, S. A., Matsumoto, A. M., & Palmiter, R. D. (1995). Noradrenaline is essential for mouse fetal development. *Nature, 374*: 643–646.

Thomas, S. A., & Palmiter, R. D. (1997). Impaired maternal behavior in mice lacking norepinephrine and epinephrine. *Cell, 91*: 583–592.

Thomayer, J. (1897). Sur la signification de quelques rêves. *Revue Neurologique, 5*: 98–101.

Thompson, D. (1942). *On Growth and Form*. Cambridge: Cambridge University Press.

Thompson, R. A. (1998). Empathy and its origins in early development. In: S. Braten (Ed.), *Intersubjective Communication and Emotion in Early Ontogeny* (pp. 144–157). Cambridge: Cambridge University Press.

Tomasello, M. (1999). *The Cultural Origins of Human Cognition*. Cambridge, MA: Harvard University Press.

Tomasello, M., Carpenter, M., Call, J., Behne, T., & Moll, H. (2005). Understanding and sharing intentions: The origins of cultural cognition. *Behavioral and Brain Sciences, 28* (5): 675–735.

Tomizawa, K., Iga, N., Lu, Y. F., Moriwaki, A., Matsushita, M., Li, S. T., et al. (2003). Oxytocin improves long-lasting spatial memory during motherhood through MAP kinase cascade. *Nature Neuroscience, 6* (4): 384–390.

Toulmin, S., & Goodfield, J. (1961). *The Fabric of the Heavens*. New York: HarperCollins.

Trevarthen, C. (1979). Communication and cooperation in early infancy: A description of primary intersubjectivity. In: M. Bullowa (Ed.), *Before Speech: The Beginning of Interpersonal Communication* (pp. 321–347). New York: Cambridge University Press.

Trevarthen, C. (1993). The self born in intersubjectivity: The psychology of an infant communicating. In: U. Neisser (Ed.), *The Perceived Self: Ecological and Interpersonal Sources of Self-Knowledge* (pp. 121–173). New York: Cambridge University Press.

Trevarthen, C., & Aitken, K. J. (2001). Infant intersubjectivity: Research, theory, and clinical applications. *Journal of Child Psychology and Psychiatry, 42*: 3–48.

Triseliotis, J., & Russell, J. (1984). *Hard to Place: The Outcome of Adoption and Residential Care*. London: Heinemann.

Tronick, E. Z. (1989). Emotions and emotional communication in infants. *American Psychologist, 44*: 112–119.

Tronick, E., Als, H., Adamson, L., Wise, S., & Brazelton, T. B. (1978). The infant's response to entrapment between contradictory messages in face-to-face interaction. *Journal of the American Academy of Child & Adolescent Psychiatry, 17*: 1–13.

Trowell, J., Joffe, I., Campbell, J., Clemente, C., Grayson, K., Barnes, J., & Almqvist, F. (in press). Childhood depression: A place for psychotherapy. *European Journal of Child and Adolescent Psychiatry.*

Tzavaras, A. (1967). *Contribution à l'étude de l'agnosie des physiognomies* [Contribution to the study of agnosia for faces]. Unpublished doctorial dissertation, Faculté de Médecine de Université de Paris.

Uddin, L. Q., Kaplan, J. T., Molnar-Szakacs, I., Zaidel, E., & Iacoboni, M. (2005). Self-face recognition activates a frontoparietal "mirror" network in the right hemisphere: An event-related fMRI study. *NeuroImage, 25* (3): 926–935.

Uexkull, J. v. (1957). A stroll through the worlds of animals and men. In: C. H. Schiller (Ed.), *Instinctive Behavior*. London: Methuen.

Uller, C., & Nichols, S. (2000). Goal attribution in chimpanzees. *Cognition, 76*: B27–B34.

U.S. Department of Health and Human Services, Administration on Children Youth and Families (2003). *Child Maltreatment 2001*. Washington DC: U.S. Government Printing Office,.

Uvnas-Moberg, K. (1998). Oxytocin may mediate the benefits of positive social interaction and emotions. *Psychoneuroendocrinology, 23*: 819–835.

Uvnas-Moberg, K., & Eriksson, M. (1996). Breastfeeding: Physiological, endocrine and behavioural adaptations caused by oxytocin and local neurogenic activity in the nipple and mammary gland. *Acta Paediatrica, 85* (5): 525–530.

van der Kolk, B., Burbridge, J., & Suzuki, J. (1997). The psychobiology of traumatic memory. In: R. Yehuda & A. C. McFarlane (Eds.), *Psychobiology of Posttraumatic Disorder* (pp. 99–113). New York: New York Academy of Sciences.

van der Kolk, B., & Fisler, R. (1994). Childhood abuse and neglect and loss of self-regulation. *Bulletin of the Menninger Clinic, 58*: 145–168.

van der Kolk, B., Greenberg, M., Boyd, H., & Krystal, J. (1985). Inescapable shock, neurotransmitters, and addiction to trauma: Toward a psychobiology of post traumatic stress. *Biological Psychiatry, 20*: 314–325.

van IJzendoorn, M. H. (1995). Adult attachment representations, parental responsiveness and infant attachment: A meta-analysis on the predictive validity of the Adult Attachment Interview. *Psychological Bulletin, 117* (3): 382–403.

van Ijzendoorn, M. H., & Bakermans-Kranenburg, M. J. (1996). Attachment representations in mothers, fathers, adolescents and clinical groups: A meta-analytic search for normative data. *Journal of Consulting and Clinical Psychology, 64* (1): 8–21.

Van Leengoed, E., Kerker, E., & Swanson, H. H. (1987). Inhibition of postpartum maternal behavior in the rat by injecting an oxytocin antagonist into the cerebral ventricles. *Journal of Endocrinology, 112*: 275–282.

van Praag, H. M. (1996). Serotonin-related, anxiety/aggression-driven, stressor related depression. A psychobiological hypothesis. *European Psychiatry, 11*: 57–67.

Varela, F., Thompson, E., & Rosch, E. (1991). *The Embodied Mind: Cognitive Science and Human Experience*. Cambridge, MA: MIT Press.

Vaughn, C., & Leff, J. (1976). The measurement of expressed emotion in the families of psychiatric patients. *British Journal of Social and Clinical Psychology, 15*: 157–165.

Vogel, G., Barrowclough, B., & Giesler, D. (1972). Limited discriminability of REM and sleep onset reports and its psychiatric implications. *Archives of General Psychiatry, 26*: 449.

Volkmar, F. R., Paul, R., Klin, A., & Cohen, D. J. (Eds.) (2005). *Handbook of Autism and Pervasive Developmental Disorders* (3rd edition). New York: Wiley.

Vygotsky, L. S. (1962). *Thought and Language*. Cambridge, MA: MIT Press.

Vygotsky, L. S. (1978). *Mind in Society: The Development of Higher Psychological Processes*. Cambridge, MA: Harvard University Press.

Vythilingam, M., Heim, C., Newport, J., Miller, A. H., Anderson, E., Bronen, R., Brummer, M., Staib, L., Vernetten, E., Charney, D. S., Nemeroff, C. B., & Bremner, J. D. (2002). Childhood trauma associated with smaller hippocampal volume in women with major depression. *American Journal of Psychiatry, 159*: 2072–2079.

Wade, W. A., Treat, T. A., & Stuart, G. L. (1998). Transporting an empirically supported treatment for panic disorder to a service clinic setting: A benchmarking strategy. *Journal of Consulting and Clinical Psychology, 66*: 231–239.

Wallis, P., & Steele, H. (2001). Attachment representations in adolescence: Further evidence from psychiatric residential settings. *Attachment and Human Development, 3* (3): 259–269.

Wapner, W., Judd, T., & Gardner, H. (1978). Visual agnosia in an artist. *Cortex, 14*: 343–364.

Ward, M. J., & Carlson, E. A. (1995). Associations among adult attachment representations, maternal sensitivity and infant–mother attachment in a sample of adolescent mothers. *Child Development, 66* (1): 69–79.

Warren, S. L., Huston, L., Egeland, B., & Sroufe, L. A. (1997). Child and adolescent anxiety disorders and early attachment. *Journal of the American Academy of Child & Adolescent Psychiatry, 36* (5): 637–644.

Wasserman, G. A., Ko, S. J., & Jensen, P. S. (2001). Columbia Guidelines for Child and Adolescent Mental Health Referral. In: *Report on Emotional and Behavioral Disorders in Youth: Evidence-Based Assessment and Interventions for the Real World, 2* (pp. 9–23). New York: Civic Research Institute.

Watson, J. S. (1972). Smiling, cooing, and "the game". *Merrill-Palmer Quarterly, 18*: 323–339.

Watson, J. S. (1979). Perception of contingency as a determinant of social responsiveness. In: E. B. Thomas (Ed.), *The Origins of Social Responsiveness* (pp. 33–64). New York: Lawrence Erlbaum.

Watson, J. S. (1985). Contingency perception in early social development. In: T. M. Field & N. A. Fox (Eds.), *Social Perception in Infants* (pp. 157–176). Norwood, NJ: Ablex.

Watson, J. S. (1994). Detection of self: The perfect algorithm. In: S. T. Parker, R. W. Mitchell, & M. L. Boccia (Eds.), *Self-Awareness in Animals and Humans: Developmental Perspectives* (pp. 131–148). New York: Cambridge University Press.

Watson, J. S. (2001). Contingency perception and misperception in infancy: Some potential implications for attachment. *Bulletin of the Menninger Clinic, 65* (3): 296–321.

Weaver, I. C., Cervoni, N., Champagne, F. A., D'Alessio, A. C., Sharma, S., Seckl, J. R., Dymov, S., Szyf, M., & Meaney, M. J. (2004). Epigenetic programming by maternal behavior. *Nature Neuroscience, 7* (8): 847–854.

Weaver, I. C., Grant, R. J., & Meaney, M. J. (2002). Maternal behavior regulates long-term hippocampal expression of BAX and apoptosis in the offspring. *Journal of Neurochemistry, 82* (4): 998–1002.

Weersing, V. R. (2005). Benchmarking the effectiveness of psychotherapy: Program evaluation as a component of evidence-based practice. *Journal of the American Academy of Child & Adolescent Psychiatry, 44* (10): 1058–1062.

Weersing, V. R., & Brent, D. A. (2006). Psychotherapy of depression in children and adolescents. In: D. J. Stein, A. Schatzberg, & D. Kupfer (Eds.), *Textbook of Mood Disorders* (pp. 421–436). Arlington, VA: American Psychiatric Publishing.

Weersing, V. R., Hamilton, J. D., & Warnick, E. (2005). *"Things Fall Apart": Transporting and Maintaining CBT for Adolescent Depression in Clinical Service.* Manuscript in preparation, Yale University.

Weersing, V. R., Iyengar, S., Birmaher, B., Kolko, D. J., & Brent, D. A. (2006). Effectiveness of cognitive-behavioral therapy for adolescent depression: A benchmarking investigation. *Behavior Therapy, 37* (1): 36–48.

Weersing, V. R., & Weisz, J. R. (2002). Community clinic treatment of depressed youth: Benchmarking usual care against CBT clinical trials. *Journal of Consulting and Clinical Psychology, 70*: 299–310.

Weersing, V. R., Weisz, J. R., & Donenberg, G. R. (2002). Development of the therapy procedures checklist: A therapist-report measure of technique use in child and adolescent treatment. *Journal of Clinical Child and Adolescent Psychology, 31*: 168–180.

Wegner, D. M., & Wheatley, T. (1999). Apparent mental causation: Sources of the experience of will. *American Psychologist, 54* (7): 480–492.

Wei, F., Wang, G. D., Kerchner, G. A., Kim, S. J., Xu, H. M., Chen, Z. F., et al. (2001). Genetic enhancement of inflammatory pain by forebrain NR2B overexpression. *Nature Neuroscience, 4*: 164–169.

Weinfield, N. S., Sroufe, L. A., & Egeland, B. (2000). Attachment from infancy to early adulthood in a high-risk sample: Continuity, discontinuity, and their correlates. *Child Development, 71* (3): 695–702.

Weinfield, N. S., Whaley, J. L., & Egeland, B. (2004). Continuity, discontinuity, and coherence in attachment from infancy to late adolescence: Sequelae of organization and disorganization. *Attachment and Human Development, 6* (1): 73–98.

Weiss, B. H., Catron, T., Harris, V., & Phung, T. M. (1999). The effectiveness of traditional child psychotherapy. *Journal of Consulting and Clinical Psychology, 67*: 82–94.

Weisz, J. R., Weersing, V. R., & Henggeler, S. W. (2005). Jousting with straw men: Comment on the Westen, Novotny, and Thompson-Brenner (2004) critique of empirically supported treatments. *Psychological Bulletin, 131* (3): 418–426.

Weisz, J. R., Weiss, B., Alicke, M. D., & Klotz, M. L. (1987). Effectiveness of psychotherapy with children and adolescents: A meta-analysis for clinicians. *Journal of Consulting and Clinical Psychology, 55*: 542–549.

Weisz, J. R., Weiss, B., & Donenberg, G. R. (1992). The lab versus the clinic: Effects of child and adolescent psychotherapy. *American Psychologist, 47*: 1578–1585.

Werner, E. E. (1997). Vulnerable but invincible: High-risk children from birth to adulthood. *Acta Paediatrica* (Suppl. 422): 103–105.

Werner, E. E., & Smith, R. S. (2001). *Journeys from Childhood to Midlife: Risk, Resilience, and Recovery*. Ithaca, NY: Cornell University Press.

Wertsch, J. V. (Ed.) (1979). *The Concept of Activity in Soviet Psychology*. Armonk, NY: M. E. Sharpe.

Westen, D., Novotny, C. M., & Thompson-Brenner, H. (2004). The empirical status of empirically supported psychotherapies: Assumptions, findings, and reporting in controlled clinical trials. *Psychological Bulletin, 130:* 631–663.

Wetherby, A. M., Prizant, B. M., & Schuler, A. L. (2000). Understanding the nature of communication and language impairments. In: A. M. Wetherby & B. M. Prizant (Eds.), *Autism Spectrum Disorders: A Transactional Developmental Perspective* (pp. 109–142). Baltimore, MD: Paul H. Brookes.

White, M. (1997). *Narratives of Therapists' Lives*. Adelaide: Dulwich Centre Publications.

Whitty, C., & Lewin, W. (1957). Vivid day-dreaming: An unusual form of confusion following anterior cingulectomy. *Brain, 80*: 72–76.

WHOSIS (2005). *Mortality Database.* World Health Organization Statistical Information System (accessed 15 March: http: //www3.who.int /whosis/mort/table1.cfm).

Wichers, M. C., Danckaerts, M., Van Gestel, S., Derom, C., Vlietink, R., & van Os, J. (2002). Chorion type and twin similarity for child psychiatric symptoms. *Archives of General Psychiatry, 59*: 562–564.

Widom, C. S. (1999). Posttraumatic stress disorder in abused and neglected children grown up. *American Journal of Psychiatry, 156* (8): 1223–1229.

Wilbrand, H. (1887). *Die Seelenblindheit als Herderscheimnung und ihre Beziehung zur Alexie und Agraphie*. Bergmann.

Wilbrand, H. (1892). Ein Fall von Seelenblindheit und Hemianopsie mit Sectionsbefund. *Deutsche Zeitschrift fur Nervenheilkunde, 2*: 361–387. (English version in: *Classic Cases in Neuropsychology*, trans. M. Solms, K. Kaplan-Solms, & J. Brown, ed. C. Code, C.-W. Wallesch, Y. Joannette & A. Lecours. Hillsdale, NJ: Lawrence Erlbaum, 1996).

Winnicott, D. W. (1960). Ego distortion in terms of true and false self. In: *The Maturational Processes and the Facilitating Environment* (pp. 140–152). New York: International Universities Press, 1965.

Winnicott, D. W. (1956). Primary maternal preoccupation. In: *Collected Papers: Through Paediatrics to Psycho-Analysis* (pp. 300–305). London: Hogarth Press, 1975.

Winnicott, D. W. (1971). *Playing and Reality*. London: Tavistock.

Winograd, T. (1975). Frame representations and the procedural–declarative controversy. In: D. Bobrow & A. Collins (Eds.), *Representation and Understanding Studies in Cognitive Science*. New York: Academic Press.

Winograd, T., & Flores, F. (1986). *Understanding Computers and Cognition*. Norwood, NJ: Ablex.

Winter, S. K. (1970). Fantasies at breast feeding time. *Psychology Today, 3*: 31–32.

Wood, A., Harrington, R., & Moore, A. (1996). Controlled trial of a brief cognitive-behavioural intervention in adolescent patients with depressive disorders. *Journal of Child Psychology and Psychiatry, 37:* 737–746.

Wood, B. L., Hargreaves, E., & Marks, M. N. (2004). Using the working model of the child interview to assess postnatally depressed mothers' internal representation of their infants: A brief report. *Journal of Reproductive and Infant Psychology*, 22 (1): 41–44.

Wooley, S., & Lewis, K. (1987). Multi-family therapy within an intensive treatment program for bulimia. In: J. Harkaway (Ed.), *Eating Disorders: The Family Therapy*. Rockville, MD: Aspen.

Woolgar, M. (1999). Projective doll play methodologies for preschool children. *Child Psychology & Psychiatry Review*, 4 (3): 126–134.

Woolston, J., Adnopoz, J., & Berkowitz, S. (in press). *Staying Home: Doing Better. A New Paradigm for Children with Serious Psychiatric illness*. New Haven, CT: Yale University Press.

Yehuda, R. (2002). Posttraumatic stress disorder. *New England Journal of Medicine, 346*: 108–114.

Yehuda, R., McFarlane, A. C., & Shalev, A. Y. (1998). Predicting the development of posttraumatic stress disorder from the acute response to a traumatic event. *Biological Psychiatry, 44*: 1305–1313.

Young, J. E. (1990). *Cognitive Therapy for Personality Disorders: A Schema-Focused Approach*. Sarasota, FL: Professional Resource Exchange.

Zajonc, R. (1980). Feeling and thinking: Preferences need no inferences. *American Psychologist, 35* (2): 151–175.

Zanarini, M. C., Vujanovic, A. A., Parachini, E. A., et al. (2003). Zanarini rating scale for borderline personality disorder (ZAN-BPD): A continuous measure of DSM-IV borderline psychopathology. *Journal of Personality Disorders, 17*: 233–242.

Zeanah, C., & Anders, T. (1987). Subjectivity in parent–infant relationships: A discussion of internal working models. *Infant Mental Health Journal, 6*: 237–250.

Zeanah, C., Benoit, D., & Barton, M. I. (1986). "Working Model of the Child Interview." Unpublished manuscript, Brown University Program in Medicine.

Zeanah, C. H., Benoit, D., Hirshberg, L., Barton, M. I., & Regan, C. (1994). Mothers' representations of their infants are concordant with infant attachment classifications. *Developmental Issues in Psychiatry and Psychology, 1*: 1–14.

Zeki, S. (1993). *A Vision of the Brain*. Oxford: Blackwell.

Zinaman, M. J., Hughes, V., Queenan, J. T., Labobok, M. H., & Albertson, B. (1992). Acute prolactin and oxytocin responses and milk yields to infant suckling and artificial methods of expression in lactating women. *Pediatrics, 89*: 437–440.

INDEX

For Product Safety Concerns and Information please contact our EU
representative GPSR@taylorandfrancis.com
Taylor & Francis Verlag GmbH, Kaufingerstraße 24, 80331 München, Germany

www.ingramcontent.com/pod-product-compliance
Ingram Content Group UK Ltd.
Pitfield, Milton Keynes, MK11 3LW, UK
UKHW021512250926
475702UK00043B/251
9780367324063